Color Atlas of Diseases and Disorders of Cattle

For Mosby:

Commissioning Editor: Jonathan Gregory/Joyce Rodenhuis
Project Development Manager: Tim Kimber
Project Manager: Jane Dingwall/Pat Miller
Design Direction: Andy Chapman

Color Atlas of
Diseases and
Disorders of Cattle

Roger W Blowey BSc BVSc FRCVS
Wood Veterinary Group
Gloucester
England

A David Weaver BSc DR MED VET PHD FRCVS

Bearsden   Emeritus Professor
Glasgow   College of Veterinary Medicine
Scotland   University of Missouri
         Columbia, Missouri
         USA

With a Foreword by
Douglas C Blood

SECOND EDITION

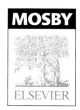

MOSBY
ELSEVIER

MOSBY
An imprint of Elsevier Limited

First edition 1991/reprinted 1997
Translations into Japanese (1994), and Danish (1999)
Second edition 2003
    Reprinted 2005

ISBN 0 7234 3205 8

British Library Cataloguing in Publication Data
A catalogue record for this book is available from the British Library

Library of Congress Cataloguing in Publication Data
A catalogue record for this book is available from the Library of Congress

Note
Medical knowledge is constantly changing. As new information becomes available, changes in treatment, procedures, equipment and the use of drugs become necessary. The editors, contributor and the publishers have taken care to ensure that the information given in this text is accurate and up to date. However, readers are strongly advised to confirm that the information, especially with regard to drug usage, complies with the latest legislation and standards of practice.

ELSEVIER   your source for books, journals and multimedia in the health sciences
www.elsevierhealth.com

Working together to grow
libraries in developing countries
www.elsevier.com | www.bookaid.org | www.sabre.org
ELSEVIER   BOOK AID International   Sabre Foundation

The publisher's policy is to use paper manufactured from sustainable forests

Printed in China

Contents

Foreword to the First Edition

Textbooks dealing with diseases of cattle have never been good sources of photographic illustrations. They have either omitted pictures altogether or included a collection of disastrous black and white photographs of very poor quality. When I heard that Wolfe were to supplement their excellent collection of colour atlases with one dealing with cattle diseases it was obvious that future books would not feel obliged to add to the existing pictorial indiscretions. This was especially so because my colleagues Roger Blowey in the UK and David Weaver in the USA were bovine clinicians of long and wide experience covering two continents.

The need for these illustrations is obvious. For students at all stages in their careers, good colour pictures can add enormously to their understanding and ability to recognise individual diseases. In recognition of this, most clinical teachers accumulate their own colour transparencies. On several occasions I have looked at my own collection with a speculative eye, but discarded the idea because, like most amateur photographs, they lack the quality that an atlas demands. Most importantly they must illustrate the clinical signs by which the particular disease is recognised. There is no point in a photograph of a thin cow with its head hung down to illustrate tuberculosis, acetonaemia or cobalt deficiency, or a dozen other diseases. What are needed are photographs containing explicit details of specific signs. The photographs also need to be models of photographic artistry, well lit, well composed, with good contrast. Roger Blowey and David Weaver have, for their part, ensured that the photographs are truly illustrative and educational, and that the captions point up the salient features of each illustration in the minimum number of well chosen words.

Many authors, including myself, must have contemplated this task because of its potentially enormous value to veterinary medicine. I congratulate Wolfe and the authors on their courage and perseverance in going ahead and getting it done.

1991

Douglas C. Blood
Professor Emeritus School of Veterinary Science University of Melbourne

Preface to the Second Edition

This second edition published in 2002, follows two printings and several translations of the first (1991) edition. On the advice of the publisher, American spelling has been used in this edition.

Some illustrations may have been deleted, others have been replaced for better pictures, and new examples have been added for such conditions as necrotic enteritis, tail necrosis, melanoma and heel ulcers. The total number of illustrations has increased from 730 to 752, making this one of the principal color publications on diseases of cattle. The major revision in this second edition however, is the inclusion of brief notes on the management of the various conditions, and we hope this will make the text considerably more useful. We have avoided making specific recommendations on drug dosages, because the availability and permissible use of products varies enormously from country to country and new products frequently enter the market.

Readers will find new illustrations of the two major cattle diseases affecting the UK in the last 10 years, namely BSE and foot-and-mouth disease, with a cross-referenced differential diagnosis. Preparation of this new edition was again a pleasure. It is directed towards veterinarians working in different fields of cattle medicine, veterinary and agricultural students and livestock producers world-wide, and we hope that it will continue to be useful.

July 2003

R. W. Blowey
A. D. Weaver

Preface to the First Edition

For centuries cattle have been the major species for meat and milk production, and in some countries they also serve an additional role as draught animals. Disease, leading to suboptimal production or death, can have a major economic effect on a community reliant on cattle. This atlas attempts to illustrate the clinical features of over 360 conditions. These range from minor problems, such as necrosis caused by tail bands (used for identification purposes), to major infectious diseases, such as foot-and-mouth and rinderpest, which can wreak havoc when introduced into countries and areas previously free of infection. In endemic areas, which all too often include developing countries short of natural resources, they can be a constant source of serious economic loss.

To emphasise the worldwide scope of cattle disease, we have deliberately sought illustrations from many countries. Over one hundred contributors (acknowledged elsewhere) have graphically given this atlas a truly global perspective. Examples come from all five continents: the Americas, Africa, Asia, Europe and Australasia.

Wherever possible, we have tried to illustrate characteristic features of disorders. This has involved the use of a substantial number of internal views of animals. Thus, while the integumentary chapter comprises almost exclusively external views, the respiratory and circulatory sections inevitably contain much more gross pathology. Where single characteristic features do not exist, we have attempted to show typically severe examples of the conditions. Some are difficult to demonstrate in still photography, and this is particularly true of nervous diseases, where the text has been expanded to include behavioural changes.

Each chapter has a brief introductory outline followed, where appropriate, by a grouping of related conditions. No attempt has been made to consider treatment or management of specific conditions, as the atlas is designed to be used alongside standard textbooks. The major emphasis is on the diagnosis and differential diagnosis of conditions, based on visual examination. This aim has been followed with the likely readership in mind: the veterinarian in practice or government service, veterinary students, livestock producers, and agricultural and science students.

We have deliberately excluded microscopic, histopathological and cytological illustrations, since space precludes the large range of illustrations that would have been necessary. Our purpose is to make the atlas comprehensive over the range of international diseases in terms of gross features. In presenting this first attempt at a comprehensive world atlas of cattle diseases, the authors appreciate that some areas may not be covered sufficiently. We welcome suggestions and submissions for improvements to a second edition. We hope that the use of this book will aid and improve the diagnosis of cattle diseases, so permitting the earlier application of appropriate treatment and control measures. We would feel amply rewarded if the atlas helped to reduce both the substantial economic losses and the unnecessary pain and discomfort endured by cattle affected by the many health problems that hinder optimal productivity.

1991
      Roger W. Blowey, Gloucester, England
A. David Weaver, Columbia, Missouri, USA

Acknowledgments

We are very grateful to our many colleagues (deceased marked[†]) throughout the world who have generously allowed us access to, and use of, their transparencies and have often spent a considerable amount of time selecting them for us. Their help has been invaluable.

Material was supplied by: Mr J.R.D. Allison, Beechams Animal Health, Brentford, England, 444, 629. Prof S. van Amstel, University of Pretoria, South Africa, 672, 673. Dr E.C. Anderson, Animal Virus Research Institute, Pirbright, England, 653–658. Dr A.H. Andrews, Royal Veterinary College, England, 96, 195. Prof J. Armour, Glasgow University Veterinary Hospital, Scotland, 162. E. Sarah Aizlewood, Lanark, Scotland, 259, 269, 475, 664. Mr I.D. Baker, Aylesbury, England, 231, 559. Dr K.C. Barnett, Animal Health Trust, Newmarket, England, 433, 435. Dr A. Bridi, MSD Research Laboratories, Sao Paulo, Brazil, 117, 119, 121, 122. Dr G.M. Buening, University of Missouri, USA, 22, 24, 60, 186, 194, 203, 219, 238, 256, 260, 373, 488, 490, 509, 510, 536, 725, Mr G.L. Caldow, Scottish Agricultural College VSD, St Boswells, Scotland, 61, 62, 63, 137, 246, 247, 396, 593, 668, 669. Dr W.F. Cates, Western College of Veterinary Medicine, Saskatoon, Canada, 541. Dr J.E. Collins, University of Minnesota, USA, 46, 47. Dr K. Collins, University of Missouri-Columbia, USA, 466. Dr B.S. Cooper, Massey University, New Zealand, 448. Dr R.P. Cowart, University of Missouri-Columbia, USA, 1. Dr V. Cox, University of Minnesota, USA, 345, 347, 398. Mr M.P. Cranwell, MAFF VI Centre, Exeter, England, 724. Dr S.M. Crispin, University of Bristol, England, 431, 440, 458. Dr J.S.E. David, University of Bristol, England, 349, 542, 543, 545–547, 549, 550, 552–556. Drs J. Debont and J. Vercruysse, Rijksuniversiteit te Gent, Belgium, 226. Prof A. De Moor, Rijksuniversiteit te Gent, Belgium, 16, 364, 409. Dept. of Surgery (Prof J. Kottman), Veterinary Faculty, Brno, Czechoslovakia, 388, 403. Dept. of Veterinary Pathobiology, University of Missouri-Columbia, USA, 22, 24, 50, 60, 186, 194, 203, 219, 256, 260, 373, 488, 490, 509, 510, 536, 725. Prof G. Dirksen, Medizinische Tierklinik II, Universität München, Germany, 734. Prof J. Döbereiner and Dr C.H. Tokarnia, Embrapa-UAPNPSA, Rio de Janeiro, Brazil, 75, 420, 421, 425, 429, 494, 723, 732, 733, 735, 736, 742. Dr A.I. Donaldson, Animal Virus Research Institute, Pirbright, England, 648–650. Dr S.H. Done, VLA, Weybridge, England, 240–242. Dr J. van Donkersgoed, Western College of Veterinary Medicine, Saskatoon, Canada, 439. Mr R.M. Edelsten, CTVM, Edinburgh, Scotland, 102, 112, 455. Dr. N. Evans, Pfizer Animal Health, New York, USA, 258. Prof Fan Pu, Jiangxi Agricultural University, People's Republic of China, 752. Prof J. Ferguson, Western College of Veterinary Medicine, Canada, 379, 399. Mr A.B. Forbes, MSD Agvet, Hoddesdon, England, 101, 115. Mr J. Gallagher, MAFF VI Centre, Exeter, England, 148, 149, 411, 416, 423, 426, 427, 481, 482, 591. Dr J.H. Geurink, Centre for Agrobiological Research, Wageningen, Netherlands, 745, 746. Dr E. Paul Gibbs, University of Florida, USA, 144, 152, 234, 239–240, 248, 497, 610, 612, 613, 614, 615, 611, 616, 617, 618, 619. Mr P.A. Gilbert-Green, Harare, Zimbabwe, 666. Dr H. Gosser, University of Missouri-Columbia, USA, 228, 728–730. [†]Dr W.T.R. Grimshaw, Pfizer Central Research, Sandwich, England, 28, 178, 221, 265, 508, 714, 715, 719, 720, 722. Dr S.C. Groom, Alberta Agriculture, Canada, 491. [†]Prof E. Grunert, Clinic of Gynaecology and Obstetrics of Cattle, Tierärztliche Hochschule Hannover, Germany, 548. Dr Jon Gudmundson, Western College of Veterinary Medicine, Saskatoon, Canada, 175, 262, 264, 419, 450. Mr S.D. Gunn, Penmellyn Veterinary Group, St Columb, England, 503. Dr S.K. Hargreaves, Director of Veterinary Services, Harare, Zimbabwe, 646, 687, 689, 704, 731. Prof M. Hataya, Tokyo, Japan, 11, 332. Prof C.F.B. Hofmeyr, Pretoria, South Africa, 535. Mr A. Holliman, VI Centre, Penrith, England, 751. Mr A.R. Hopkins, Tiverton, England, 521, 584. Mr A.G. Hunter, CTVM, Edinburgh, Scotland, 702. Dr P.G.G. Jackson, University of Cambridge, England, 748. Dr L.F. James, USDA Agricultural Research Service, Logan, USA, 737. Mr P.G.H. Jones, European Medicines Evaluation Agency, England, 163, 257. Prof Peter Jubb, University of Melbourne, Australia, 422. Prof R. Kahrs, University of Missouri-Columbia, USA, 144, 234, 239, 532. Mr J.M. Kelly, University of Edinburgh, Scotland, 474. Mr D.C. Knottenbelt, University of Liverpool, England, 136, 436, 480, 533. Dr R. Kuiper, State University of Utrecht, Netherlands, 111, 204, 205. Dr A. Lange, University of Pretoria, South Africa, 693, 694. Dr L. Logan-Henfrey, International Laboratory for Research on Animal Diseases, Kenya, 690–692. [†]Mr A. MacKellar, Tavistock, England, 679–682, 684. Mr K. Markham, Langport, England, 3, 18, 66, 87, 222, 298, 662. Dr M. McLellan, University of Queensland, Australia, 472, 685, 688. Mrs M.F. McLoughlin, Veterinary Research Laboratories, Belfast, N. Ireland, 711. Dr C.A. Mebus, APHIS Plum Island Animal Disease Center, USA, 670. Dr M. Miller, University of Missouri-Columbia, USA, 165, 227, 229, 251. Mr R.J. Monies, VLA, Truro, England, 255. Dr A. Morrow, CTVM, Edinburgh, Scotland, 107, 108, 114, 674. Dr C. Mortellaro, University of Milan, Italy, 317. Prof M.T. Nassef,

Assiut University, Egypt, 110. Dr D.R. Nawathe, University of Maiduguri, Nigeria, 652.
Dr S. Nelson, University of Missouri-Columbia, USA, 52. Dr S. Nicholson, Louisiana State
University, USA. Dr P.S. Niehaus, Jerome, Idaho, USA, 371. Dr J.K. O'Brien, University of
Bristol, England, 129, 156, 341, 438, 484. Dr G. Odiawo, University of Zimbabwe, Zimbabwe,
695–697. †Dr O.E. Olsen, South Dakota State University, USA, 738. Mr D.J. Dr Peter Ossent,
University of Zürich, Switzerland, 282. Prof A.L. Parodi, École Nationale Vétérinaire d'Alfort,
France, 417, 418. †Prof H. Pearson, University of Bristol, England, 10, 13, 212, 216, 270, 514,
526–528, 581, 713. Dr Lyall Petrie, Western College of Veterinary Medicine, Canada, 71, 100,
155, 197, 517, 518. Mr P.J.N. Pinsent, University of Bristol, England, 55, 72, 208, 363, 721.
*Mr G.C. Pritchard, VLA, Bury St Edmunds, England, 592. Dr José Ramos-Vara, VMDL,
University of Missouri-Columbia, USA, Prof G.H. Rautenbach, MEDUNSA, South Africa, 743.
Dr C.S. Ribble, Department of Population Medicine, University of Guelph, Guelph, Ontario,
Canada, 9. Dr A. Richardson, Harrogate, England, 6. Dr J.M. Rutter, CVL, Weybridge, England,
242. Dr D.W. Scott, New York State College of Veterinary Medicine, USA, 89, 91. Dr G.R.
Scott, CTVM, Edinburgh, Scotland, 665, 667, 671. Dr P.R. Scott, University of Edinburgh,
Scotland, 469. Mr A. Shakespeare, Dept. of Entomology and Dept. of Helminthology,
Onderstepoort, VRI, South Africa, 103, 104, 105, 224, 225. Dr M. Shearn, Institute for Animal
Health, Compton, England, 623, 625, 627, 630. Dr J.L. Shupe, Utah State University, USA,
739, 749, 750. Dr Marian Smart, Western College of Veterinary Medicine, Saskatoon, Canada,
428. Mr B.L. Smith, MAFTech Ruakura Agricultural Centre, New Zealand, 740, 741. Mr S.E.G.
Smith, Hoechst UK Ltd, Milton Keynes, England, 44, 506. Mr J.B. Sproat, Castle Douglas,
Scotland, 5, 7, 499, 707. †Mr T.K. Stephens, Frome, England, 8, 73, 80, 85, 86, 146, 158, 217,
263, 283, 299, 304, 333, 354, 434, 446, 451, 464, 557, 590, 597, 601, 622, 631. Prof M.
Stöber, Clinic for Diseases of Cattle, Tierärztliche Hochschule Hannover, Germany, 489, 496.
Dr S.M. Taylor, Veterinary Research Laboratories, Belfast, N. Ireland, 161, 223. Prof H.M.
Terblanche, MEDUNSA, South Africa, 529, 580. Dr E. Teuscher, Lausanne, Switzerland, 698,
699, 700, 701. Mr I. Thomas, Llandeilo, Wales, 493. †Dr E. Toussaint Raven, State University of
Utrecht, Netherlands, 318. Mr N. Twiddy, MAFF VI Centre, Lincoln, England, 410, 470, 501.
Dr C.B. Usher, MSD Research Laboratories, Sao Paulo, Brazil, 118, 120. Veterinary Medical
Diagnostic Laboratory, University of Missouri-Columbia, USA, 555, 660. Dr W.M. Wass, Iowa
State University, USA, 30, 31. †Mr C.A. Watson, MAFF VI Centre, Bristol, England, 29.
Mr C.L. Watson, Gloucester, England, 651. Dr D.G. White, Royal Veterinary College, England,
19, 109, 272, 358, 359, 683, 716. Dr R. Whitlock, University of Pennsylvania, USA, 2, 21, 113,
168, 169, 196, 200, 206, 230, 337, 346, 357, 360, 372, 381, 383, 387, 415, 502, 709, 710, 718.
Dr W.A. Wolff, University of Missouri-Columbia, USA, 261, 266, 643. Dr Kazunomi Yoshitani,
Nanbu Livestock Hygiene Center, Hokkaido, Japan, 12.

Numerous illustrations have been published previously by the Farming Press Ltd in *A
Veterinary Book for Dairy Farmers*; 25, 474, 526, 528 and others by the *Veterinary Record* and
In Practice; 442 and 491 by the *Canadian Veterinary Journal*; 745 and 746 by Stikstof,
Netherlands; 535 by Iowa State Press; 615 by W B Saunders and 526 and 527 by Baillière
Tindall in *Veterinary Reproduction and Obstetrics*.

Again, gratitude is due to many clinical and pathological colleagues for useful advice and
their readiness to be slide-quizzed; Julia Harvey, Somerset, is thanked for a mountain of
secretarial help, as is Catherine Girdler in the Wood Veterinary Group Practice. Norma Blowey
showed endless patience, food and coffee during the joint revision sessions in Gloucester.
Considerable help with the text has been given by colleagues at the Centre of Tropical
Veterinary Medicine, University of Edinburgh, notably Dr G.R. Scott, Mr Martyn Edelsten and
Mr A.G. Hunter, while Dr David Taylor of the Glasgow University Veterinary School revised the
microbiological nomenclature. Mr George L. Caldow and Dr Sheila Crispin were particularly
helpful with their provision of slides and comments on sections of the text.

chapter 1

Congenital disorders

Introduction

Congenital defects or diseases are abnormalities of structure or function that are present at birth. Not all congenital defects are caused by genetic factors. Some are due to environmental agents acting as teratogens. Examples include toxic plants (e.g., *Lupinus* species in crooked calf disease), prenatal viral infections (e.g., bovine virus diarrhea (BVD) resulting in cerebellar hypoplasia and hydrocephalus), and mineral deficiencies in dams of affected calves (e.g., manganese causing skeletal abnormalities).

Hereditary bovine defects are pathologically determined by mutant genes or chromosomal aberrations. Genetic defects are classified as lethal, sublethal and subvital (including compatibility with life). Although typically occurring once or twice in every 500 births, a massive range of congenital disorders affecting different body systems has been identified in cattle, primarily as a result of records kept by artificial insemination (AI) organizations and breed societies. Economic losses are low overall, but abnormalities may cause considerable financial loss to individual pedigree breeders. Most congenital abnormalities are evident on external examination. About half of all calves with congenital defects are stillborn. Many of these stillbirths have no clearly established cause.

Examples of congenital defects are given by affected system. Some are single skeletal defects, others are systemic skeletal disorders such as chondrodysplasia. Certain congenital central nervous system (CNS) disorders may not manifest their first clinical effects until weeks or months after birth, e.g., cerebellar hypoplasia, spastic paresis and strabismus, respectively.

If several neonatal calves have similar defects, an epidemiological investigation is warranted. This should include the history of the dams (their nutrition and diseases, any drug therapy during gestation, and any movement of the dams onto premises with possible teratogens), and any possible relationship of season, newly introduced stock, as well as pedigree analysis.

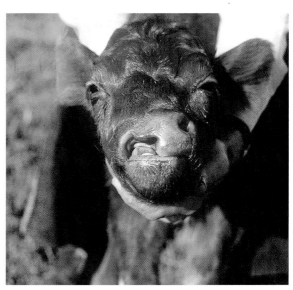

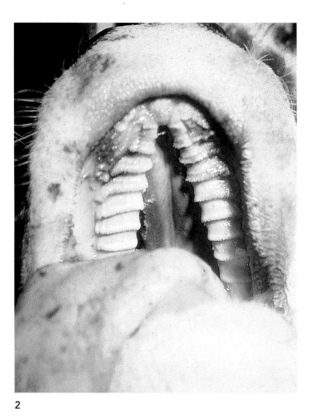

2

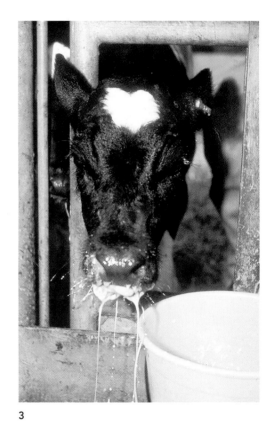

3

Congenital ocular defects are considered elsewhere (Chapter 8), as are umbilical hernia (**39**), cryptorchidism (**522**), pseudohermaphroditism (**544**) and cerebellar hypoplasia (**144**).

Cleft lip ('harelip', cheilognathoschisis); cleft palate (palatoschisis)

Definition: a failure of midline fusion during fetal development can lead to defects that affect different parts of the skeleton.

Clinical features: two obvious cranial abnormalities are illustrated here. A cleft lip in a young Shorthorn calf is shown in **1**, in which a deep groove extends obliquely across the upper lip, nasolabial plate and jaw, involving not only skin but also bone (maxilla). This calf had extreme difficulty in sucking milk from the dam without considerable loss through regurgitation.

A congenital fissure or split of varying width is seen occasionally in the hard palate, or in both the hard and soft palates of neonatal calves (**2**). The major presenting sign is nasal regurgitation, as seen in the Friesian calf (**3**). An aspiration pneumonia often develops early in life from inhalation of milk, and in some while they are still nursing. Cleft palate is often associated with other congenital defects, particularly arthrogryposis (**15**). The Holstein calf (**2**) was a 'bulldog' (see **6**). Other midline defects include spina bifida (**18**) and ventricular septal defect (**38**).

Meningocele

The large, red, fluid-filled sac (**4**) is the meninges protruding through a midline cleft in the frontal bones. The sac contains cerebrospinal fluid. The calf, a 4-day-old Hereford crossbred bull, was otherwise healthy. An inherited defect was unlikely in this case (see also **18**).

Salivary mucocele

Definition: extravasation of saliva into subcutaneous tissues.

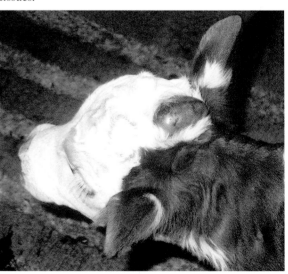

4

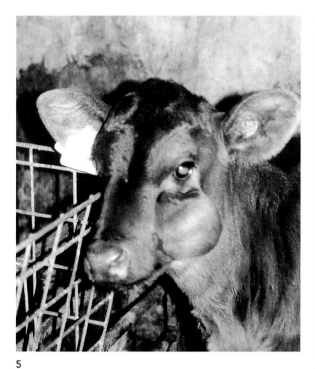

5

within 2 weeks and the calves then walk normally. Other organ abnormalities are not seen.

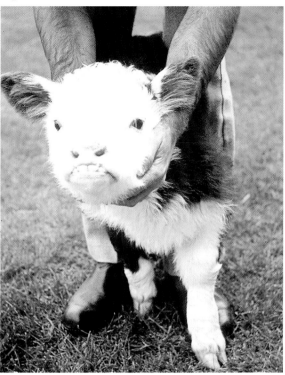

6

Clinical features: this Limousin x Friesian heifer (5) had shown this soft, painless, fluctuating swelling since birth.

Achondroplastic dwarfism ('bulldog calf') or dyschondroplasia

Definition: a failure of cartilaginous growth usually as an inherited defect.

Clinical features: the Hereford calf (6) demonstrates a brachycephalic dwarfism. The head is short and abnormally broad, the lower jaw is overshot and the legs are very short. The abdomen was also enlarged. The calf had difficulty in standing, was dyspneic as a result of the skull deformity ('snorter dwarf'), and a cleft palate was also present. A 2-week-old Simmental crossbred suckler calf (7) shows severe bowing of all four legs, especially forelegs, stunting, and a slightly dished face, and euthanasia was indicated. Born in May from a winter-housed dam fed only silage, extra feed appeared to reduce the incidence of achondroplasia from 40/200 to 5/200 offspring in successive years.

Bulldog calves are often born dead (8). This Ayrshire has a large head and short legs, but also has extensive subcutaneous edema (anasarca). Dwarfism is inherited in several breeds, including Hereford and Angus.

A related condition is congenital joint laxity and dwarfism (CJLD), which is a distinctive congenital anomaly in beef cattle in Canada. The newborn calf (9) has a crouched appearance, short legs, metacarpo-phalangeal hyperextension and sickle-shaped hind legs. Many calves are disproportionate dwarfs. The joints become stable

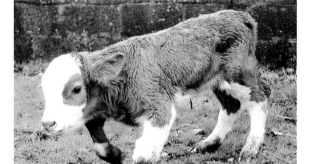

7

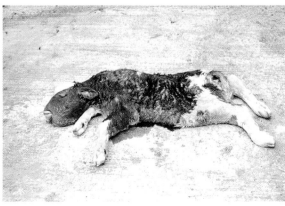

8

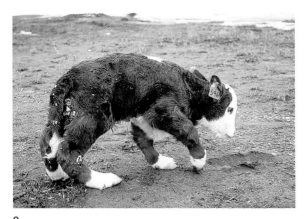

9

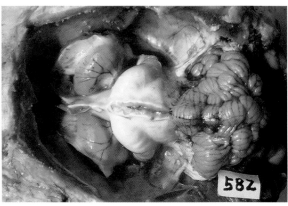

11

Schistosomus reflexus

One calf of twins was a normal live calf and the other was a schistosomus reflexus (**10**). The hindquarters are twisted towards the head, the ventral abdominal wall is open and the viscera are exposed. This anomaly usually causes dystocia.

Hydranencephaly

In hydranencephaly the cerebral hemispheres are absent and their site is occupied by cerebrospinal fluid. The fluid has been drained from this specimen (**11**) after removal of the meninges. Hydranencephaly and arthrogryposis occur

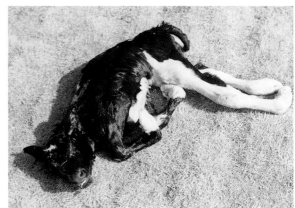

12

as a combined defect in epidemic form following certain intrauterine viral infections, e.g., Akabane virus (**12**). This calf with both arthrogryposis and hydranencephaly died shortly after birth.

Hydrocephalus

The cranium (**13**) is enlarged due to pressure from an excessive volume of cerebrospinal fluid within the ventricular system. Though usually congenital in calves, it also can occur as a rare acquired condition in adult cattle, through infection or trauma. In one form of bovine hydro-

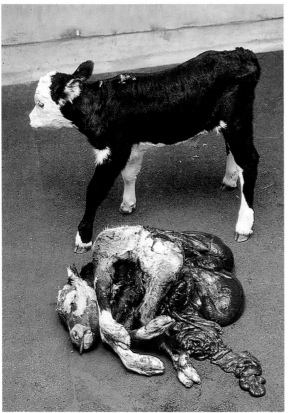

10

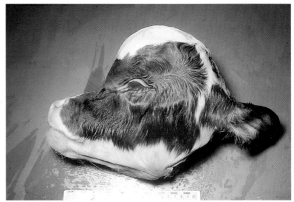

13

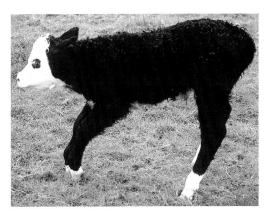

14

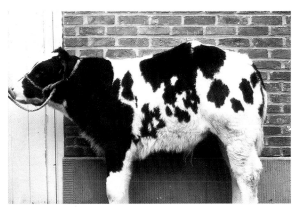

16

cephalus there is achondroplastic dishing of the face and a foreshortened maxilla ('bulldog', see 6).

Contracted tendons

Considered as the most prevalent musculoskeletal abnormality of neonatal calves, congenital contraction of the flexor tendons in this neonatal Hereford crossbred calf (14) has caused excessive flexion of the carpal and fetlock joints in the forelimbs. The hind legs are placed under the body to improve weightbearing. The affected joints may be manually extended. Pectoral amyotonia is frequently present. Some forms of the condition are inherited through an autosomal recessive gene. Rarely, cases are associated with cleft palate (2).

Management: mild cases recover without treatment. Moderate cases can be splinted, and severely affected calves may need surgery (tenotomy of one or both flexors).

Arthrogryposis

Arthrogryposis (15) is an extreme form of contracted tendons, in which many joints are fixed in flexion or extension (ankylosed). Frequently, two, three or all four limbs are involved in various combinations of flexion and extension. This calf has torticollis. The left foreleg is rotated about 180° (note the position of the dewclaws) and the right hind leg is sickle-shaped. Many such fetuses cause dystocia if carried to term. Some cases involve an

in utero viral infection, e.g., BVD (p. 43), Akabane virus (see p. 4), or the CVM (complex vertebral malformation) gene.

Vertebral fusion and kyphosis

Fusion of most of the cervical, thoracic and lumbar vertebrae in this 2-week-old Holstein calf (16) was associated with a shortened neck and increased convex curvature of the spine (kyphosis). The etiology is unknown. Kyphosis may also be an acquired condition (see 357).

Atresia ani and hypoplastic tail

Congenital absence of the anus (17) is manifested clinically by an absence of feces and the gradual development of abdominal distension. A small dimple may indicate the position of the anal sphincter. Some calves have a soft bulge from the pressure of accumulating feces. Calves usually show marked colic within 3 days. A fistula may develop between the rectum and urogenital tract, in this case with the pelvic urethra (see also 43). This calf also has a 'wry tail' or hypoplastic coccyx.

Spina bifida

Severe posterior paresis is seen in this Friesian neonate (18). The red, raised and circumscribed protuberance in

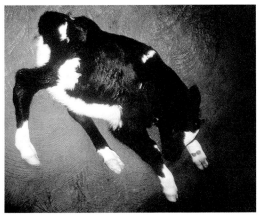

15

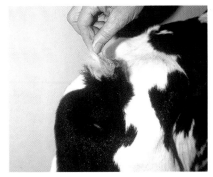

17

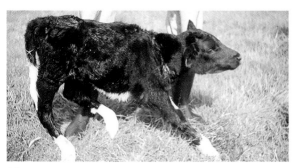

18

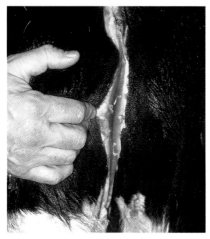

19

Segmental jejunal aplasia, atresia coli

To the right, the proximal jejunum (A) is grossly distended with fluid, as the calf (20), a 1-week-old Charbray, initially suckled normally. The distal jejunum (B) is empty owing to jejunal aplasia and stenosis. Meconium was present in the large intestine. The calf had developed progressive abdominal distension from 4 days old.

Other cases of intestinal aplasia can involve the ileum, colon and rectum, producing similar signs. Atresia coli calves appear normal at birth, rapidly develop abdominal distension and die within 1 week, with the small intestine and cecum grossly distended and the colon empty. However, proximal intestinal obstruction tends to produce a more acute and rapidly progressive condition. In some cases the intestine opens into the abdominal cavity, causing peritonitis and death within 48 hours.

Differential diagnosis: mesenteric torsion (216), intussusception (217) and perforated abomasal ulcer (57).

Syndactyly ('mule foot')

The claws of both forelegs of this Holstein bull calf (21) are fused. This congenital defect is due to homozygosity of a simple autosomal recessive gene with incomplete penetrance. It is the most common inherited skeletal defect of US Holstein cattle, but also occurs in several other breeds. One or more limbs may be affected.

the sacral region involves a myelomeningocele (protrusion of both cord and meninges). The congenital defect is due to an absence of the dorsal portion of the spine (compare 4).

Hypospadia

In this rare, male congenital anomaly, the urethra opens onto the perineum below the anus (19). The rudimentary penis is seen as a pink groove. There is urine staining of the inguinal region below.

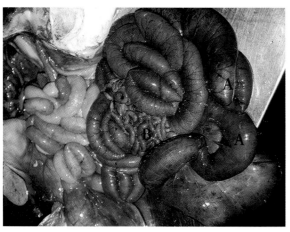

20

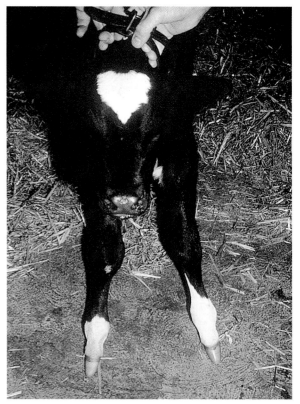

21

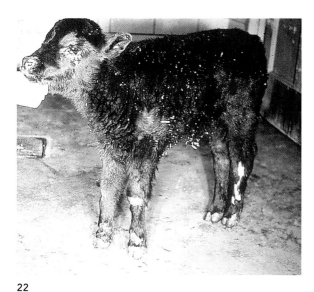

22

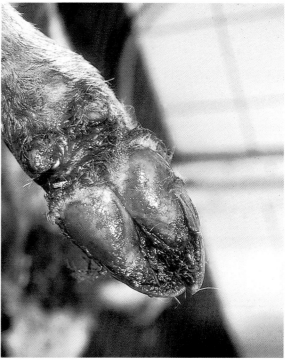

23

Epitheliogenesis imperfecta

Epitheliogenesis imperfecta is a congenital absence of the skin, in this case (22) involving the digital horn, seen most clearly in the hind feet. In a young Holstein calf (23), the extensive loss of digital horn, which involved all four limbs, is obvious. It is a rare sublethal defect in various breeds, inherited as a simple autosomal recessive gene. Large epithelial defects can involve the distal parts of the limbs as well as the muzzle, tongue and hard palate. Bleeding and secondary infection can lead to septicemia and early death.

Hypotrichosis

In one form of this inherited condition, viable hypotrichosis, the coat hair is thin, wavy and silky (24). The wrinkled skin (A) is only 2–3 cells thick. The calf has several areas of abraded skin including the carpus and the elbow. A simple autosomal recessive trait is recorded in Herefords. In

another form, lethal hypotrichosis, calves, usually hairless, are born dead or die shortly afterwards.

Parakeratosis (adema disease, lethal trait A46)

Parakeratosis is an inherited defect, which in Friesian-type cattle is associated with a poor intestinal uptake of zinc. Calves develop conjunctivitis, diarrhea and increased susceptibility to infection, and eventually die unless treated. This calf (25) was normal at birth, but developed a generalized parakeratosis at 5 weeks old. The skin of the

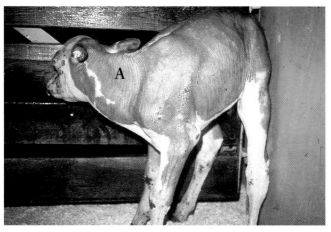

24

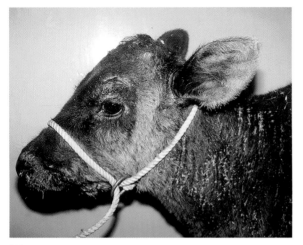

25

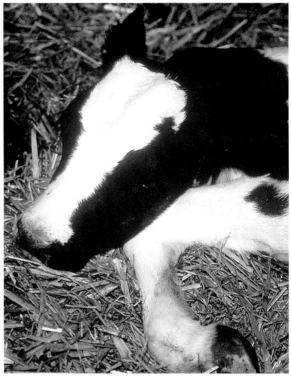

head and neck has become thickened with scales, cracks and fissures. Above the eye, the underlying surface is raw.

Differential diagnosis: dermatophilosis (106), severe lice infestation (pediculosis) (93). Diagnosis confirmed by response to Zn therapy.

Management: calves should be culled (lethal trait).

27

Baldy calf syndrome

Baldy calf syndrome is associated with hypotrichosis. The autosomal recessive trait is lethal in male Holsteins, while heifers show signs within a few weeks. This Hereford-cross calf (26) was severely depressed, with pyrexia, poor appetite, lacrimation and nasal discharge. Areas of alopecia appeared over the head and neck. A congenital disorder

that is mainly seen in Holsteins, most cases are destroyed owing to chronic unthriftiness. Both baldy calf syndrome and parakeratosis (25) respond to oral zinc supplementation, but relapse when stopped.

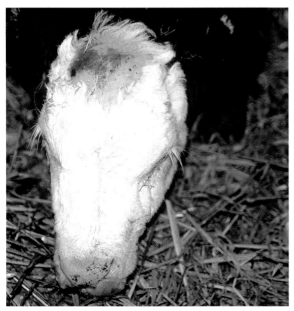

26

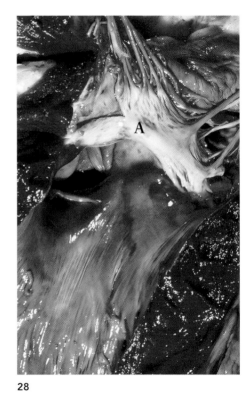

28

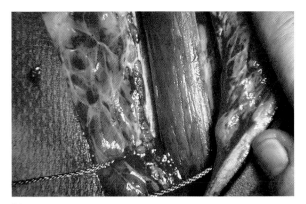

31

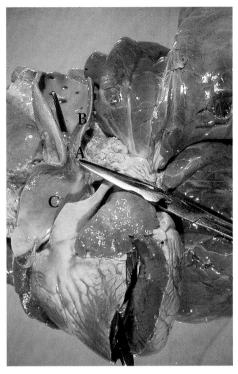

29

Ventricular septal defect (VSD)

This 2-day-old Friesian calf had a VSD (27). It was lethargic and dyspneic, especially on exercise, had pronounced tachycardia, and showed hyperemia of the muzzle. It died 2 days later. Small defects may produce few clinical effects except a loud systolic murmur. Affected calves commonly have difficulty drinking their milk and may develop severe dyspnea and/or rumen bloat from esophageal groove failure.

In a severe case revealed at postmortem, note the patency of the ventricular septum (28). The position of the left atrioventricular (AV) valves (A) shows that the opening

involves the membranous portion of the septum. Blood is usually shunted left to right. VSD may be combined with other cardiovascular anomalies.

Patent ductus arteriosus (PDA)

The heart of a crossbred Charolais bull calf (29), which suddenly collapsed with signs of severe tachypnea when 18 days old, shows an opening (A) (internal diameter 2.5 mm) between the aortic trunk (B) and the pulmonary artery (C). This opening usually closes soon after birth. If it remains patent, unoxygenated blood can pass from the pulmonary trunk into the aorta, producing signs similar to a VSD. Scissors point to the PDA. Forceps have been placed between the left ventricle (bottom) and the aorta to show normal blood flow.

Erythropoietic porphyria ('pink tooth')

Etiology and pathogenesis: the teeth (30) and ribs (31) are brownish-red owing to an abnormal accumulation of uroporphyrin I. Porphyria results from a deficiency of the enzyme uroporphyrinogen III cosynthetase.

Clinical features: the major signs, which include retarded growth, discoloration of the teeth and urine, pale mucosae, and photodermatitis, vary considerably with the age of the cattle and the season. This rare condition is inherited as a simple autosomal recessive gene. Diagnosis is aided by demonstration of ultraviolet (UV) fluorescence of the teeth.

Differential diagnosis: photosensitization due to other causes (see pp. 24, 214, 215).

Management: affected cattle, if their retention can be justified economically for fattening, should be permanently housed.

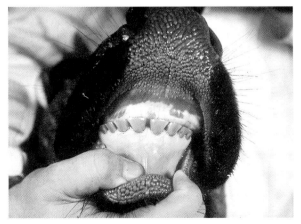

30

chapter 2

Neonatal disorders

Introduction

This chapter covers disorders of the calf from birth until postweaning. The first section deals with navel ill, umbilical hernia and general conditions of the navel. Later sections cover different forms of diarrhea and alopecia, with a miscellaneous group including calf diphtheria and joint ill. According to the presenting signs, other diseases of the young calf are considered in the relevant chapters, for example, lice, ringworm and skin diseases are to be found in Chapter 3, respiratory problems in Chapter 5, and meningitis in Chapter 9.

A calf mortality rate of 5% of live births is considered to be a 'normal' figure. Much higher losses may occur where husbandry and management are poor. There are many reasons why the young calf is particularly susceptible to disease: its defense mechanisms are not fully developed; it will be going through the transition from passive to active immunity; it may have several changes of diet; moreover, the navel provides an additional route by which infection may enter the body. Many calf diseases are exacerbated by failure to provide adequate housing, management or colostral intake.

Conditions of the navel

Umbilical eventration

Clinical features: umbilical eventration is seen in a small proportion of calves immediately after birth. The prolapsed intestines (jejunum) may be fully exposed, as in the Friesian (32), or contained in a sac of peritoneum. Opening the sac in a Charolais calf revealed a congested intestine (33). Often the exposed intestine ruptures when the calf moves. The prognosis is then hopeless. In more advanced and exposed cases the intestinal loops turn a deep red color owing to ischemic necrosis.

Management: except in the very recent (<3 hours) case surgery is rarely warranted.

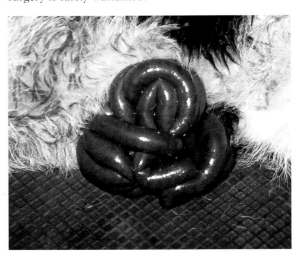

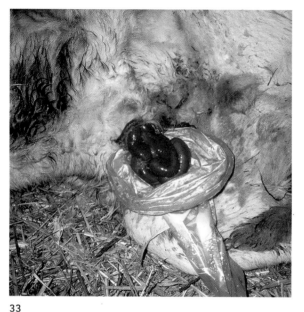

33

Navel ill (omphalophlebitis)

Definition: inflammation, usually by infection of the tissues of the umbilicus.

Clinical features: lacking skin or any other protective layer, the moist, fleshy navel cord is particularly prone to infection until it dries up, normally within 1 week of birth. In the first calf (**34**) (shown at 3 days old) the enlarged and still moist navel cord is seen entering an inflamed and swollen umbilical ring. Navel ill is uncommon at this age.

The more typical case is pyrexic, with a swollen, painful navel exuding a foul-smelling creamy-white pus (**35**). Culture usually reveals a mixed bacterial flora including *Escherichia coli*, *Proteus*, *Staphylococcus* and *Arcanobacterium pyogenes*. This case persisted for several weeks.

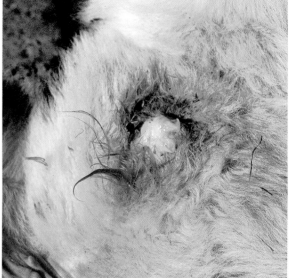

35

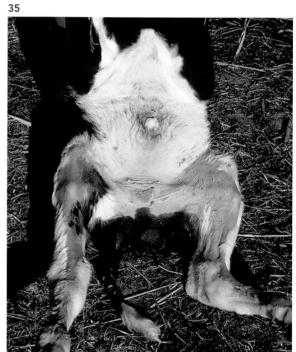

36

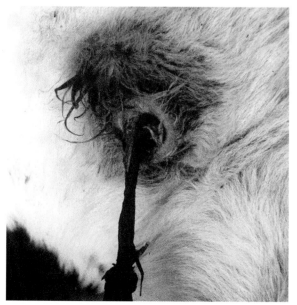

34

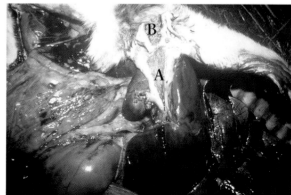

37

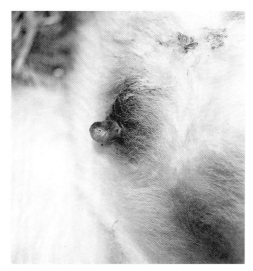

38

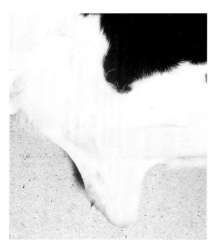

39

Alopecia on the medial aspects of the thighs (**36**) is due to a combination of urine scald and excessive cleansing of the navel by the owner. Some cases show no gross discharge, but the tip of the swollen navel will be moist and malodorous.

In other cases an intra-abdominal abscess may develop in the omphalic (umbilical) vein. In **37**, A shows the intra-abdominal abscess in the grossly distended umbilical vein, adjacent to the navel B. Spontaneous rupture of the abscess can lead to death from peritonitis (as in this calf). Occasional cases involve the urachus to produce a cystitis.

Septicemia can result in localization of infection in the joints (**73 & 74**), meninges, endocardium or end-arteries of limbs.

Differential diagnosis: umbilical hernia (**39**), eventration (**32**) and granuloma (**38**).

Management: cleansing, removal of necrotic tissue, drainage, including deep flushing of intra-abdominal lesions, systemic antibiotics. Prevention involves improved hygiene at calving, routine use of topical dressings to disinfect and desiccate the moist navel cord, optimal colostral intake.

Umbilical granuloma

A small, nonpurulent mass of granulation tissue protrudes from the navel of this 2-week-old crossbred Hereford (**38**). It is only slightly painful and the calf is not pyrexic, but the condition will not resolve until the mass is removed by ligation at its base.

Umbilical hernia

Clinical features: a large, soft, painless and fluctuating swelling can be seen cranial to the prepuce in this 3-month-old Friesian male calf (**39**). Hair has been clipped from the skin overlying the hernial sac, within which the small intestine and the fibrosed navel cord were palpable. Both were easily reducible through the large umbilical ring. Although present from birth, many hernias are not noticed until the calf is at least 2–3 weeks old. A proportion of cases are inherited.

Differential diagnosis: navel abscess (**40**), urolithiasis and ruptured urethra (**513**).

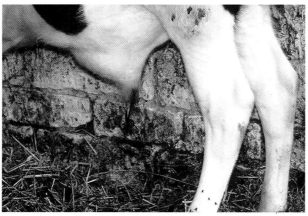

40

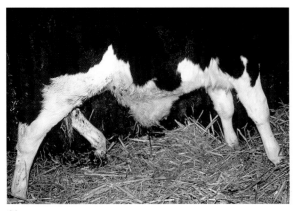

41

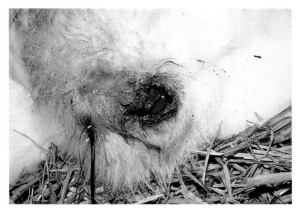

42

Management: small hernial rings often close within 6 months. Large rings require surgery.

Umbilical abscess

Clinical features: the swelling in this 4-month-old Friesian male (**40**) is cranial to the prepuce (compare urolithiasis (**513**), where it is caudal) and appeared spontaneously. The mass was initially hard, hot and painful. Pyrexia led to systemic illness. Parenteral antibiotics resulted in a change to a more fluctuating swelling, which was successfully lanced and drained.

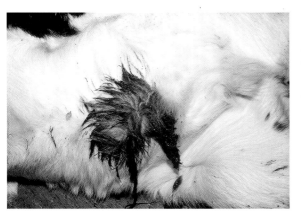

43

A hernia and an umbilical abscess can occur together. Occasionally, navel ill or navel abscess produces a localized peritonitis that erodes through the rumen wall to produce a rumenal fistula. **41** shows a 3-month-old Friesian male with a grossly enlarged navel sac, soiled anteriorly. Rumen contents leaked through the fistula, shown in close-up in **42**.

Differential diagnosis: navel ill (**34**), umbilical hernia (**39**) and rectourethral fistula (**43**).

Management: careful investigation is needed to define any intra-abdominal involvement. Exploratory surgery, with guarded prognosis.

Conditions of the gastrointestinal tract

Rectourethral fistula

Note the very soiled hair around the navel and prepuce, and the discolored urine in this 2-day-old Holstein male (**43**).

Differential diagnosis: this uncommon condition may be confused with navel ill and pervious urachus.

Management: spontaneous resolution does not occur. Surgical correction is usually impossible.

Navel suckling

Navel suckling (**44**) is a common vice in group-housed, bucket-fed calves, which are often in poor condition and have intercurrent diseases. The calf being sucked has an enlarged navel which could be infected. There is hair loss around the navel, indicating a chronic problem. The ears, tail and scrotum can also be suckled.

Management: rear calves in single pens until 1 week postweaning. Feed milk from teats, not bucket. Control intercurrent disease.

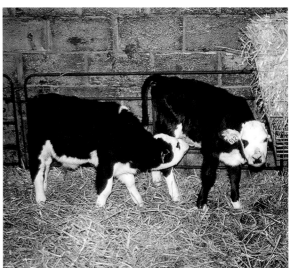

44

Calf scour

Etiology and pathogenesis: enteritis and diarrhea in calves are major causes of death in the first few weeks of life. A wide range of agents can be involved, some producing diarrhea with or without dehydration, others leading to systemic involvement. Diarrhea in the first few days of life is commonly caused by bacterial infections, for example, *E. coli* or *Clostridium perfringens*. Their toxins lead to hypersecretion from the intestine and subsequent fluid loss, seen as diarrhea. Viral infections (rotavirus and coronavirus) and *Cryptosporidia* typically occur at 10–14 days (as maternal colostral antibody wanes) and are considered to be the major causes of calf scour. Diarrhea occurs because the intestinal wall is damaged, preventing reabsorption of fluid. *Salmonella* scouring can occur at any age.

The role of other agents (e.g., parvovirus, Breda virus, a calici-like virus, and astrovirus, BVD and IBR viruses) in the calf scour syndrome has not been well defined.

Management: hygiene, colostrum and good feeding practices are very important for control. Vaccines are available against *E. coli*, rotavirus, coronavirus and *Salmonella*. It is not possible to differentiate fully between the various causes of scour on the basis of gross appearance alone, although the following illustrations give a few guidelines.

Rotavirus, coronavirus and cryptosporidia

Clinical features: the majority of calves become infected with rotavirus, coronavirus and *Cryptosporidia*, but normally only those subjected to a heavy challenge or concurrent disease show clinical signs. The cross-bred Limousin calf (**45**) is bright and alert, but has a pasty yellow diarrhea around the tail. Both rotavirus and *Cryptosporidia* were identified in the feces. Increased mucus may be passed. There may be tenesmus with *Cryptosporidiae*. More advanced cases (**46**) show dehydration and general systemic involvement such as sunken eyes, a dry muzzle, hyperemia of the nares and a purulent nasal discharge. At postmortem 2 days later, the colon was thickened, corrugated and exuding blood (**47**). *Cryptosporidia*,

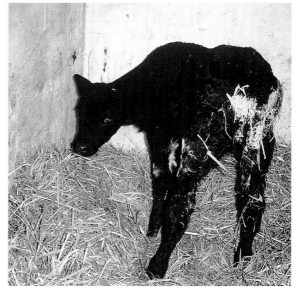

45

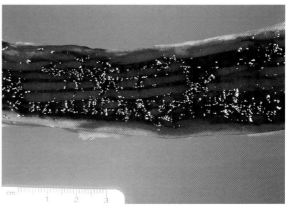

47

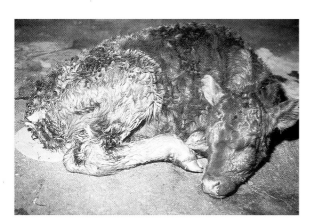

46

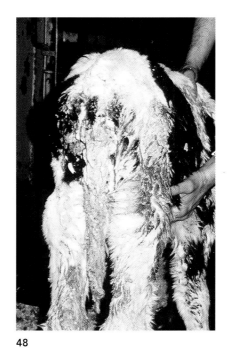

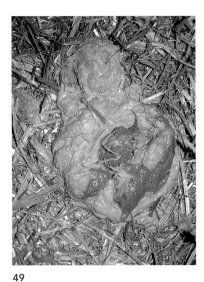

49

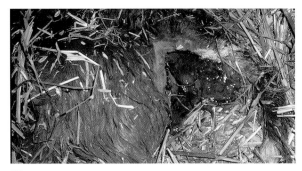

51

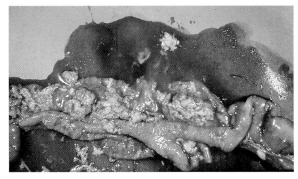

52

rotavirus, coronavirus and enterotoxigenic *E. coli* (responsible for the hemorrhagic colitis) were all isolated.

White scour

Clinical features: 'white scour' occurs when intestinal damage is such that partially digested white milk is passed in the feces. Note the characteristic white fecal soiling of the flanks and tail in this 3-week-old Holstein heifer (**48**). Originally considered to be part of the colibacillosis syndrome, it is now known that white scour can result from a range of agents, including rotavirus. Voluminous, white, rotavirus-positive feces can be voided during an explosive outbreak in a calf unit (**49**).

Enterotoxemia

Clinical features: *Clostridium perfringens* enterotoxemia normally affects calves in the first few days of life. The small intestine on the left of **50** shows a dark-red ischemic necrosis. Other areas are gas-filled, which is indicative of gut stasis and gas formation. Following sudden death, type C enterotoxin was demonstrated.

Salmonellosis

Definition: a widespread contagious disease caused by *Salmonella* spp., localized in almost any organ, leading to enteritis, septicemia, arthritis and meningitis. *S. enterica*, serotype *Typhimurium* is most common, but many other serotypes may be involved.

Clinical features: a 1-week-old crossbred Hereford calf (**51**) is moribund and passing dysenteric feces, a mixture of blood, mucus and intestinal mucosal lining. Classically, a postmortem revealed a diphtheritic enteritis (**52**), with thickening of the mucosa. However, not all calves are affected so severely. Although *Salmonella enterica*, serotype *Typhimurium* was isolated from the dysenteric feces of the affected 3-week-old Friesian calf (**53**), it was only mildly ill. Other cases show slight intestinal inflammation, the main changes being lung congestion and epicardial and renal hemorrhages. Animals recovering

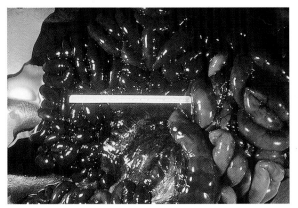

50

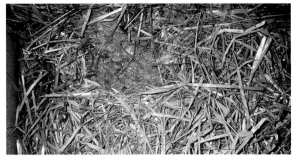

53

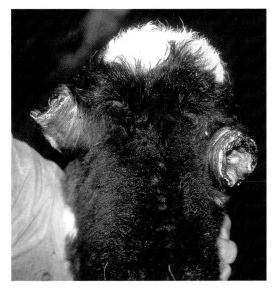

54

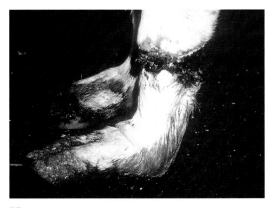

55

from peracute septicemia (especially *S. dublin*) may occasionally develop necrosis of the extremities, particularly in the ear tips, tail and legs. The 4-month-old Friesian (**54**) was recovering from a nonspecific pyrexia 6 weeks previously. Enteritis had not been observed, and is often not involved, but later ear-tip necrosis produced a bilateral slough of more than half of the pinna. *S. dublin* was isolated from the feces. In the 4-month-old crossbred Hereford (**55**), circumferential skin necrosis immediately

above the hind fetlocks has produced gangrene and necrosis of the extremities. There may be over-extension at the fetlocks, probably due to flexor tendon rupture. Salivation is a pain response.

Differential diagnosis: *E. coli* septicemia (p. 15), coccidiosis (**60**), ergot poisoning (**415**), constricting wire around leg (**412**).

Management: treatment should include fluids and electrolyte solutions given orally or in severe cases intravenously. Prophylaxis includes isolation of diseased calves, improved hygiene and adequate colostral intake in the first 6 hours after birth. Dam vaccination protects against enteritis, septicemia and abortion, and also reduces *Salmonella* excretion rates in both dam and calf. Calves may also be vaccinated. Thorough cleansing and disinfection between batches, including 'all in/all out' systems and vermin control are important in eliminating reservoirs of *Salmonella*. The zoonotic risk to man should be borne in mind.

Abomasal ulceration

Clinical features: abomasal ulceration may be associated with acute onset abomasal bloat in milk-fed calves. Affected calves develop severe abdominal pain and shock, with a right-sided tympany. Nevertheless the majority are subclinical and possibly associated with irregular feeding and early consumption of dry feed.

The 2-week-old Friesian (**56**) was moribund, with drooping ears, sunken eyes and regurgitated rumen contents on its lips. It died within hours and a postmortem revealed an acute abomasitis with two perforated ulcers (**57**), each with a creamy-white necrotic lining. Death was due to acute peritonitis (**58**). Fibrin and food coat the serosal surface of an inflamed and dilated small intestine. Abomasal ulcers are also seen in adult cattle (**207, 208**), in veal calves and in thriving beef calves, 2–4 months old, at pasture.

Differential diagnosis: includes salmonellosis (**51**), BVD, peritonitis and intestinal obstruction.

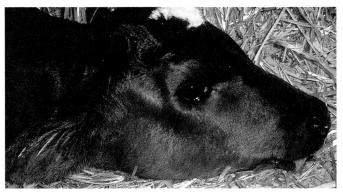

56

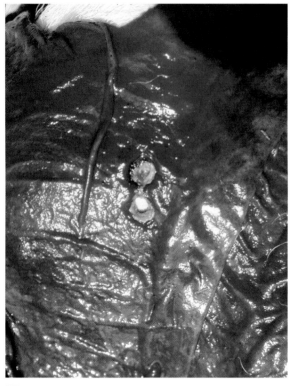

57

Management: metaclopramide has been given to control abomasal bloat. NSAIDs, anti-inflammatory drugs and antibiotics aid control of inflammation and ulceration.

Prevention: avoid overfeeding, sudden dietary changes and excessive milk flow rates through teats.

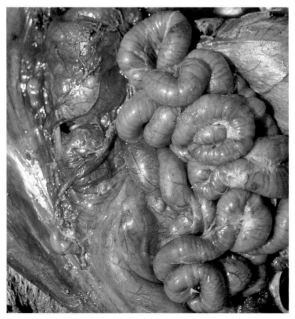

58

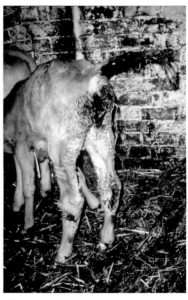

59

Coccidiosis

Definition: coccidiosis is an infection of the lower small intestine, cecum, colon and rectum, caused by the protozoan parasite *Eimeria zuernii* or *E. bovis*.

Clinical features: it is usually associated with calves crowded in unhygienic conditions. Adult animals (e.g., suckler cows) may be carriers, though oocysts may survive many months in the environment. The incubation period is 17–21 days. Affected calves are dull, pyrexic and typically produce watery feces, usually mixed with blood. Tenesmus (**59**), with continued straining and passing of small quantities of blood and feces, is a characteristic sign. The anal sphincter is open, exposing the rectal mucosa. Hair loss on the inside of the leg results from fecal soiling. Another calf (**60**) shows a thickened and inflamed colonic mucosa. Blood on the surface of freshly passed feces is a normal feature of some calves, but it occurs more often following stress, e.g., transport, or sale through a livestock market.

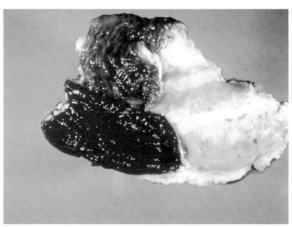

60

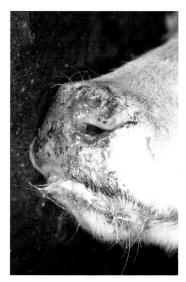

61

Differential diagnosis: diagnosis depends on demonstration of oocysts on fecal flotation or direct smear. Differentials include salmonellosis (51–53), BVD (145) and necrotic enteritis (see below).

Management: treatment includes oral decoquinate, amprolium or sulfaquinoxaline, and with parenteral sulfonamides in advanced cases. Prevention is by coccidiostats and management changes such as improved feeding methods to avoid fecal contamination.

Necrotic enteritis

Clinical features: this relatively recently recognized disease of groups of 2–3-month-old suckled beef calves in the UK has an unknown etiology. The major signs are tenesmus with diarrhea or dysentery, prominent nasal and oral lesions, grossly typical of mucosal disease but calves have no BVD antigen. Typical crusty muzzle changes are seen in **61**, while postmortem exposes the extent of pharyngeal and laryngeal necrosis (**62**). The serosal surfaces of the small intestine (**63**) show fibrin overlying extensive hemorrhagic areas. These changes extend into the muscular

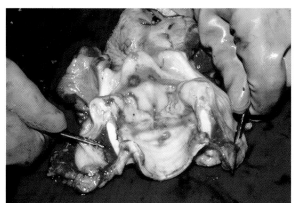

62

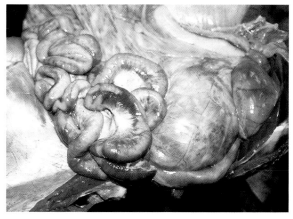

63

and mucosal layers. Other internal viscera also have hemorrhages (e.g., kidney, abomasum, lungs).

Differential diagnosis: coccidiosis (59), abomasal ulceration (56), salmonellosis (51). The postmortem findings are diagnostic (62, 63).

Management: supportive therapy.

Ruminal tympany and digestive scour ('peri-weaning calf diarrhea')

Definition: accumulation of gas in the rumen in the milk-fed calf, and an associated low-grade scour.

Clinical features: scour and chronic ruminal tympany that occur immediately pre- and postweaning commonly result from feeding errors that lead to incomplete esophageal groove closure. Milk entering the rumen may produce bloat with severe colic. Inadequate intakes of concentrates pre-weaning may also retard ruminal development. High-starch

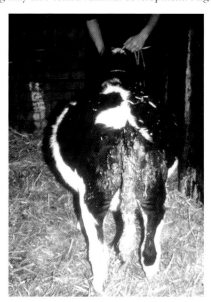

64

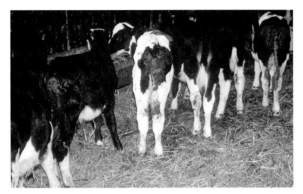

65

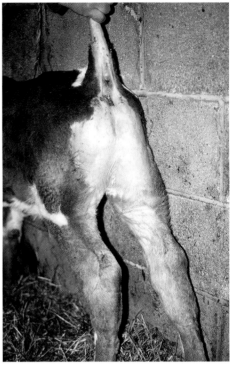

67

and low fiber diets leading to rumen acidosis predispose to peri-weaning diarrhea, as will irregular feeding, poor rumen development, and anti-nutrient factors such as excessive levels of wheat gluten and trypsin inhibitors in soya. Most outbreaks have a high morbidity but low mortality. The 4-week-old Hereford cross calf (64) shows severe ruminal tympany, with soiling of the tail and perineum, associated with chronic diarrhea which often accompanies the condition. Bloat also occurs in older cattle (see 197). The 7-week-old white Friesian calf in the center of 65 is in poor condition, with its tail and perineum matted with feces. This is typical of the peri-weaning calf diarrhea syndrome. These calves were fed unsuitable protein in a concentrate intended for adult cattle and remained stunted for many months. Infection with *Giardia* and *Campylobacter* species has been implicated in some cases.

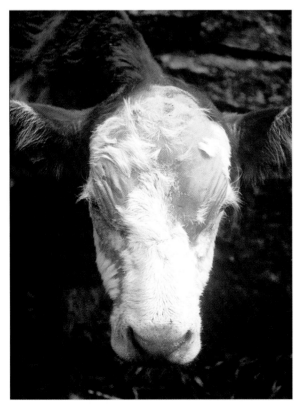

66

Differential diagnosis: digestive upsets, coccidiosis, enteric salmonellosis.

Management: optimal rumen development by feeding well-balanced high-quality rations. 'Coarse mix' rations may produce fewer problems than pellets from a reduced eating rate and increased chewing and salivation. Improved hygiene.

Conditions of the skin

Alopecia

Three distinct types of alopecia or hair loss in calves are illustrated.

Idiopathic alopecia

Spontaneous hair loss often occurs over the head, as in the crossbred Hereford calf (66). Less commonly, the whole body may be involved. Milk allergy and vitamin E deficiency are suggested causes. Most cases recover slowly over 1–2 months, without treatment.

Alopecia post-diarrhea

In the Charolais calf (67), fecal soiling following severe rotavirus scour has totally denuded the perineum and ventral surface of the tail. Following recumbency, there may also be further hair loss over the hock and lower abdomen, including the navel. Urine scald may also be a contributory cause (36).

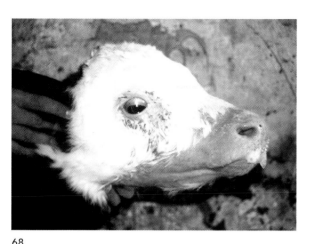

68

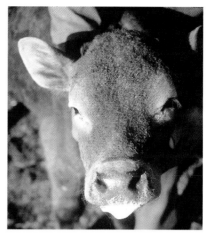

70

Alopecia on the muzzle

Alopecia of this type is seen in calves fed milk substitute and results from fat globules adhering to the skin over the muzzle. The causes include inadequate mixing of milk substitute, feeding it at too low a temperature, and calves that drink slowly. Hair loss on this 3-week-old crossbred Hereford (68) extends from the muzzle onto the nasal arch. The underlying pink skin shows secondary scab formation.

Management: ensure milk substitutes are thoroughly mixed according to manufacturer's instructions, and fed at the correct temperature.

Miscellaneous disorders

Diphtheria (oral necrobacillosis, necrotic laryngitis)

Definition: an ulcerative necrosis of the cheek, tongue, pharynx or larynx caused by *Fusobacterium necrophorum*.

Clinical features: diphtheria can produce a range of clinical signs. The Charolais calf (69) is a mild case in-volving the cheek and producing an external swelling and oral mucosal ulceration. If the tongue is involved, calves salivate excessively (70). They may drool and regurgitate partially masticated food. 71 shows a deep ulcerative area on the tongue that has been cleaned to remove necrotic debris and food. A few calves develop laryngeal diphtheria, manifested as a severe dyspnea, stridor ('roaring' breathing) and pyrexia. Such calves otherwise remain surprisingly bright and continue to feed, thus differentiating the condition from pneumonia. Normally, there is no palpable external laryngeal swelling. Contact ulcers of the laryngeal cartilages may be the initial lesions. A fetid odor is often apparent.

Postmortem examination (72) reveals a caseous infection (A), typically located bilaterally between the vocal processes (B) and the medial angles of the arytenoid cartilages (C), where it restricts air passage.

Differential diagnosis: pharyngeal and laryngeal trauma, severe viral laryngitis (IBR), actinobacillosis, laryngeal edema or abscessation.

Management: therapy with parenteral antibiotics is very effective except in the laryngeal form, where therapy may be needed for 2–3 weeks. A tracheotomy may be necessary in severe cases. Anti-inflammatory drugs may be helpful.

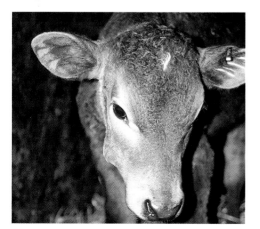

69

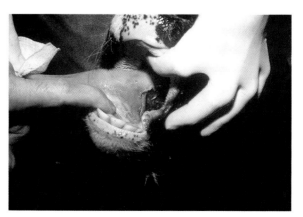

71

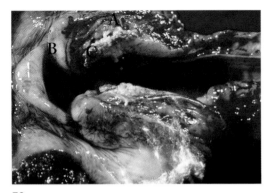

72

Joint ill

Clinical features: septicemic infection entering the navel at birth (see Navel ill) may localize in joints to produce arthritis and severe lameness, especially in colostrum-deficient calves. In the Friesian calf (**73**) the carpus is swollen as a result of intra-articular fibrinopurulent material and a periarticular soft tissue reaction. These changes are seen in the opened carpal joint in **74**. Affected calves are pyrexic. The hock, carpus and stifle are most commonly involved. Polyarthritis is often fatal. Joint ill is first seen at 3–4 weeks old (later than navel ill) and typical cases have no residual evidence of navel infection.

Differential diagnosis: physeal separation (379), fractures (377).

Management: prompt, aggressive and prolonged (7–10 days) treatment with broad-spectrum antibiotics, along with anti-inflammatory drugs for a few days. Joint lavage may be useful. Implantation of gentamycin beads into the joints has recently given good results.

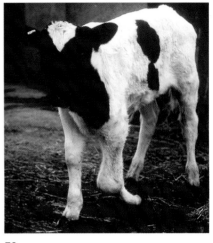

73

Iodine deficiency goiter

Clinical features: pregnant cows have an increased iodine requirement and deficient animals may give birth to still-born or weakly calves with enlarged thyroids (>20 g), known as goiter. A subcutaneous swelling is clearly visible over the larynx in this 2-week-old Zebu calf from Brazil (**75**), but in the vast majority of cases there are no external signs and the thyroid glands must be dissected and weighed. Edema and hair loss may also occur. Iodine-deficient soils occur in granite areas, mountainous regions and areas distant from the sea.

Management: mild cases respond to treatment with iodized salt. Stabilized iodized salt should be fed to dams in all areas suspected to be iodine-deficient, or where the diet contains high levels of goitrogens such as brassicas.

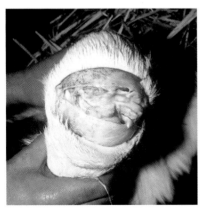

74

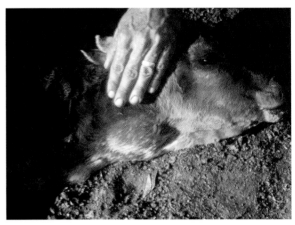

75

chapter 3

Integumentary disorders

Introduction

Skin is the largest organ of the body and performs a wide range of functions. It is mechanically protective against physical injury and provides a barrier against infections, many of which only become established when surface integrity has been compromised by physical or environmental trauma. Sense receptors detect touch and pain. Vitamin D is synthesized under the influence of ultraviolet light. Skin has a primary function in heat control, insulating against heat and cold, and, through sweating, it acts as a thermoregulator. The depth and thickness of hair coat is the main factor affecting insulation.

The major breeds of cattle in Europe and North America are derived from *Bos taurus* and have a limited ability to sweat. Cattle derived from *Bos indicus* (Brahman, USA; Africander, Africa), such as the Santa Gertrudis, can sweat copiously for long periods, although there are considerable differences in sweat production from different regions of the body surface.

Visual appraisal of the skin is easily carried out and a wide range of disorders is recognized. Anaphylactic reactions can produce urticaria. Photosensitization may result from a range of intoxications including St. John's Wort, *Lantana* and facial eczema (see also Chapter 13, **731**, **740–742**). Parasitic (lice and mange), fungal (ringworm), bacterial infections (skin tuberculosis) and fly infestations (myiasis and warbles) all produce skin changes which are discussed in this chapter. The final section deals with physical conditions such as hematomas, abscesses, frostbite and other traumatic incidents. Many skin changes are secondary to other diseases and these are described in the relevant chapters, for example, gangrene secondary to mastitis (see **600**) or ergot poisoning (see **415**), or subcutaneous swellings associated with urolithiasis (see **513**) or umbilical (navel) conditions (**39**).

Cutaneous urticaria (urticaria, angioneurotic edema, 'blaine')

Definition: a vascular reaction of the skin, thought to be an as yet unidentified plant or immunological

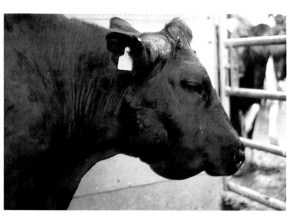

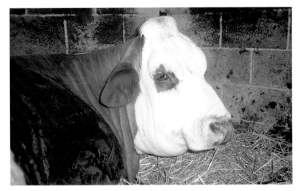

77

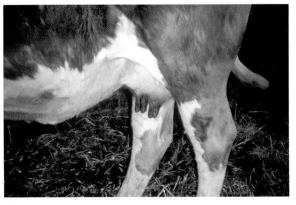

79

hypersensitivity, leading to development of multiple wheals.

Clinical features: urticaria is sudden in onset. Cases are sporadic. The Friesian cow (**76**) has raised plaques of edema (wheals) over the face and shoulders. The eyelids and muzzle are swollen. Although looking depressed, she was eating well and, like many such mild cases, recovered within 36 hours. The Simmental cow (**77**) was much more advanced, pyrexic and in considerable pain. The head, grossly enlarged due to subcutaneous edema, was often rested on the ground. The skin of the muzzle was

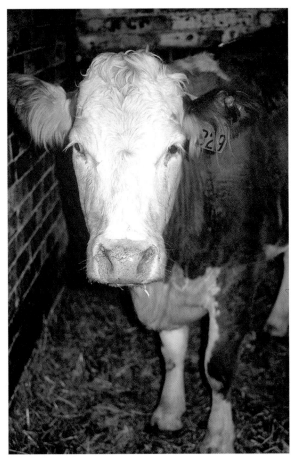

78

hyperemic. Localized areas sloughed a few weeks later. Some cases are allegedly due to snake bites or bee stings, but remain unproven.

Management: mild cases resolve spontaneously. More severe cases benefit from rapidly acting corticosteroids or NSAIDs. There is no known prevention.

Photosensitization (photosensitive dermatitis)

Etiology and pathogenesis: photosensitization has a worldwide occurrence. Photoreactive agents accumulating under the skin convert ultraviolet light into thermal energy, leading to inflammatory changes that initially produce skin swelling and, later, a possible slough. Only white or lightly pigmented skin is affected, since black skin prevents absorption of sunlight. The initial photoreactive agent may have been ingested (primary photosensitization), or may be produced as a result of liver damage (secondary, hepatogeneous). In cattle the principal photoreactive agents are porphyrins and phylloerythrins, the latter being a normal breakdown product of chlorophyll that is not metabolized

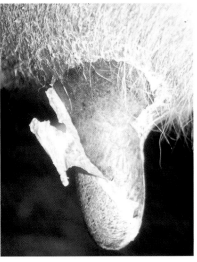

80

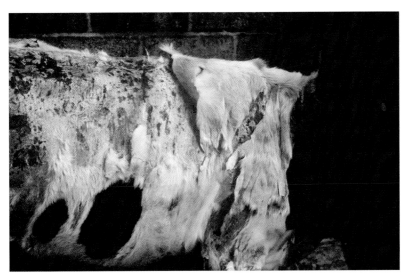

81

further. Liver damage may result from ingestion of a wide range of drugs, plants or chemicals.

Clinical features: in the early stages, affected animals show marked discomfort and pyrexia, with erythema and encrustation around the margins of the nostrils (78) and erythema of the teats (79), as in this Simmental cow. The teats are very painful and may later blister and slough (80), making milking almost impossible. The thickness of the skin slough, in this case only moderate, depends on the degree of initial damage. The primary febrile phase, edema and thickening of the white skin had passed unnoticed in the heifer in 81, and she was presented with sloughing of dry, hard areas of white skin and with a new epidermis forming beneath. Seven weeks later (82) the new skin was well-developed. Hair regrowth was possible owing to the preservation of hair follicles deeper in the epidermis. Areas of granulation tissue may retard healing (83), especially over bony prominences such as the pelvis. A dry dermatitis persisted in this cow for a further 2 years. The condition also occurs in *Lantana* poisoning (731)

and facial eczema (740–742). Serum biochemistry or hepatic biopsy may aid confirmation of liver damage.

Differential diagnosis: foot-and-mouth disease (646–650), bluetongue (659), bovine herpes mammillitis (610) and vesicular stomatitis (617, 618). Early cases, where skin edema may be difficult to detect, strongly resemble colic.

Management: during active photosensitization, cattle should be kept in the shade or preferably housed. Parenteral corticosteroids and NSAIDs may be helpful in early stages to reduce the extent of skin slough. B vitamins may help in cases with hepatic damage. Secondary skin infection and fly strike should be controlled. Skin lesions heal well despite extensive necrosis, leaving residual scarring and wrinkling.

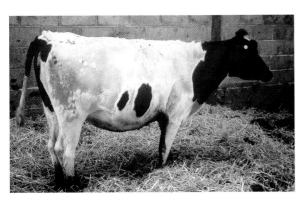

82

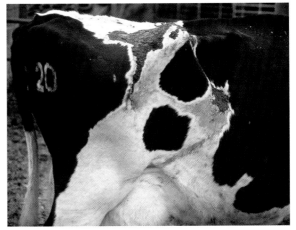

83

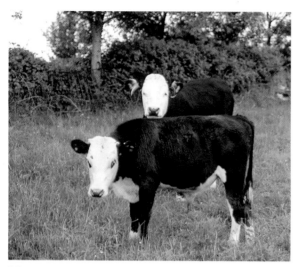

84

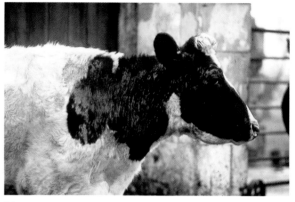

86

Brown coat color

Copper deficiency affects several systems (see **423–427**), but classically causes loss of coat color. However, copper deficiency is not the only cause of brown coat color. Animals turned out to spring grazing may retain their winter coat (**84**), particularly younger calves and first-lactation heifers. Although grazing the same pasture, the older animal at the rear is not affected.

Differential diagnosis: molybdenum toxicosis (**752**), retention of winter coat associated with ill-thrift.

Parasitic skin conditions

Cattle are affected by four genera of mange mites, i.e., *Sarcoptes*, *Chorioptes*, *Psoroptes* and *Demodex*, six species of lice, skin helminths (*Stephanofilaria* and *Parafilaria*), myiasis (screw-worm) and various fly infestations. Parasitic skin infestations are most commonly encountered in housed

cattle in winter. Many such conditions cannot be differentiated on clinical examination alone and laboratory tests are necessary. Often several conditions coexist, e.g., mange, ringworm and lice may occur simultaneously on cattle in poor condition. The appearance and location of mange lesions are generally characteristic for the particular mite, although specific diagnosis depends on microscopic examination of the mouthparts.

Mange
Sarcoptic mange (scabies)

Caused by *Sarcoptes scabiei* var. *bovis*, lesions are typically seen over the head, neck and hindquarters (**85**). Note the hair loss and severe thickening of the skin in **86**. The white areas show secondary damage due to rubbing. In severe cases there may be almost total hair loss. The close-up view (**87**) shows the dry, scaly appearance of the thickened skin.

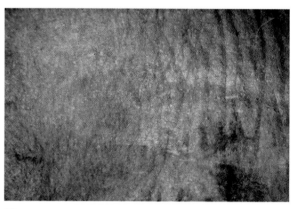

87

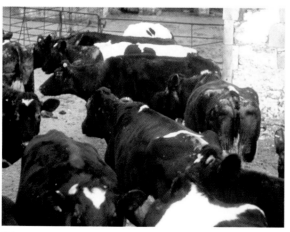

85

Chorioptic mange

Chorioptic mange is the most common type of mange in cattle. The fold of skin beside the tail is the characteristic

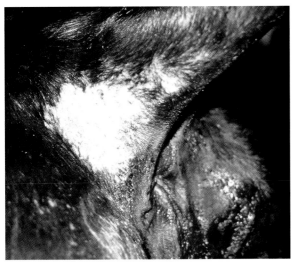

88

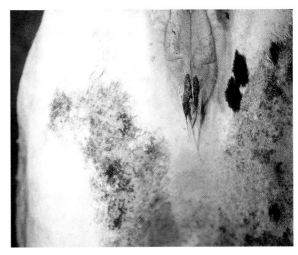

89

site for infestation by *Chorioptes bovis* (88). Lesions comprise a thick encrustation overlying an area of moist, serous exudate. They are intensely irritant. In more advanced cases (89) red, pustular lesions may spread down the perineum.

Psoroptic mange

Note the skin thickening and hair loss in the cow (90), extending from the vulva to the udder. The condition may start at the withers and spread over the whole body. Pruritus may be marked. Psoroptic mange (*Psoroptes ovis*) is notifiable in North America, where eradication programs have been in progress for many years. One type of mite that causes this type of mange is *Psoroptes natalensis*.

Demodectic mange (follicular mange)

Small papules are seen on the white skin of this cow (91), from which a thick, white, waxy material containing large numbers of mites can be expressed. Another case (92) shows papules over the skin of the shoulder. Some nodules become secondarily infected with *Staphylococci*. The condition is generally mild, with a spontaneous recovery. Extensive hair loss is rare.

Management of mange: as mite eggs take 2 weeks to hatch, two pour-on O-P treatments, 2–3 weeks apart, are needed or two injections of ivermectin. Alternative drugs are single doses of doramectin or eprinectin, both of which have greater persistence.

Lice (pediculosis)

Clinical features: sucking lice (for example, *Haematopinus eurysternus* and *Linognathus vituli* and, in North America, *Solenopotes capillatus*) are slower moving than biting lice

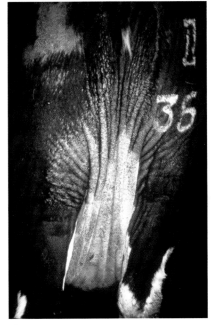

90

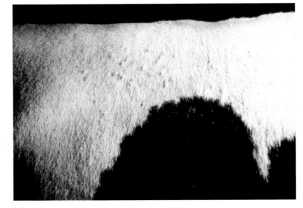

91

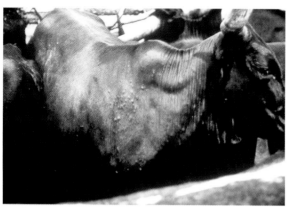

92

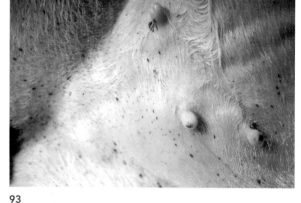

93

(*Damalinia [Bovicola] bovis*). In addition to pruritus (the only lesion due to biting lice), sucking lice may produce severe anemia, loss of condition and even death. Pediculosis is most prevalent in the winter months. Parting the hair along the back may reveal small, brown lice just visible to the naked eye. They are often more easily seen on the hairless skin of the groin (**93**). Note the variation in their size.

Clinically, infestations are manifested by rubbing, biting, scratching, and thickening of the skin. In **94** the calf's tongue is protruding and its head is held on one side, a stance typical of pruritus. In early cases the hair develops vertical lines on the neck, and small, hairless areas with white scurf may arise from biting. In more advanced cases the skin is thickened round the face and the vertical hair lines on the neck are thrown into thick folds, as in this adult Ayrshire cow (**95**). Some calves may be stunted and anemic. Ringworm often occurs in association with lice: early lesions are seen on the shoulder in **94**. Pale beige-colored oval lice eggs ('nits'), glued onto the hair shafts, can often be seen with the naked eye, particularly on the ear (**96** near tag). In older animals the coat may be matted with lice eggs.

Management: national regulatory agencies control insecticide usage in cattle. Organochlorine compounds are very effective but their use is prohibited in many countries.

Eggs hatch over a period of 2–3 weeks. Two treatments, 2 weeks apart, can be very effective, e.g., phosmet or coumaphos pour-on or as dips, or permethrin synergized with piperonyl butoxide and tetrachlorvinophos as sprays or pour-on. Single pour-on applications of doramectin are also very effective. Badly infested cattle may benefit from multivitamins.

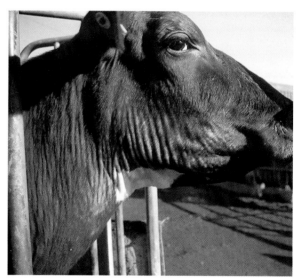

95

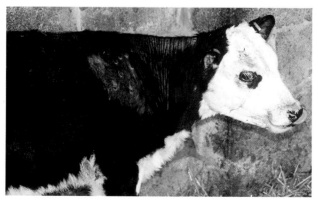

94

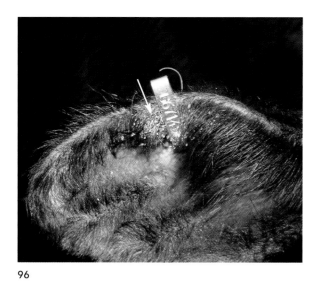

96

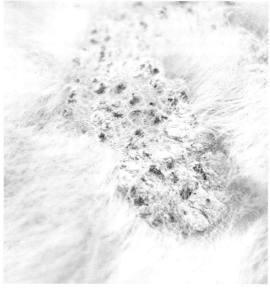

98

Ringworm (dermatophytosis)

Definition: ringworm is a fungal infection of the superficial, dead, keratinized tissues of the hair and skin, of which *Trichophyton verrucosum* is the most common cause in cattle. Occasionally, *Microsporum* species may be involved. Ringworm is an important zoonosis.

Clinical features: dermatophytosis is most commonly recognized in calves but is not uncommon in dairy cows. Lesions are commonly seen over the head and neck (97), but they may occur on any part of the body. They consist of circular areas of alopecia in which the skin is thickened and often markedly encrusted. The initial stages show progressive alopecia and erythema of the skin, with encrustation developing later. Lesions expand from the periphery and several smaller areas may coalesce (98). Older animals may show generalized small discrete lesions (99). After hair loss these tend to be erythematous and lack the dry scaly appearance seen in 97.

Ringworm causes irritation and if affected calves rub against posts or feed troughs, they deposit spores that can remain infective for up to 4 years.

Management: spontaneous recovery is commonly seen. Valuable individual animals may be treated by firstly removal of the crusted material and then whole body application of a wash or spray of natamycin or oral dosage with the fungistatic antibiotic griseofulvin. An effective live attenuated vaccine is available.

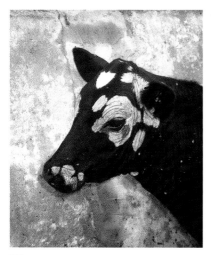

97

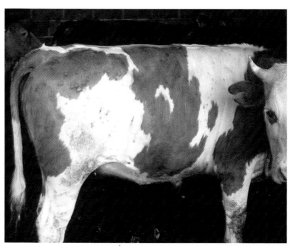

99

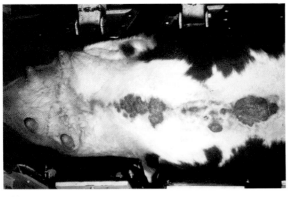

100

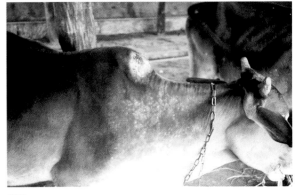

102

Skin helminths

Cattle are affected by four genera of skin helminths, *Onchocerca*, *Pelodera* (*Rhabditis bovis*), *Stephanofilaria* and *Parafilaria*.

Cutaneous stephanofilariasis

Microfilariae of *Stephanofilaria stilesi* are introduced into the skin of the ventral midline by the horn fly (*Haematobia irritans*) as it feeds, producing large, circular areas of dermatitis, seen here on the ventral abdomen (**100**). Recent lesions are moist, with blood or serous exudate, whilst long standing areas are characterized by alopecia and hyperkeratosis.

Stephanofilarial otitis (parasitic otitis)

Caused by *Stephanofilaria zaheeri*, parasitic otitis is most prevalent in older cattle in humid weather. Note the painful erythematous inflammation on the inside of the ear of this Zebu cow from India (**101**). In East Africa a free-living nematode, *Rhabditis bovis*, can also produce a purulent otitis that may lead to middle ear involvement.

Stephanofilarial dermatitis (hump sore)

Transmitted by flies, *Stephanofilaria assamensis* produces an irritant dermatitis. The raw, granulating area seen on the hump of this cross-bred Jersey cow from Bangladesh (**102**) results in lost milk production, reduced working capacity and hide damage. Exotic cattle are affected more than indigenous breeds.

Parafilarial infection

Clinical features: Parafilarial infection is common in parts of Asia, Africa and Europe. Transmitted by flies of the *Musca* genus, *Parafilaria bovicola* produces painful subcutaneous lesions that may impede the productivity of draught animals, but, more importantly, can lead to serious economic losses from carcass trimming of beef cattle at slaughter. The female worm perforates the host's skin and oviposits into blood dripping from the wound. A typical 'bleeding spot' is illustrated on the chest wall of this South African bull (**103**). (The fecal soiling on the crest wall of the neck is coincidental.) Flies feeding on the blood, which may continue to flow for several hours, ingest eggs containing microfilariae. A typical female worm nodule is shown in **104**, closely adherent to the hide.

Management: fly control, including impregnated ear tags, is important in prevention.

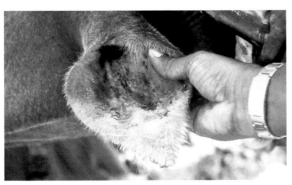

101

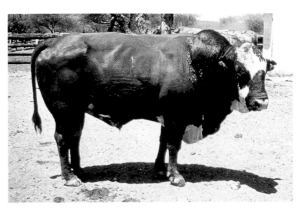

103

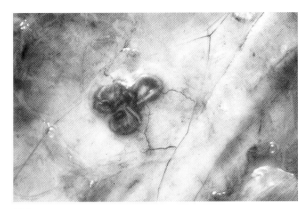

104

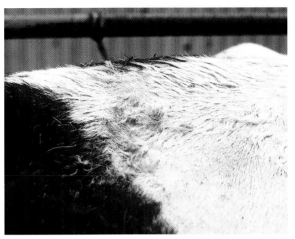

106

Besnoitiosis

A sporozoan parasite of the family Sarcocystidae, *Besnoitia besnoiti* can cause a systemic illness of fever, diarrhea and lymphadenopathy, or, as in this case (**105**), a dry sclerodermatitis. The South African bull shows intense thickening of the skin (elephant skin appearance) and complete hair loss over the affected areas. In advanced cases the skin may crack, predisposing the animal to secondary bacterial infection or myiasis, and a resulting weight loss. Mortality is low. Besnoitiosis has been reported in Southern Europe, Africa, Asia and South America. Biting flies or ticks may transmit *B. besnoiti* mechanically. Initial signs may be limited to a few cysts in the scleral conjunction.

Diagnosis: initial signs of scleral conjunctival and nasal mucosal cysts followed by fever and painful ventral swellings (anasarca), later by sclerodermatitis. Crescent-shaped bradyzoites can be seen in skin or conjunctival scrapings.

Management: isolation and symptomatic treatment of affected cattle; reduction of biting insects and ticks; possible use of a live tissue culture-adapted vaccine.

Other bacterial and viral skin disorders
Dermatophilosis (cutaneous streptothricosis)

Definition: skin lesions caused by infection with the bacterium *Dermatophilus congolensis*, and sometimes erroneously called 'mycotic dermatitis' following exposure to prolonged periods of wet weather.

Clinical features: in temperate climates lesions are mild, as in the Friesian cow (**106**), which has non-pruritic, raised clumps of hair (which can be easily lifted off) with a light brown, waxy exudate at the base. In warmer climates, particularly during periods of high humidity and increased fly and tick activity, zoo-spores dormant in the epidermis may become active in almost epidemic proportions to cause more severe skin damage, with secondary inflammation. This cow from Antigua (**107**) shows small, raised, nodular skin tufts, especially over the neck and shoulders. More advanced lesions (also West Indian origin) coalesce to form plaques (**108**) with an almost wart-like appearance. Chronic severe cases can lead to emaciation.

Differential diagnosis: warble fly (**115,116**), lumpy-skin disease (**666**), mud fever (**322**).

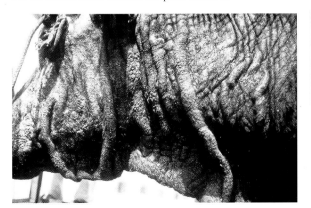

105

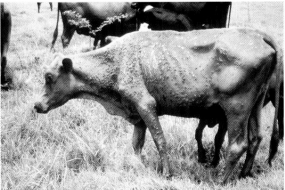

107

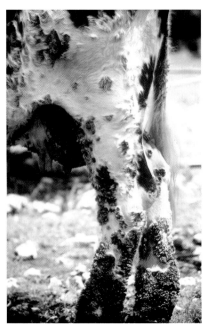

108

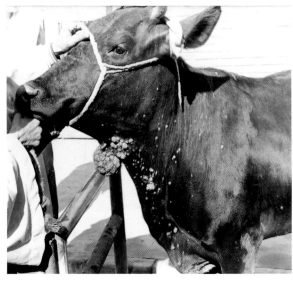

110

Management: housed cattle can be provided with self-grooming facilities such as wall brushes. Provide shelter from rain. Severe cases may benefit from parenteral antibiotics.

Fibropapillomatosis (papillomatosis, warts)

Clinical features: warts, predominantly seen in 6–18-month-old cattle, appear as fleshy lumps on the head and neck. Large, pendulous warts may also be seen along the brisket and sternum. Their size varies enormously, from 5 cm in diameter (**109**) to small nodules, only just visible above the hair of the skin. They sometimes occur in the neck region of adult draught cattle, seen here in the neck region of an Egyptian native Balady cow (**110**). Warts also occur on teats (**620–622**), penis (**523**), and in the bladder (**722**), when they are associated with bracken poisoning. Skin warts are caused by papovaviruses. Five species have been reported, including three distinct

species on teats. Warts are most commonly seen in larger groups of young cattle. Flies and lice may be important in transmission.

Management: most warts, even penile lesions, resolve spontaneously with age following development of viral immunity. Pedunculated warts may often be pulled off, sometimes following ligation of the pedicle. Some success has been claimed for simple autogenous vaccines. Extensive areas may develop secondary infection which can benefit from washing and superficial disinfection.

Skin tuberculosis (atypical mycotuberculosis)

Clinical features: typical indurated nodules, running along the path of corded lymphatics beneath the skin, are visible running obliquely across the shoulder and on the lateral aspect of the foreleg (**111**). The lesions contain nonpathogenic, acid-fast bacteria and may affect the reaction to the tuberculin skin test for TB. Some consider these chains of subcutaneous nodules are typical for animals infected with Bovine Immunodeficiency Virus (BIV) but this is unlikely.

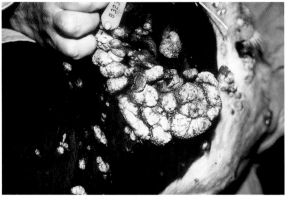

109

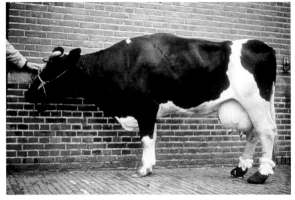

111

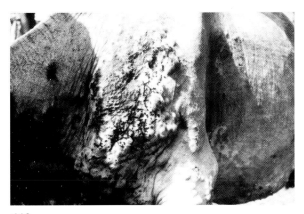

112

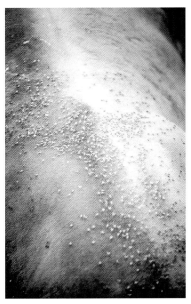

114

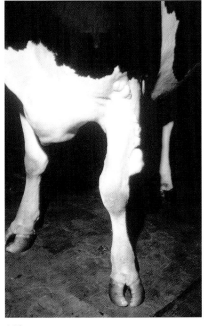

113

granulomatous proliferating lesion over the skin of the shoulder.

Ulcerative lymphangitis (pseudotuberculosis)

Caused by *Corynebacterium pseudotuberculosis*, ulcerative lymphangitis is primarily a condition of sheep and goats, although cattle can be affected. Large, caseous nodules occur in the lymphatics of the forelimb (**113**) and may involve drainage lymph nodes.

Differential diagnosis: skin tuberculosis (**111**), bovine farcy (**112**).

Fly infestations

A wide range of fly species feeds on cattle, the most common being horn flies, buffalo flies (*Haematobia irritans*) seen on the skin of the back in **114**, head flies (*Hydrotea irritans*) and face flies (*Musca autumnalis*). In addition to

Differential diagnosis: ulcerative lymphangitis (**113**) and bovine farcy (a purulent lymphangitis and lymphadenitis caused by *Nocardia farcinica*) (**112**), seen here as a pyo-

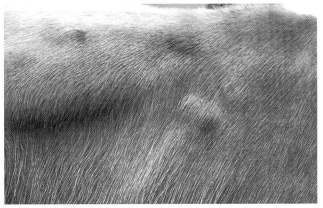

115

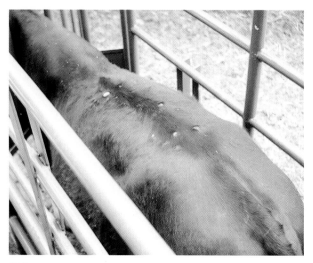

116

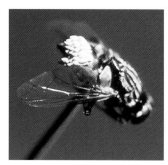

117

causing annoyance, and therefore restricting feed intake, these flies may also produce anemia and transmit disease, for example, *Parafilaria* and *Moraxella bovis* in infectious bovine keratoconjunctivitis (IBK).

Warble fly

Definition: warble fly or 'warbles' comprises a range of syndromes caused by migrating larvae of *Hypoderma*

and *Dermatobia* species. Skin damage is the most common, but spinal paralysis, choke from esophageal inflammation and anaphylactic reactions can also occur.

Clinical features: there are two species of warble fly (heel fly): *Hypoderma bovis* and *H. lineatum*. Both lay eggs on the hair of the lower legs. Emerging larvae penetrate the epidermis and migrate subcutaneously to the skin of the back, which they puncture for breathing holes, and then encyst. Encysted larvae in the subdermal tissues produce smooth skin swellings (**115**) known as warbles. Over a period of 4–6 weeks, warble larvae undergo three molts, the light cream to dark brown third-stage larva then emerging through the breathing hole to fall to the ground to pupate. A late third-stage larva (**116**) has been manually expressed onto the skin, over the anterior chest. A cluster of five larval breathing holes, with larvae feeding beneath, is present in the skin, dorsal to the lumbar spine. Losses due to warbles arise from damage to the most valuable part of the hide, from reduced grazing due to fear of the adult fly, and rare cases of paralysis resulting from hypersensitivity to dead larvae in the spinal canal.

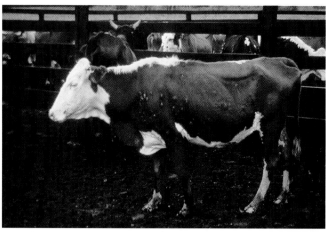

118

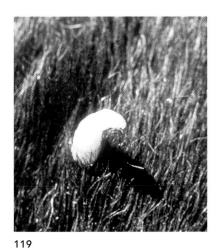

119

Management: systemic insecticides, e.g., organophosphorus compounds (contraindicated in lactating cattle) or avermectins. Warble fly infestation is a notifiable disease in many countries, including Britain, and specific control measures must be followed.

Tropical warble fly: *Dermatobia hominis*

Clinical features: *Dermatobia hominis* is known as the tropical warble fly. It is distributed only between southern Mexico and Argentina in South America, where it is a major problem. Human infection can also occur. The adult lays its eggs on a range of other insects (49 different species have been recorded), which then transmit the eggs to cattle when feeding on them. Eggs are visible between the wings of the fly, *Musca domestica*, in **117**. On hatching, larvae rapidly burrow through the skin and encyst to form a subcutaneous nodule, the warble. Firm warble nodules are seen on the Hereford crossbred cow from Brazil (**118**), especially over the shoulders and flanks. (Warbles of *Hypoderma* are seen only along the back, **116**.) After feeding for 40–50 days, the mature larvae emerge (**119**) and fall to the ground to pupate. Severe pain and irritation, with secondary infection, may occur as the larvae emerge, as seen in the Zebu cow in **120**.

Management: as for warble fly; some cattle strains show resistance to *D. hominis*.

Screw-worm or myiasis

Clinical features: the parasites known as screw-worms are the larvae of the blowflies *Cochliomyia hominivorax* and *Chrysomyia bezziana*. The adult fly lays eggs on wounds, the navel of neonates, or on tick-damaged areas (**675**). **121** shows an early infestation. More advanced lesions (**122**) may be filled with larvae of mixed ages, some of which will be mature and ready to leave and pupate in the soil. A profuse, foul-smelling exudate with extensive skin damage is typical. The disease is of major importance in South America and has been reported in North Africa and Southern Asia.

Differential diagnosis: vital to differentiate screw-worm from other fly larvae. Mature larvae are pink, 1–2 cm long and have rows of fine dark spines on the anterior part of each segment. Transport to laboratory in 70% alcohol.

Management: notifiable disease in some countries which have eradication campaigns. Local and systemic (spray, dip) treatment with organophosphorus compounds and avermectins.

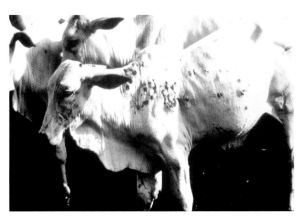

120

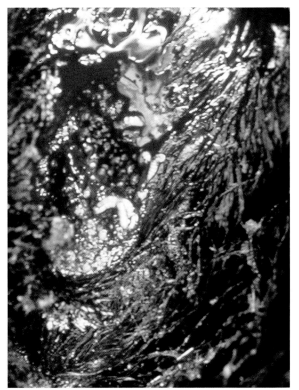

121

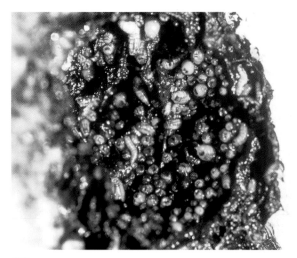

122

Traumatic and physical conditions

In addition to being the largest organ of the body, the skin is also the most exposed. Injury is common, particularly when cattle are housed in poorly designed, overcrowded buildings and handled roughly. Damp, dirty conditions may compromise the skin defenses. When such factors are combined with inadequate bedding and projections from housing, abscesses or more severe injuries can result. Cattle can withstand wide extremes of temperature, although frostbite does occur. Hematomas are commonly the result of physical injury, whilst other subcutaneous swellings may result from hernia or rupture.

Hematoma

Clinical features: hematomas are initially soft, painless, fluctuating, fluid-filled swellings that appear suddenly. Common sites are points with no muscle cover where skin trauma against bone can occur, e.g., over the pelvic prominences (**123**), spine (**124**), the lower flank (**125**) and shoulder. Occasional hematomas spread into the pelvic

cavity, increasing intrapelvic pressure and interfering with urination and defecation. The case in **124** occurred as a result of being trapped under a cubicle (free stall) division, and the flank hematoma (**125**) followed a horn gore. Without rupturing, the majority of smaller hematomas resolve to leave thick skin folds. Sometimes a hematoma becomes infected and develops into an abscess. Occasionally, hematomas burst, releasing the blood clot.

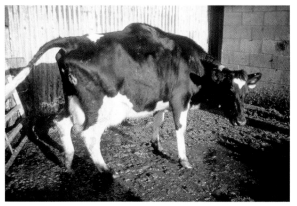

124

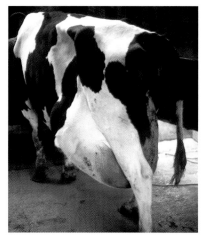

125

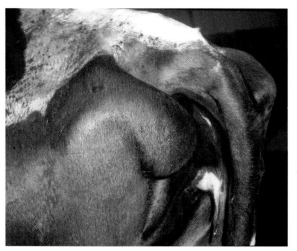

123

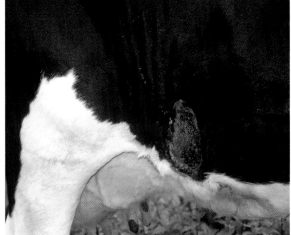

126

In one such case (126), characteristic thick folds of skin can be seen cranial to the stifle.

Differential diagnosis: abscess, flank rupture, hernia.

Management: minimal interference is best for most cases, as spontaneous resolution occurs. Some hematomas develop into abscesses and need drainage. Occasional cases are so extensive that culling is necessary.

Prevention: identify, then minimise points of trauma.

Bursitis of the neck

In **127**, hair loss at the cranial aspect of the lesion indicates that the bursitis was caused by continually pushing against a feed barrier. Like a hematoma, the swelling is soft, painless and fluctuating, but it develops more slowly. Aspiration disclosed a clear fluid. Bursitis also occurs on the hock (**389**) and carpus (**403**) as a result of inadequately bedded cubicles.

Management: individual lesions are best left to resolve spontaneously, having first removed the animal from the source of trauma. If several cattle are affected, then structural changes may be indicated, e.g., improving cubicle bedding.

Skin abscesses

Clinical features: abscesses are generally hard, hot, and slightly painful swellings that develop and enlarge slowly, thus differentiating them from a hematoma (**123**) or a hernia (**130**) which usually appear suddenly. The Hereford steer (**128**) has a sterile abscess on its neck, caused by the injection of a vaccine. Injecting a 40% solution of calcium borogluconate subcutaneously can lead to a hard, fluid-filled, sterile swelling developing over a period of 3–6 weeks. The popliteal region is a common site for abscessation, as seen in the Friesian cow (**129**). A large, fluctuating swelling is seen on the left leg, lateral to the stifle. The abscess is often deep in the muscle and may slowly enlarge over several months.

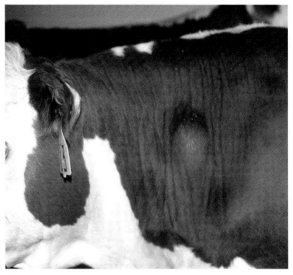

128

Management: abscesses are best left to develop until one part of the capsule is obviously softer, and then lanced at this point, drained and flushed to achieve resolution. Repeated pressure irrigation is also useful.

Flank hernia

Clinical features: the flank hernia in the Ayrshire cow (**130**) developed suddenly, probably as a result of a horn gore by another cow, 2 months before presentation. Other cases occur spontaneously, especially in older cows in late pregnancy, where pressure of intra-abdominal contents will be a predisposing factor.

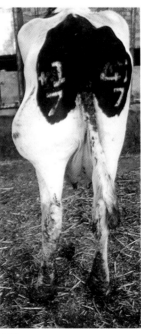

129

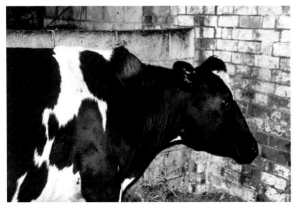

127

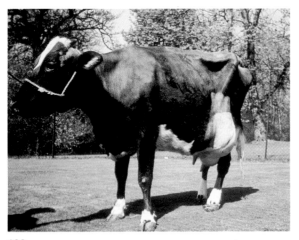

130

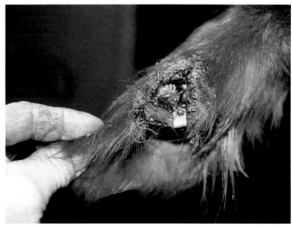

132

Management: large flank hernias in adult cattle can rarely be successfully treated by surgery, and tend to enlarge in late pregnancy, reducing in size after calving.

Rupture of prepubic tendon

The udder has dropped ventrally and the sac of skin and muscle anterior to it contains abdominal organs (**131**). Hydrallantois had resulted in the excessive abdominal distension and subsequent rupture.

Management: repair is hopeless, and culling is indicated.

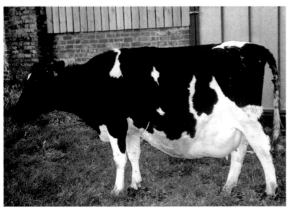

131

Infected ear tag

Infection of an ear tag occurs when insufficient space is allowed for growth of the ear margin, or when the tag is inserted too close to the ear base. In **132** granulation tissue and a wet, purulent exudate have developed around the tag. Such areas are painful and subject to myiasis.

Management: the tag must be removed and the area cleansed, whereupon the residual wound heals rapidly.

Ear necrosis from frostbite

The tips of both ears of the Limousin cow (**133**) are missing: the cause was neonatal frostbite. Scrotal frostbite is illustrated in **541**.

Differential diagnosis: septicemia, e.g., associated with peracute salmonellosis (**55**), fescue toxicity (**414**) and ergot poisoning (**415**), can produce similar changes in the extremities.

Skin necrosis following caustic dehorning paste

Excessive use of caustic dehorning paste produced the scab-covered skin slough extending from the horn bud towards the eye of this Limousin calf (**134**).

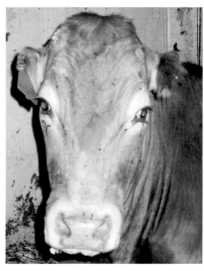

133

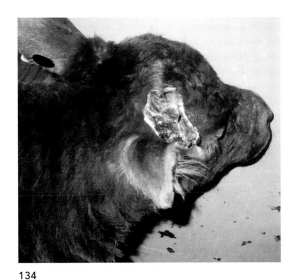

134

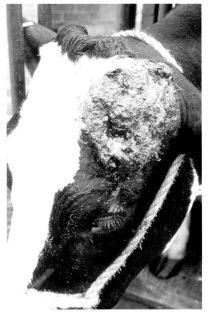

136

Ingrowing horn

Etiology and pathogenesis: the horn tip in **135**, which has now been removed, had penetrated through the skin into the underlying dermis, producing this painful, festering wound, which could develop secondary myiasis. This has serious welfare implications. Some cases develop as a result of apparently normal horn growth in older cattle, others are the result of earlier horn damage.

Management: check the space between horn tip and skin in any suspect case. The horn tip is non-sensitive and can be removed without local anesthetic.

Horn core carcinoma

Definition: a squamous cell carcinoma of the mucosa of the frontal sinus, developing in horned or dehorned breeds, especially common in the Indian subcontinent.

Clinical features: a severe case of horn core cancer is shown in **136**, a 6-year-old Holstein cow in the UK, which had been dehorned at 2 years old. The tumor grew slowly

at first, was worried by flies and suddenly showed this massive enlargement. The frontal sinus was filled with neoplastic and granulation tissue. Metastases were present in regional nodes.

Differential diagnosis: in early stages it may resemble a frontal sinusitis.

Management: incurable.

Tail-tip necrosis

Clinical features: tail-tip necrosis (**137**) is seen as a group problem in steers, heifers and beef bulls in over-crowded accommodation with slatted floors. The typical tail-tip damage is seen close-up in **137**. The tip is trampled causing initial trauma followed by suppuration and the risk of ascending infection and septicemic spread to other

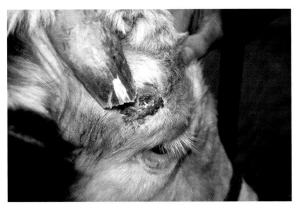

135

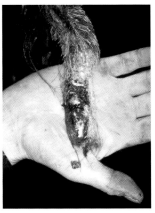

137

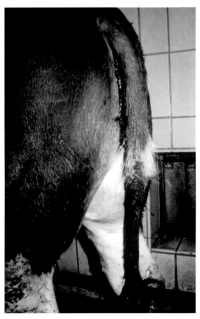

138

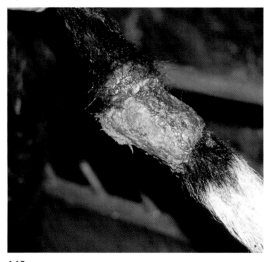

140

Prevention: appropriate husbandry changes to reduce overcrowding, and improved bedding.

Tail sequestrum

Clinical features: tail fractures can occur as the result of rough handling, or trauma, for example when a tail is stood on by another cow in overcrowded yards, or occasionally, when it is caught in a gate or similar. Simple fractures result in a deviation of the tail at the point of fracture and appear to cause little discomfort. Complicated fractures and those involving a bony sequestrum often result in a chronic discharging sinus and discomfort, as in **139**. Amputation is the only treatment option.

Fecolith

Etiology and pathogenesis: Fecoliths (hard accumulations of dry feces on the tail, developing during

organs. Tail necrosis in a beef bull (**138**) resulted in an ascending *Arcanobacterium pyogenes* infection, and involvement of the proximal coccygeal nerve supply has resulted in tail paralysis. Risk factors include slatted concrete floors, close confinement, and humid conditions. The tail is repeatedly trapped between the hock and floor as the animal makes several attempts to stand. Individual cases may be seen in dairy cows. Injuries may arise from similar causes, or result from rough handling and restraint. Diagnosis is easy.

Management: affected animals should be detected early and undergo amputation of the tail, with antibiotic therapy.

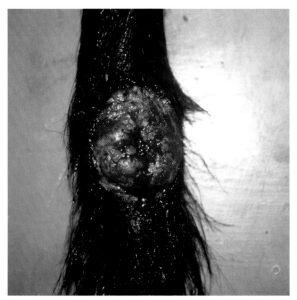

139

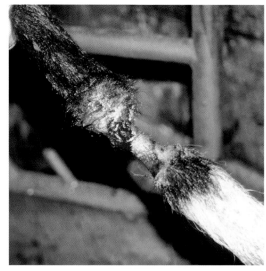

141

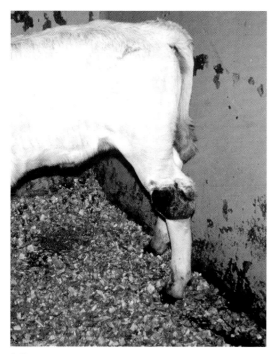

142

bouts of diarrhea) can occur spontaneously, or may develop around tail marker tape. As the fecal mass dries, it contracts, constricts the blood flow and produces swelling and ulceration, as seen on the left of the fecolith in **140**. When removed, the full extent of the ischemic necrosis is apparent (**141**). The tail tip eventually sloughed. Similar injuries can be caused by marker tape applied incorrectly.

Management: fecoliths are most easily removed by first cracking the dry fecal ring between two hard surfaces. Tail tape should be removed when no longer needed.

Melanocytoma (melanoma)

Definition: sporadic bovine tumor arising from melanocytes in the skin or subcutis, often in younger cattle, occasionally congenital.

Clinical features: this discrete benign melanoma on the left hock of a 3-week-old Charolais crossbred heifer (**142**) was present at birth. It is lobulated, extending both medially and laterally. Gray or black and painless, it presents an obvious cosmetic blemish.

Management: many are amenable to surgery, such as this case, which did not recur in the succeeding 2 years.

Alimentary disorders

Introduction

Chapter 4 illustrates those conditions with primary alimentary signs. It excludes congenital (e.g., cleft palate) and acquired neonatal conditions (e.g., calfhood enteritis). The first section comprises infectious and contagious diseases: bovine virus diarrhea/mucosal disease (BVD/MD) complex, vesicular stomatitis, papular stomatitis (all of which have rather similar gross features), and paratuberculosis. The second section covers the alimentary parasitic conditions: ostertagiasis, and small and large intestinal parasitism (for coccidiosis, see **59, 60**). The remaining conditions are listed by anatomical site (oral cavity to anus), irrespective of their traumatic, nutritional or other etiology.

Viral diseases

Three viral diseases present problems clinically in differential diagnosis: bovine virus diarrhea/mucosal disease (BVD/MD), vesicular stomatitis, and bovine papular stomatitis. In some regions, further differential diagnosis from foot-and-mouth disease and rinderpest may be necessary (see **646–657**). The pathogenicity and economic importance of these vesicular viral diseases vary greatly. Accurate differentiation is essential and usually depends on laboratory studies.

Bovine virus diarrhea/mucosal disease (BVD/MD)

Definition: major infectious disease caused by a pestivirus.

Clinical features: BVD/MD is a major viral disease worldwide. Congenital defects such as cerebellar hypo-

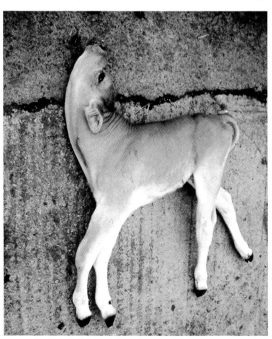

143

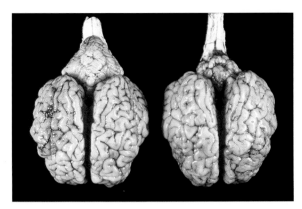

144

plasia and cataracts (432) may develop in the progeny of females infected during early pregnancy. BVD/MD causes diarrhea and unthriftiness in young cattle. Erosive stomatitis and rhinitis occur, together with similar lesions on other mucous membranes.

In utero infection in the first trimester can produce early embryonic death and infertility, or congenital abnormalities such as in the Piedmontese calf in **143**. Though alert, and suckled with difficulty, it was unable to stand. Although relatively normal at rest, this posture of extensor spasm and opisthotonus was adopted on minimal stimulation, for example when attempting to feed. Cerebellar hypoplasia was confirmed at postmortem examination. **144** shows a normal brain (left) and the affected brain (following inoculation of the dam at 150 days' gestation).

In utero infection in the second trimester, before the age of immunological competence of the fetus, can lead to the birth of a persistently infected calf which is BVD antigen +ve, but antibody –ve. Such animals may be either clinically normal or stunted, but they continually excrete

virus. At a later date, usually 3–30 months old, super-infection with a non-cytopathic strain of BVD virus leads to a syndrome of mucosal disease, with ulceration throughout the gastrointestinal tract. Clinically these animals present signs of oral, intestinal and respiratory involvement. Erosions and hyperemia around the nares, lips and gums are seen in **145**.

The specimen in **146** shows numerous erosive and hemorrhagic lesions over the entire hard palate. Secondary bacterial infection of the lesions produces the necrotic ulcers seen in the caudal pharynx and rima glottidis (**147**). Necrosis and abscessation surround the epiglottis. The laryngeal mucosa is also hemorrhagic. Pus lies between the arytenoids, making respiratory efforts difficult and painful. Similar necrotic ulcers may extend over the hard palate, down the esophagus and into the abomasum. The esophagus may have patchy, linear areas of hemorrhage, edema and erosions. Erosions may be seen on the edematous

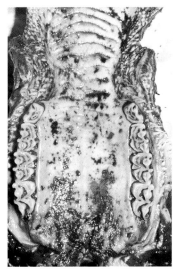

146

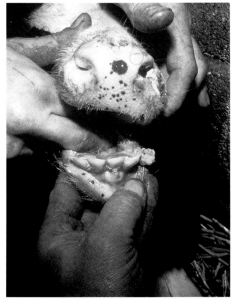

145

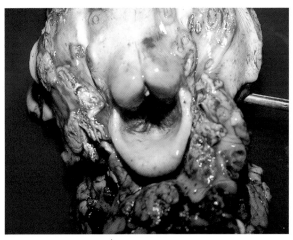

147

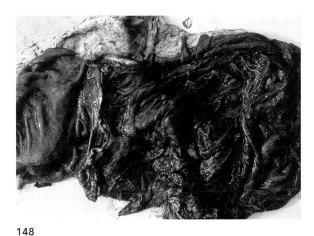

148

and hyperemic edges of the abomasal rugae (148). Small intestinal erosions can lead to mucosal sloughing and the production of casts that pack the intestinal lumen (149). A secondary bacterial infection may be responsible for the enlarged nodes. Erosions may also occur around the coronary band and in the interdigital cleft (150).

The two cattle in 151 are both 18 months old. The nearer heifer, with an abnormal, rust-colored coat, is stunted as a result of chronic, persistent infection (antigen positive,

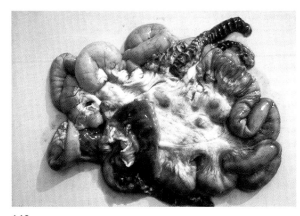

149

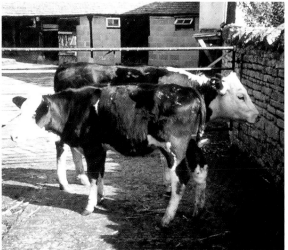

151

antibody negative) due to maternal infection with BVD virus acquired in early pregnancy. Many of the mucosal changes are so severe as to leave the chronic, persistent infective case emaciated (as in the crossbred animal in 152) and a constant source of infection to susceptible contact cattle.

In some herds primary BVD in non-immune cattle can also produce severe enteric signs and an increased mortality, especially in dairy cows, although most primary infections in younger animals are subclinical.

Differential diagnosis: salmonellosis, paratuberculosis (157), winter dysentery (159, 160) and other causes of acute enteritis in individuals. Bovine papular stomatitis (155), vesicular stomatitis (154), FMD (646–650) and other causes of oral ulceration.

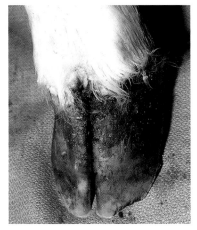

150

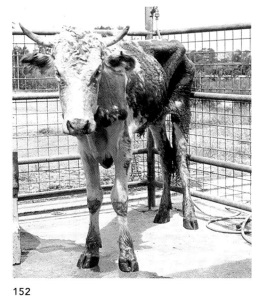

152

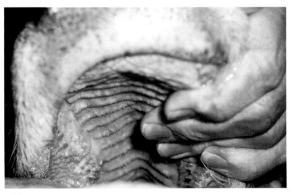

153

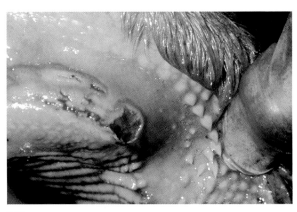

154

Management: long-term program needed for effective control: persistently infected virus-positive cattle should be identified by blood-testing and culled, as they represent the major source of virus. Screen all purchased stock. Double-fence neighboring cattle. Vaccinate prior to service to prevent the development of persistently infected offspring.

Vesicular stomatitis

Definition: caused by a rhabdovirus (two strains: New Jersey and Indiana) causing vesicular formation in various superficial tissues. It is probably spread by insect vectors.

Clinical features: the Charolais calf shows blanched areas on the rugae of the hard palate, dental pad and gums (**153**). These pale areas are vesicles that rupture after some days (**154**). Secondary infection is rare. Vesicular stomatitis has only been confirmed in North and South America. Many animals may be simultaneously affected on one farm, showing excessive salivation, together with oral and possibly teat lesions. Teat lesions (**617**) in vesicular stomatitis can cause problems with milking. Secondary lesions may involve the claws.

Differential diagnosis: foot-and-mouth disease (**646–650**) and bovine papular stomatitis (**155, 156**). Diagnosis by

ELISA or CF, and if negative, following passage, virus neutralization tests.

Management: suspect cases should be immediately reported to State authorities. (List A disease of Office International des Epizooties (OIE).)

Bovine papular stomatitis (BPS)

Definition: mild disease caused by a parapox virus classified as a 'paravaccinia virus' which generally has no adverse effect on the calf.

Clinical features: shallow papules and vesicles are seen on the muzzle, hard palate and gums of these young cattle (**155, 156**). Papules develop a distinct roughened center that sometimes expands to merge with adjacent vesicles. Teats are not affected. Immature cattle, sometimes an entire group, are usually involved and recovery is rapid. Systemic effects are rare.

Differential diagnosis: foot-and-mouth disease (**646–650**) and vesicular stomatitis (**153, 154**).

Management: specific treatment is rarely necessary.

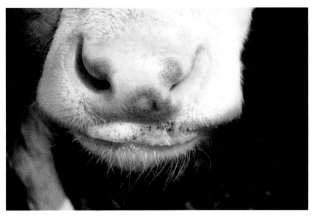

155

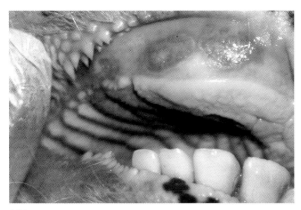

156

Johne's disease (paratuberculosis)

Definition: chronic wasting disease caused by *Mycobacterium avium paratuberculosis* (formerly *M. johnei*).

Clinical features: Johne's disease causes progressive weight loss, leading to eventual emaciation, although animals may remain alert and continue to eat. This chronic wasting disease is characterized by a profuse, watery diarrhea as seen in an 8-year-old Santa Gertrudis cow (**157**). When compared with normal ileum (**158**), the mucosa in a clinically overt case (A) shows numerous, thick, transverse rugae that cannot be smoothed out by stretching. Local intestinal lymph nodes are usually enlarged and pale, and may contain granulomatous areas. The usual age range is 3–9 years for the onset of clinical signs, which may be insidious, or develop suddenly after

calving. Carrier animals excrete for many months prior to this. Infection is introduced into healthy herds by subclinical carriers. Young calves become infected *in utero*, via colostrum, or by oral ingestion. Age immunity develops by 4–6 months old.

The disease may be potentially zoonotic (Crohn's disease).

Differential diagnosis: salmonellosis, severe parasitism, BVD.

Management: no effective treatment is known. Suspect cows should be tested (ELISA, CF, AGID) and culled if positive. Biopsy and histopathology of intestinal lymph nodes is an effective method of diagnosis. Vaccines have limited efficacy in control. There is no test to detect accurately subclinical carriers, and heifers from infected dams should be culled. Reduce spread of infection by hygiene at calving and possibly by pasteurization of pooled colostrum.

Winter dysentery (winter diarrhea)

Definition: etiology uncertain, although coronavirus has recently been implicated.

Clinical features: a watery diarrhea (**159**) lasting about 3 days, winter dysentery causes a sporadic problem in adult dairy cattle. Spontaneous recovery usually takes place after a few days.

Some animals show profuse intestinal hemorrhage, passing large quantities of fresh blood in feces (**160**), and suffer a severe production drop, though deaths are rare. Seroconversion to coronavirus can be used for diagnosis, although many animals in a herd are already seropositive.

Repeated outbreaks are possibly due to the presence of carrier animals.

Differential diagnosis: Johne's disease (**157**), rumenitis or overeating (**192**), BVD, salmonellosis, bovine influenza A (diarrhea with respiratory signs), PPH (**501**).

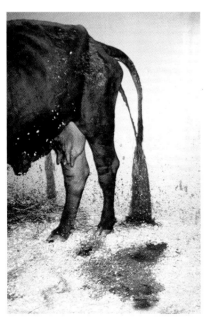

157

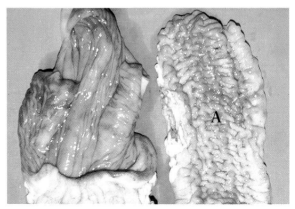

158

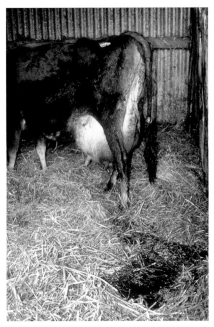

159

Management: fresh water and palatable feed should be available. The value of intestinal astringents and protectants is disputed. No vaccine is available.

Gastrointestinal parasitism

Introduction: the major gastrointestinal parasites of cattle are the stomach (abomasal) worms *Haemonchus placei* (barber's pole worm or large stomach worm, 18–30 mm long male), *Ostertagia ostertagi* (medium or brown stomach worm, 6–9 mm long), and *Trichostrongylus axei* (small stomach worm, 5 mm long). In tropical regions, other species, e.g., *Mecistocirrus digitatus* (up to 40 mm long), are significant. Severe infestations of *Haemonchus* can cause marked anemia, while the major effect of *Ostertagia* and *Trichostrongylus* is a severe, protein-losing gastroenteropathy, characterized by a profuse, watery diarrhea. All three species have the facility for their

embryonated eggs or infective larvae to survive in feces for weeks or months at lower temperatures (e.g., over winter) or in drought conditions, until a favorable environment returns.

Of the three species, *Ostertagia ostertagi* is overall the most pathogenic and economically important in most temperate regions of the world, including Great Britain and much of the USA. As with most gastrointestinal parasites, the most severe effects are seen in growing animals. Nevertheless, it can be a devastatingly debilitating disease in susceptible adults.

Ostertagiasis

Clinical features: cattle are most commonly affected with a chronic, persistent diarrhea and weight loss during their first season at pasture. Type I disease caused by *Ostertagia ostertagi* results from the ingestion of large numbers of L_3 larvae from herbage, starting 3–6 weeks before the onset of clinical signs. Small nodules that are 1–2 mm in diameter are present on and between the abomasal folds on the mucosal surface (**161**). In severe cases a 'Morocco leather' or 'cobblestone' appearance is evident (**162**). Higher magnification of a severe case shows the thickened ridges and the white worms (**163**). Marked edema of the gastrointestinal wall is often present. Type II disease occurs when larvae ingested in the autumn lie dormant in the abomasal glands (as L_4), and then emerge *en masse* in late winter or early spring to produce a profuse scour and weight loss in housed cattle. Note the weight loss, chronic diarrhea and tenesmus in an older Charolais heifer (**164**).

Oesophagostomum infection

Clinical features: clinical signs tend to be much less severe than with *Ostertagia*. Heavy worm burdens in calves cause anorexia, severe, dark diarrhea and weight loss. In older animals the nodules affect gut motility. These nodules may be palpated *per rectum*. The worms measure 12–15 mm and the head is angled to the body.

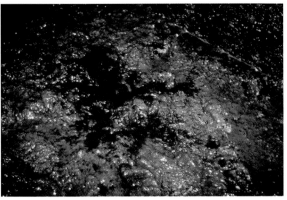

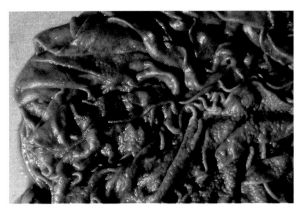

160

161

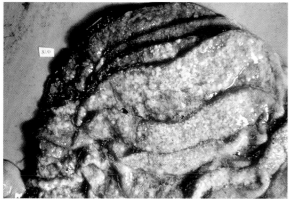

162

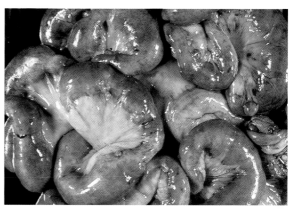

165

165 shows the serosal surface of the distal small intestine. Numerous caseated and calcified nodules indicate the presence of *Oesophagostomum radiatum* (nodular worm 12–15 mm long) in an older, resistant animal.

Management of Ostertagiasis and *Oesophagostomum* infection: in a clinical outbreak, all animals in the group should be treated with an appropriate broad-spectrum anthelmintic. The group should be moved to a 'clean' pasture, and adequate nutrition should be ensured. Strategic management techniques have

been developed as preventative measures, varying with worm types, climate, management systems and economic considerations. In the UK the most common control is anthelmintic therapy of first-season calves from turn-out to late June, by which time all over-wintered larvae will have died.

Dental problems
Excessive incisor wear

Dental problems are not a common cause of clinical disease in cattle. Occasionally, when the temporary incisors are being replaced by the permanent dentition, 2–3-year-old heifers show difficulty in prehension (**166**) leading to excessive salivation and weight loss. Diets such as heavily impacted self-feed silage leading to excessive incisor wear (**167**) may cause progressive weight loss. The crowns have almost disappeared, resulting in impairment of the animal's foraging ability.

Management: heifers should ideally be milked as a separate group during their first lactation and be given easy-access feed.

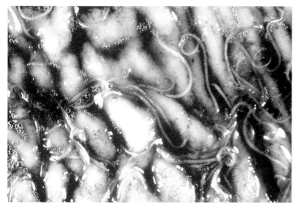

163

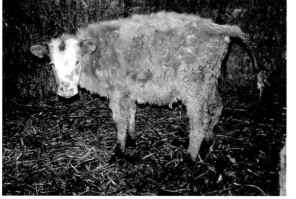

164

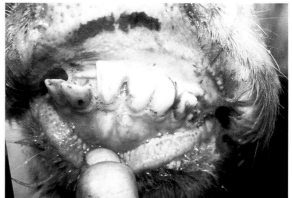

166

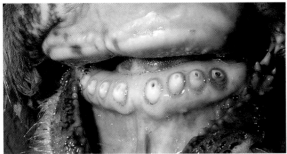

167

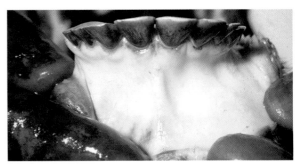

169

Fluorosis

Fluorosis (**168**) leads to mottling and excessive wear of temporary teeth during their development. The more severe fluorine-induced discoloration (**169**) should be differentiated from the staining caused by ingestion of some forms of grass silage. Other signs of fluorosis are seen in **749** and **750**.

Irregular molar wear

Irregular molar wear can sometimes cause masticatory problems. When eating or ruminating, this 8-year-old bull (**170**) occasionally kept the jaws apart as a result of 'locking' the overgrown lingual edge of the upper molars and premolars against the buccal edge of the mandibular cheek teeth. The length of the bilaterally symmetrical overgrowth was about 1 cm. **170** shows the typical open 'locked' position.

Mandibular fracture

Clinical features: mandibular fractures can occur in calves being kicked by cows or occasionally from iatrogenic trauma, e.g., from farm machinery. In the mature Friesian cow (**171**) with the symphysial fracture, the central incisor was displaced. There was little separation of the two halves of the mandible. A considerable quantity of saliva is being lost. In this case the cause was unknown, and full recovery occurred without treatment.

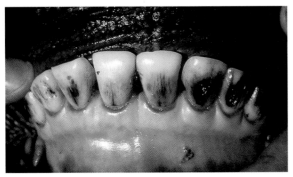

168

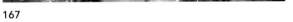

170

Management: a recent mandibular symphysial fracture may be stabilized by figure-of-eight wiring or use of a resin block across the incisor teeth. Milk-fed calves commonly continue to suckle and recover without treatment.

Discrete swellings of the head

Actinobacillosis, actinomycosis and local abscessation related to *Arcanobacterium pyogenes* can present similar clinical features in some cattle. Typically, however, actinobacillosis affects the soft tissues, especially the tongue, while actinomycosis involves bone. Abscessation related to tooth root infection is rare in cattle. A curious disorder or vice of habitual tongue playing, not involving any oral pathology, is shown in **172**. This Guernsey cow lost a considerable volume of saliva through drooling.

Actinobacillosis ('wooden tongue')

Clinical features: *Actinobacillus lignieresii* preferentially colonizes the soft tissues of the head, especially the tongue. External swelling beneath the jaw may be seen (**173**). It typically causes a localized, firm swelling of the dorsum (D), as in this dairy cow (**174**) and firm, easily palpable, sub-epithelial masses elsewhere. Other parts of the head, such as the nares or facial skin, are sometimes alone affected. Infection may pass down the esophagus, and lesions in the esophageal groove typically cause vomiting

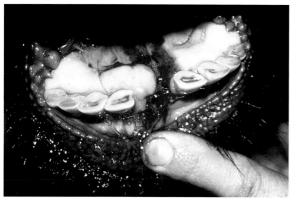

171

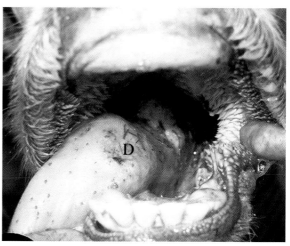

174

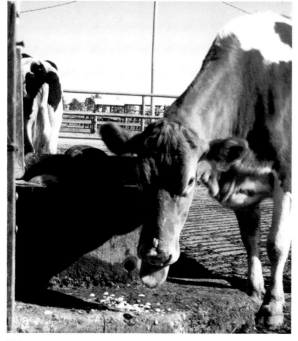

172

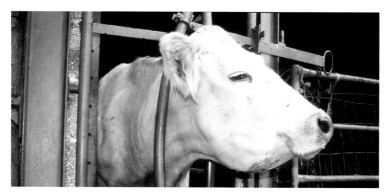

173

exposure to a concentrated infective dose of organisms, which are part of the normal flora of the upper GI tract. Such massive lesions are particularly liable to bleed and ulcerate. Most cases tend to occur in mature cattle of dairy breeds.

Differential diagnosis: tooth abscess, actinomycosis, foot-and-mouth disease, snakebite (**176**, showing thickening and ulceration 4 days later).

Management: systemic antibiotics are effective, but prolonged therapy (7–10 days) may be needed. Provide clean feed and water, and avoid access to muddy streams.

Actinomycosis ('lumpy jaw')

Clinical features: actinomycosis (*Actinomyces bovis*) causes a rarefying periostitis of the maxilla and the mandible, with a surrounding soft-tissue reaction. The Guernsey cow in **177** has a right maxillary swelling and several granulomatous masses have typically broken through the skin. The cow experienced no apparent interference with mastication for 18 months after the swelling was first seen. The crossbred Hereford cow with 'lumpy

of rumen contents. Other areas of the body (e.g., the limbs, **175**, face or flanks) develop cutaneous actinobacillosis. Skin infection usually follows trauma and

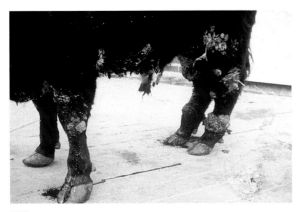

175

jaw' (**178**) had moderate difficulty in chewing. A large, fist-sized, proliferating mass lies over the angle of the mandible. Despite secondary infection, body condition remained good. Dysphagia is usually due to malalignment of molar teeth. A lateral radiograph (**179**) of a 2-year-old heifer with mandibular actinomycosis (in considerable discomfort and rapidly losing weight) shows massive periosteal new bone formation (A) and cavitation (B).

Differential diagnosis: mandibular abscess (**184**) and actinobacillosis (**172–175**).

Management: actinomycosis has a poor prognosis despite attempts at debridement and prolonged (7+ days) systemic use of β-lactam antimicrobial drugs (e.g., synthetic penicillins and cephalosporins).

Malignant edema (necrotic cellulitis)

Etiology: malignant edema is caused by *Clostridium septicum* and results from contaminated wounds in any superficial part of the body, although the head and neck are most commonly affected.

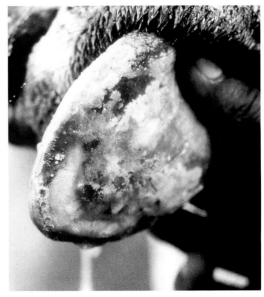

176

Clinical features: anorexia, pyrexia and toxemia develop rapidly along with local lesions. In this cow (**180**), infection entered the masseter area of the right cheek to cause a rapidly enlarging and unilateral soft tissue swelling, especially obvious around the right nostril. There was pronounced salivation. The brisket is enlarged with edematous fluid (**181**). Despite prompt, prolonged antibiotic therapy, infection spread to the forelegs and, as in many cases, was fatal. Gas formation is rare.

Differential diagnosis: cutaneous urticaria (blaine) (**76**) and abscessation (**184**).

Management: prolonged and aggressive parenteral penicillin plus NSAIDs may cure some early cases. Some

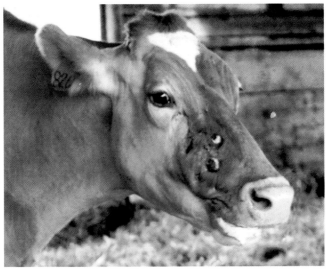

177

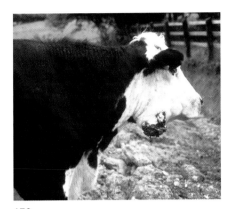

178

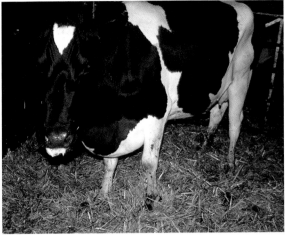

181

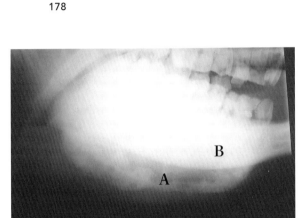

179

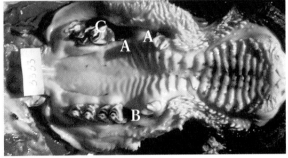

182

benefit from drainage of foci. Although clostridial vaccines are available, most cases are sporadic and herd vaccination is rarely indicated.

Alveolar periostitis (*Cara inchada*, 'swollen face')

Definition: severe periodontal disease associated with secondary bacterial infection in young cattle of unknown etiology.

Clinical features: alveolar periostitis is a major problem in some parts of South America, such as Brazil. Periodontal disease affects the sockets of the upper premolars and molars in calves following a severe gingivitis and secondary bacterial infection (*Arcanobacterium pyogenes* and *Prevotella melaninogenica*). The first sign is uni- or bilateral swelling of the cheek as a result of impaction by pasture grass. Postmortem examination

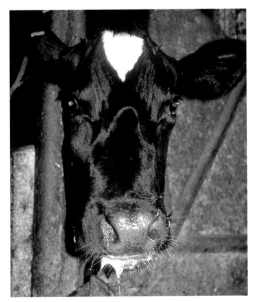

180

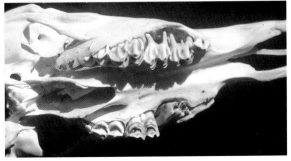

183

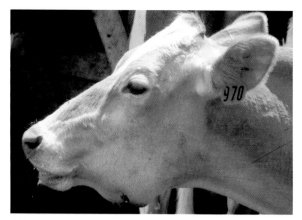

184

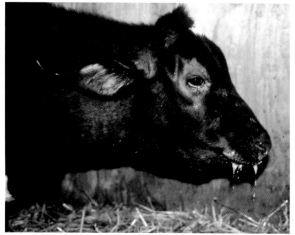

185

reveals loss or marked displacement of several temporary teeth, particularly premolars two and three, and a massive periosteal and osteolytic reaction in the related maxilla (182, 183). On pastures of guinea grass (*Panicum maximum*), which causes traumatic damage to the gingiva, the condition leads to malnutrition and sometimes death. The 18-month-old mixed Zebu steer from the Mato Grosso (182) has lost the right second and third upper premolars (A) and the left second premolar (B). Loss of the surrounding cement has led to deep pockets on the labial side of the right arcade (C). The steer was severely emaciated. 183 shows a similar type of animal. A striking, chronic, ossifying periostitis affects the region around the roots of P2 and P3, explaining the likelihood of tooth loss.

Submandibular abscess

Clinical features: caused by *Arcanobacterium pyogenes*, a smooth and localized soft-tissue swelling, discharging pus, lies over the horizontal ramus of the left mandible (184). It developed rapidly over 3 weeks and resolved slowly.

Differential diagnosis: actinomycosis (177), actinobacillosis (173), and fracture of the mandible (171).

Management: surgical drainage and flushing. Systemic antibiotics may be unnecessary.

Pharyngeal and retropharyngeal swellings

Introduction: pharyngeal and retropharyngeal swellings can range from being innocuous to rapidly fatal. Careful external and oral/pharyngeal examination is essential. A swelling may be indicative of systemic disease elsewhere, such as right heart failure manifested as submandibular and retropharyngeal edema (268). The swelling may involve retropharyngeal and parotid lymph nodes in a neoplastic reaction (712). Severe reactions in the submucosal tissues of the pharynx, with potentially dire consequences to the airway and possibly death, can result from ingestion of neat caustic soda (NaOH) from improperly mixed caustic

wheat, or anthelmintic bolus gun injuries. The introduction of a small amount of irritant material (e.g., poloxalene for bloat control) through an accidental puncture wound, or other forms of extensive lacerations to the pharyngeal wall, cause severe edema, cellulitis and pose a major problem (see below).

Drenching gun injury

Clinical features: perforation of the pharyngeal wall by a drenching gun caused a septic cellulitis leading to the grossly enlarged submandibular and parotid regions (185). One consequence of this cellulitis was a malodorous, purulent nasal and oral discharge. The heifer was pyrexic and anorexic. Postmortem examination of another case (186) revealed masses of inspissated pus beneath the pharyngeal and laryngeal mucosae, which had caused respiratory embarrassment (inspiratory stridor). Note the congestion of the mucosal surface of the epiglottis.

Incorrect dosing techniques can result in anthelmintic boluses penetrating the pharyngeal mucosa, migrating

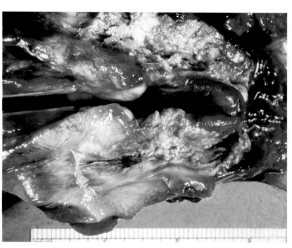

186

down the neck and producing severe respiratory distress due to foreign body reaction and airway obstruction.

Management: aggressive and prolonged antibiotics and anti-inflammatories are needed, but effective therapy is very difficult in severe cases with extensive septic cellulitis. Respiratory obstruction is possible (emergency tracheotomy) or rumen tympany (trocarization), but most cases fail to respond and culling is the usual economic option.

Retropharyngeal abscess

Clinical features: a discrete and relatively painless fluctuating, tennis ball-sized mass lies in the retropharyngeal region (**187**). The spread of infection (compare **185**) was limited by the development of a fibrous capsule. Abscess-ation in this region is commonly caused by ingestion of sticks and thorns, although it may be the result of ac-cidental pharyngeal damage from drenching or balling guns, probangs or other rigid instruments (see above).

Management: most abscesses eventually develop superficial softer areas for drainage, though deep-seated abscesses can be hazardous due to the proximity of other structures, e.g., carotid artery, jugular vein or parotid salivary gland.

Esophageal disorders

Esophageal obstruction (choke)

Clinical features: a potato is lodged two-thirds of the way down the cervical esophagus to the left of the hand (**188**). The animal was uncomfortable and drooling as a result of its inability to swallow saliva. Since eructation was impeded, it also had rumen tympany. Common sites of esophageal obstruction are just dorsal to the larynx and at the thoracic inlet. In cattle, esophageal foreign bodies tend to be solid objects, such as apples, large portions of turnips or beets, or corncobs (maize). Other

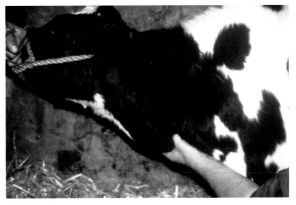
188

suspicious signs of esophageal obstruction include extension of the head and neck, dyspnea, occasional coughing, and chewing movements. A cervical esophageal foreign body is readily palpated externally.

Differential diagnosis: acute rumenitis (**192–196**), traumatic reticulitis, oral lesions and rabies (**495–497**).

Management: some foreign bodies can be pushed towards the pharynx by external manipulation and, using a gag, removed manually. Any severe ruminal tympany should be relieved by trocarization. Other conservative therapy (spasmolytics, e.g., acepromazine, or sedative and muscle relaxants, e.g., xylazine) is preferable to attempts to push the object downwards with a probang.

Megaesophagus

Definition: chronic dilatation and atony of the esophagus.

Clinical features: the entire cervical esophagus (**189**) is grossly distended (about 5–6 cm in diameter). Contrast radiography revealed a similar distension of most of the thoracic esophagus. The abnormality had been first observed at 1 year of age. Clinical signs included frequent regurgitation. The 15-month-old Charolais heifer was observed for 1 year and almost completely recovered. Megaesophagus is rare and, although usually congenital, this case was probably secondary to a systemic infection.

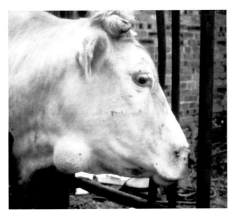
187

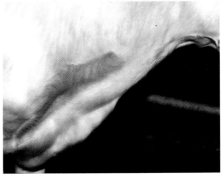
189

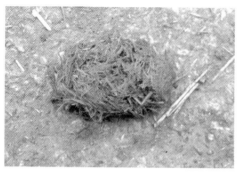

190

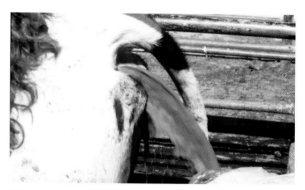

192

Differential diagnosis: esophageal obstruction.

Management: diet.

Rumen and reticulum

Rumen acidosis (rumenitis)

Definition: ruminal inflammation resulting from excessively rapid fermentation following overeating of grain (corn), or other high-starch/low-fiber diets.

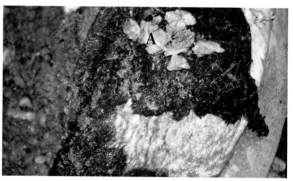

193

Clinical features: low-grade rumen acidosis can present clinically as rumen atony, cud regurgitation (190) and a matted sweaty coat. Passage of loose yellow feces as in this animal (191) leads to extensive soiling of the tail and hindquarters. Tail swishing often produces fecal soiling along the back. More severe overeating can result in rapid carbohydrate fermentation, severe rumenitis, metabolic acidosis and a subsequent laminitis (337). Affected cattle are very dull, weak, ataxic or recumbent. A light-colored diarrhea containing grain particles may be seen (192). Ruminal pH is usually very acidic (pH < 5.5). 193 shows areas of sloughed ruminal epithelium and intense serosal hemorrhage in a 10-month-old Simmental bull which died 24 hours after unlimited access to fodder beet. Whole fragments of undigested fodder beet are clearly visible (A). Four to six days after a grain overload, mycotic or

fusobacterial rumenitis may be seen (194), comprising sharply defined, thick oval lesions that are often red or dark. A close-up view of a more chronic rumenitis (195) shows a rumen fold separating the disorganized and necrotic rumenal papillae (A) from more normal papillae (B). In rumenitis colonized by *Fusobacteria* and fungi, healing eventually occurs after sloughing of the necrotic layers, contraction of the ulcer, and peripheral epithelial regeneration, resulting in stellate scar formation. The rumen is, however, left with a reduced absorptive capacity, and a secondary hepatic abscessation may result.

The omasum in 196 shows a fungal infection (most likely due to *Aspergillus* species) following the accidental ingestion of moldy feed, e.g., cereals or beans. Changes are most

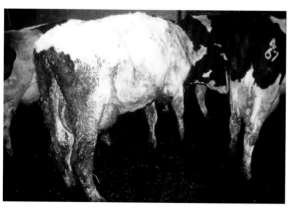

191

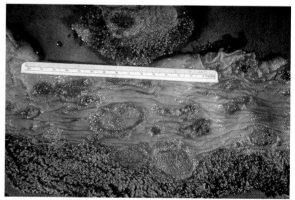

194

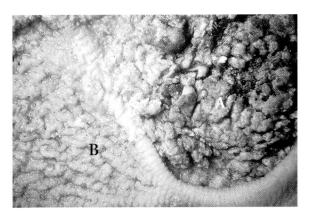

195

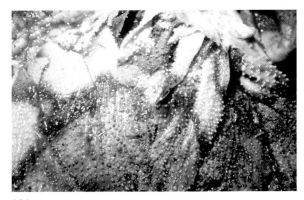

196

common in the ruminoreticulum (**194**) and omasal involvement is rare.

Differential diagnosis: winter dysentery, bloat and diarrhea from other causes, e.g., influenza A.

Management: cases of mild acidosis will resolve without treatment. More severe cases require oral antibiotics (to reduce rumen fermentation), NSAIDs (to suppress laminitis) and antacids and B vitamins (since ruminal vitamin B synthesis is depressed by acidosis). Advanced cases with a metabolic acidosis benefit from i.v. sodium bicarbonate infusion and even evacuation of rumen contents (rumenotomy or esophageal flushing).

Prevention is based on dietary management. Cattle on ad-lib cereals should always have access to palatable fiber (e.g., straw) and never be allowed to get hungry. High-yielding dairy cows need adequate digestible and long fiber to balance a high-starch diet. Ideal concentrate:fiber ratio should never exceed 60:40.

Rumen tympany ('bloat')

Definition: accumulation of gas in a distended rumen. The gas may be free or present as a foam. (See also bloat in younger calves, **64**.)

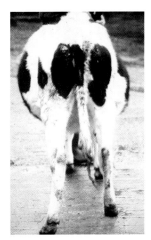

197

Clinical features: the Holstein heifer in **197** has an obvious distension of the left paralumbar fossa. The swelling may extend above the level of the lumbar spine, as seen in the Hereford steer (**198**). Both of these animals had a gaseous as opposed to a foamy (or frothy) bloat. Extreme cases may die from increased intra-abdominal pressure leading to cardiac and respiratory failure, often with inhalation of rumen contents.

Differential diagnosis: distinguish gas bloat from frothy bloat; esophageal obstruction (**188**), an esophageal groove mass (**199**), traumatic reticulitis (**203**) and rumenal atony. (For bloat in a calf, see **64**.)

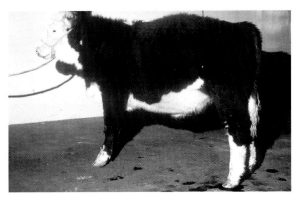

198

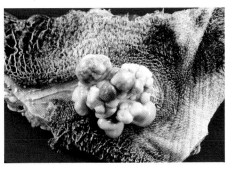

199

Management: frothy bloat responds well to oral surfactants such as paloxalene. Gas bloat can usually be relieved by stomach tube, but extreme cases require trocarization. Prevention depends on avoidance of causative agents.

Ruminal neoplasia

Clinical features: this pedunculated mass (199) is a benign papilloma. Lying at the proximal end of the esophageal groove, it caused partial obstruction of the lower esophageal sphincter, resulting in an intermittent ruminal tympany. Esophageal groove obstructions often lead to vomiting.

Differential diagnosis: exploratory rumenotomy may be needed to differentiate neoplasia from actinobacillosis of the esophageal groove, chronic reticuloperitonitis or reticular wall abscessation. (See 203 for another ruminoreticular neoplasm (fibroma).)

Abdominal pain

In comparison with the horse, such signs of pain as seen in this heifer (200) are uncommon. The forefeet are placed further forward than normal, presumably in an attempt to reduce tension on the abdominal viscera. The head is turned towards the flank. The tail is slightly elevated (indicative of tenesmus) and the heifer is kicking at the belly with a hind foot. The stance suggests an intestinal problem. Posterior abdominal pain can result in tenesmus that may not necessarily reflect an alimentary origin, for example, babesiosis (679–684), cystitis (519) or urethritis (514).

Traumatic reticulitis (reticuloperitonitis)

Definition: perforation of reticular wall and parietal peritoneum (usually diaphragm) with development of localized or generalized peritonitis.

Clinical features: Cattle with acute reticuloperitonitis are pyrexic, slightly bloated and typically grunt during reticular movements unless there is ruminoreticular stasis. Affected cattle may rapidly become dehydrated,

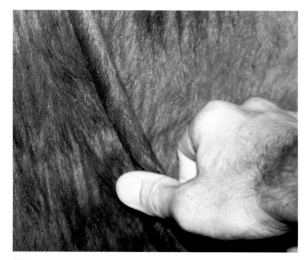

201

one sign of which is obvious skin 'tenting' (201): the skin fold remains for 3–10 seconds or more (indicating approximately 6–12% dehydration). They appear dejected, have an arched back, raised tail, sunken eyes as a result of the dehydration, weight loss, and an empty flank and 'tucked up' belly due to lack of rumen fill (202). They are often reluctant to move due to abdominal pain.

This section of the reticular wall illustrates the typical wires (203) that may perforate the wall to cause a localized or generalized peritonitis (219, 220), hepatic abscessation (229), or may travel cranially to produce a septic pericarditis (271). An incidental abnormality in this reticulum (203) was a discrete pedunculated fibroma (A). Wires contained within fragmenting car tyres, originally used to keep grass silage sheets in place or left in a field corner, are a frequent source. Herd outbreaks may arise when an entire tyre is accidentally chopped up in the feed wagon.

Differential diagnosis: left (211) or right (213) displaced abomasum, abomasal ulceration with perforation (207), cecal dilation (215), bacterial endocarditis (269), rumen acidosis (194, 195) and other digestive upsets.

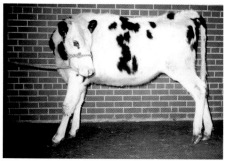

200

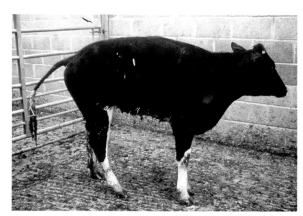

202

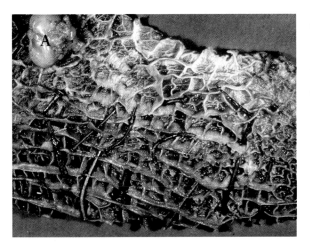

203

Management: prognosis is good in early acute case following rumenotomy and removal of penetrating wire in reticulum. Alternative medical management involves antibacterials for several days, elevation of the forequarters, and oral administration of a magnet which is useful both for prophylaxis and treatment.

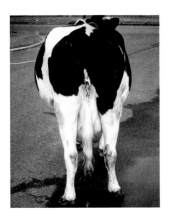

204

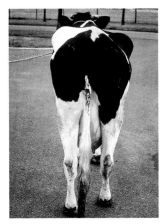

205

Abomasum
Forestomach or abomasal obstructive syndrome (vagal indigestion, Hoflund syndrome)

Definition: the cause of vagal indigestion, or Hoflund syndrome, is a functional disturbance of the normal motility of the forestomachs or the abomasum, or of all compartments.

Clinical features: the silhouette of the abdominal wall shows a massive, left-sided swelling due to an accumulation of fluid, primarily in the ruminoreticulum (**204**). After pumping out 90 liters, the flanks became almost symmetrical (**205**). The distension is characteristically in the upper left and lower right flanks, resulting in the so-called 'ten-to-four' appearance. **206** is a typical example.

Ruminoreticular distension that results from vagal dysfunction due to chronic reticuloperitonitis is the most common form. Severe ruminal distension is most marked in the left sublumbar fossa and low down in the right flank (so-called 'papple-shaped', i.e., pear x apple).

Discrete omasal obstruction (as opposed to secondary abomasal obstruction) due to reticuloperitonitis is rare. When compared with **204**, the abdominal silhouette of the 2-year-old Holstein bull in **206** is similarly asymmetrical, showing distension of the upper left (ruminoreticulum) and lower right (omasum, and to a lesser extent ruminoreticulum) flanks. The cause of the omasal obstruction was secondary impaction due to a reticular wall abscess (foreign body: wire) and a localized reticuloperitonitis. Mechanical causes, such as neoplastic infiltration near the pylorus, can lead to similar effects. Diagnosis depends on exploratory laparotomy.

Differential diagnosis: chronic traumatic reticulitis, peritonitis, rumen tympany, abomasal impaction and obstruction of the reticulo-omasal orifice.

Management: diagnosis of the specific cause involves an exploratory laparotomy and rumenotomy. Evacuation of rumen contents may improve motility temporarily.

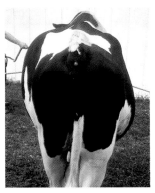

206

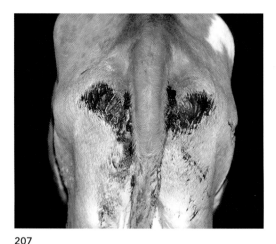

207

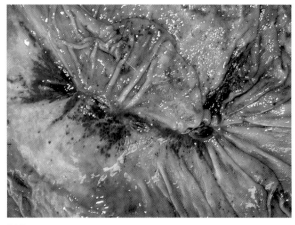

209

Symptomatic treatment is necessary. The prognosis is often poor.

Abomasal ulceration

Clinical features: abomasal ulceration occurs in mature dairy and beef cattle and in calves (56–58). Some cases in adults are the result of primary diseases such as infiltrative lymphosarcoma, and systemic infections such as BVD and malignant bovine catarrh. In high-yielding dairy cows, although the cause is unknown, ulcers are usually associated with stress and high concentrate rations. Multiple abomasal ulcers may occur in calves (57). There are four types of ulcer, Type I being that which causes no clinically apparent disease. Type II is a bleeding ulcer that, if persistent, results in progressive anemia. Types III and IV cause an acute localized or generalized peritonitis with signs of pain and Type IV is almost always fatal. Animals are dull, with a drop in yield, often a subnormal temperature and general signs of anemia.

The Guernsey cow in 207 had abdominal pain due to a Type III (perforating) abomasal ulcer causing a localized peritonitis. She passed black, tarry feces containing much digested blood (207). Cows sometimes die following severe blood loss into the abomasal lumen. Postmortem examination (208) reveals numerous ulcers, several filled with blood (A), and a diffuse abomasitis. The pathology is similar to that of the calfhood disease (56–58), with localized or generalized peritonitis as possible sequelae. Healing abomasal ulcers (209) show scar tissue causing contraction of the abomasal wall in a stellate pattern. Some bleeding was still occurring.

Differential diagnosis: traumatic reticulitis, abomasitis and abomasal lymphoma (lymphosarcoma) (210).

Management: depending on the symptomatology, broad-spectrum antibiotics are indicated in perforating ulcers, while fluid therapy including blood may be given to dehydrated animals and cases of bleeding ulcers. Unfortunately fluids increase blood pressure and in many cases will precipitate further hemorrhage from the ulcer.

Abomasal lymphoma (lymphosarcoma)

Etiology and pathogenesis: adult lymphosarcoma is caused by the bovine leucosis virus (BLV). The tumor incidence varies widely. Enzootic leucosis affects mature cattle, and other tissues commonly affected include lymph nodes, heart and retrobulbar tissue (466).

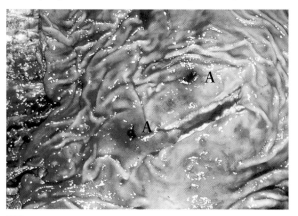

208

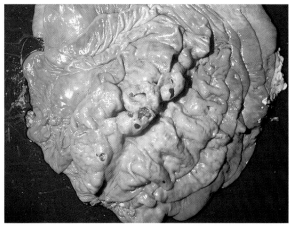

210

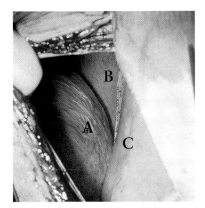

211

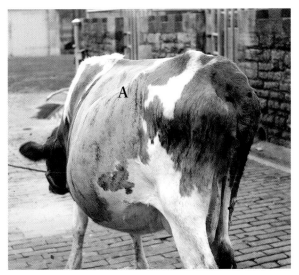

212

This specimen from an old Holstein cow shows thickened and irregular abomasal rugae as a result of lymphoma infiltration (**210**). The discrete, dark, punched-out areas are ulcers, indicating that the two conditions can occur together. Neoplastic infiltration was widespread.

Management: diagnosis requires ultimately histological confirmation. Control in a herd is difficult but regular serology may facilitate removal of positive carriers. See also **712–718**.

Abomasal surgical conditions

Introduction: in areas of intensive management, left and, to a lesser extent, right abomasal displacements are common conditions in dairy cattle. Right abomasal torsion can be a serious secondary complication of right abomasal displacement. Most cases of mechanical displacement of this type occur in high-yielding cows in early lactation, and are preceded by a period of ruminal and abomasal atony. Many cows will have had periparturient problems such as retained placenta, ketosis, metritis, mastitis and dietary-induced rumen acidosis in the preceding weeks.

Left displaced abomasum (LDA)

Clinical features: the displaced abomasum is situated almost entirely beneath the rib cage on the left, where it can be detected by percussion and auscultation. The caudal, dorsal portion may extend behind the last rib to form a palpable, soft swelling which can on rectal examination be distinguished from the underlying rumen in the para-lumbar fossa. In **211** the abomasum (A) may be seen through a left paralumbar vertical incision lying between the cranial edge of the incision and the spleen (B), which is cranial to the visible portion (C) of the rumen wall. LDA presents with variable clinical signs, often sudden onset of loss of appetite for concentrates and precipitous drop in yield. Other cows have moderate inappetance, weight loss and a secondary ketosis. With this slow loss of condition due to partial inappetance, the bulge (A) of

the abomasum may then become more obvious in the left flank (**212**).

Differential diagnosis: right displaced abomasum, cecal torsion, primary ketosis.

Management: conservative correction by rolling, confinement to a loose box and a high roughage intake can cure up to 30% of cases. Surgical abomasopexy by one of several techniques is the preferred option.

Right displaced abomasum (RDA)

Clinical features: clinical signs are similar to left displacement, but a tympanitic abomasum is detectable by percussion on the right side. In this Guernsey cow (**213**) the distended abomasum is seen through a vertical right flank paralumbar incision about 7 cm caudal to the

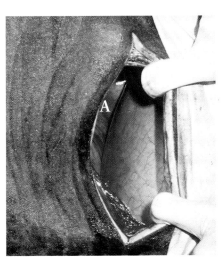

213

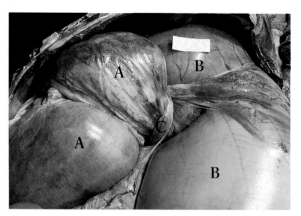

214

last rib. The remainder of the abomasum is located medial to the costal arch. The greater omentum containing the descending duodenum (A), is seen caudal to the abomasal swelling.

Differential diagnosis: left displaced abomasum, abomasal, intestinal or cecal torsion, ketosis, abomasal ulceration.

Management: mild cases of RDA may slowly respond to medical therapy (meclofenamic acid, spasmolytics) and dietary management. More advanced cases require surgical drainage and abomasopexy. After removal of the large volumes of gas and fluid, most cases recover slowly.

Abomasal torsion

Clinical features: abomasal torsion with dilatation is clinically severe, and affected cows are dull, sometimes recumbent, totally anorexic, dehydrated, in shock and have an empty rectum. The dilated abomasum can be percussed on the right flank and may be palpable *per rectum*. A postmortem specimen (**214**) of the abomasum (A), ruminoreticulum (B) and duodenum (C) shows a complex torsion of both the abomasum and omasum. Typically, the cow was found in extreme shock. The abomasal fluid volume exceeded 90 liters (normal volume: 10–20 liters).

Management: most cases should be culled. Any attempt at treatment involves correction of the fluid imbalance and right-sided abomasal drainage followed by attempted reposition of the abomasum.

Large intestine

Cecal torsion

Clinical features: affected cows are dull, partially anorexic and have a depressed yield. Onset may be slow and subtle. The dilated cecum can be percussed in the caudal upper right flank and be palpated *per rectum*

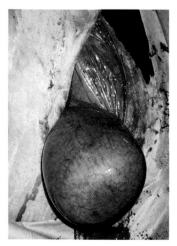

215

('loaf of bread' shape). Following cecal displacement and distension, the Holstein cow (**215**) developed an acute (painful) abdomen within 48 hours. The enlarged cecum was appreciable on rectal palpation. The cecal apex has been prolapsed through a dorsal and caudal right flank laparotomy incision (**215**), but most of the cecum still lies within the abdominal cavity. The peritoneal surface is slightly congested. Many cases of simple cecal dilatation are asymptomatic.

Differential diagnosis: right displaced abomasum, ketosis.

Management: many cases respond to spasmolytics and dietary control. Surgical drainage may be needed when viability of the cecal wall should be checked.

Jejunal torsion and intussusception ('twisted gut')

Definition: twisting of jejunum on itself and telescoping of small intestinal segment.

Clinical features: intussusception has a sporadic incidence but is the most common cause of small intestinal obstruction in cattle. Occurring at any age, it initially causes severe abdominal pain. Progressive shock develops. The rectum is totally void of feces. In larger cattle torsion may be detectable on rectal examination as a tight mesenteric band passing obliquely across the abdomen. In **216** the darker loop of small intestine (A), showing marked congestion and subserosal hemorrhage, particularly on the mesenteric border, is the segment of bowel through which the intussusception has passed. Dilated proximal intestine is seen at B. The point of invagination of the intussusception, which is not visible in this picture, lies tightly knotted deeply below the position of the fingers.

Another case (**217**) illustrates the severe and complex nature of bovine intussusception. The site of intussusception is clearly visible (A). Several jejunal loops have undergone

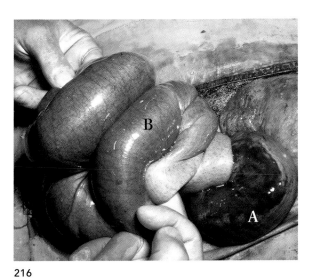

216

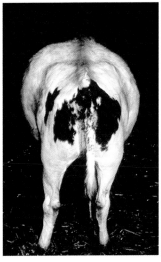

218

torsion (dark gas and fluid-filled loops to right, (B). Affected animals often have a grossly distended abdomen (218) due to fluid accumulation in the prestenotic small intestinal loops, abomasum and ruminoreticulum.

Management: early cases are sometimes amenable to surgical correction (resection and anastomosis). Most cases however should be culled. Logical preventive measures to reduce the alleged initiating factor for intussusception (intestinal irritation) are parasite control and dietary management.

Peritonitis

Clinical features: inflammation of the peritoneal cavity may be localized or generalized, acute or chronic. It is commonly secondary to contamination of the abdominal cavity, e.g., secondary to traumatic reticulitis or cesarian section. In active disease, guarding of the abdomen results in a stiff gait (see p. 58). The bovine peritoneum and greater omentum have a remarkable facility to wall off leaks of

bowel contents and localized areas of abscessation. This process often results in few or no complications in the cranial part of the abdomen. Adhesions developing in the caudal part can cause progressive bowel obstruction. In **219** the visceral and parietal peritoneum (rumen, jejunum and greater omentum) is covered with a fibrinous and purulent exudate, typical of early generalized peritonitis. The changes are more advanced and chronic in another case (**220**), resulting from septic reticuloperitonitis (see also 203).

Typical cases of active peritonitis are dull, pyrexic, often partially anorexic and have a reduced milk yield. More chronic cases are in poor bodily condition. Rectal examination reveals an empty rumen, and a typical 'doughy' feel to attempts to palpate abdominal viscera.

Other common causes of peritonitis are perforated abomasal ulcers, either in calfhood (58) or in adult life (208), and rupture of the small intestine following uncorrected intussusception or small intestinal torsion. Neonatal peritonitis may occur following the rupture of a distended small intestine proximal to an atretic bowel (20).

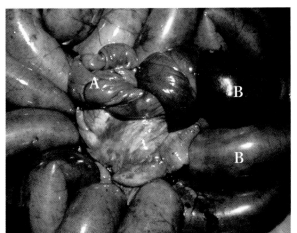

217

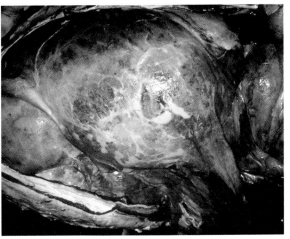

219

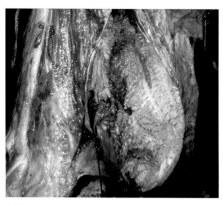

220

Diagnosis: peritonitis may be suspected from the clinical signs and rectal palpation. Abdominal paracentesis may yield suspect fluid for cytological and cultural examination.

Management: fluid therapy, aggressive broad-spectrum antimicrobial therapy, NSAIDs. Most cases are best culled.

Ascites

Definition: abnormal accumulation of serous (edematous) fluid in the abdominal cavity.

As with peritonitis, this fluid eventually leads to a pear-shaped silhouette (**221**). Ascitic fluid is serous or edematous in nature and is usually sterile. This old Galloway cow had hepatic cirrhosis resulting from chronic severe fascioliasis. Compare intestinal obstruction (**218**). The abdomen is rarely painful on palpation, unlike peritonitis (p. 63). Diagnosis is confirmed by abdominal tap (sterile needle).

Differential diagnosis: peritonitis, hydrops amnii, hydrops allantois, abomasal impaction.

Management: most cases are incurable and should be culled.

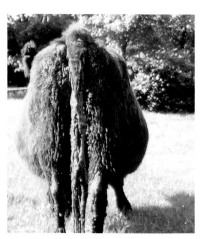

221

Hepatic diseases

Introduction: clinical signs of liver disease are variable and relate to the wide range of functions carried out by the liver. These include bile production, synthesis of specific plasma components, detoxification, storage, and a variety of metabolic processes.

Its large functional reserve results in the signs of disease usually becoming evident only when hepatic damage is extensive. There are few characteristic signs of malfunction and diagnosis often presents a major challenge to the clinician. Several specific diseases of the liver cause reduced weight gain and slaughterhouse condemnation of the liver (abscessation, fluke infestation). Ancillary diagnostic aids include enzyme estimation (sorbitol dehydrogenase (SDH), glutamate dehydrogenase (GDH), γ-glutamyl transferase (GGT)) and percutaneous hepatic biopsy.

Examples of the hepatic diseases illustrated below include necrotic hepatitis caused by *Clostridium novyi* type B (*oedematiens*), hepatic abscessation secondary to rumenitis (*Fusobacterium necrophorum*), and fascioliasis resulting from severe parasitism. Although not specifically involving the liver, other forms of fluke are also included in this section. Fatty liver syndrome produced by ill-defined nutritional and metabolic imbalance is described in Chapter 9 (**476**), and photosensitization secondary to hepatic disease in Chapter 3 (**78–83**).

Fascioliasis (common liver fluke infection)

Clinical features: low-grade fluke infestation produces nonspecific clinical signs such as poor condition, reduced performance (growth and milk yield and quality), and anemia. On postmortem the liver becomes fibrotic with enlargement, the bile ducts become grossly thickened, and mature *Fasciola hepatica* flukes occupy the lumen (**222, 223**). The walls may eventually become calcified.

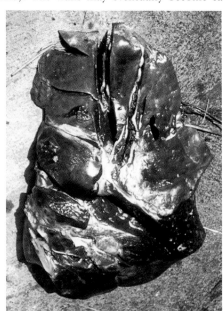

222

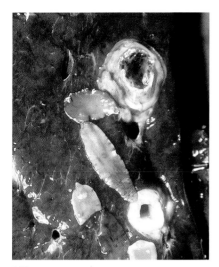

223

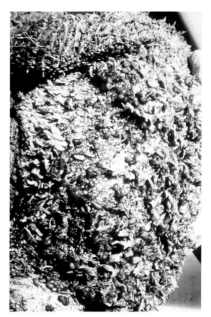

224

The visceral surface becomes irregular and granular in appearance. The associated fat in ligamentous attachments is lost, leaving little but the grayish peritoneal surface as emaciation develops. Clinical cases become hypoproteinemic, developing ventral and submandibular edema. Ascites (**221**) is a common result.

Diagnosis: in subacute and chronic disease, variable numbers of eggs may be detected in feces. An absence of fluke eggs does not eliminate the presence of fluke. Plasma GGT is elevated in cattle with bile duct damage. Serology will detect antibodies to fluke. Postmortem appearance is diagnostic.

Management: grazing management and flukicidal drugs. However some drugs kill only adult flukes, others a wider range of stages of the life cycle. Many are not licensed for use in dairy cattle, so control can be difficult.

Paramphistomiasis (rumen flukes)

Clinical features: even the relatively large numbers of soft, pink, pear-shaped, adult flukes seen attached to the rumen wall (**224**) cause few clinical signs, particularly in older cattle. However, immature stages attached to the duodenum may lead to unthriftiness, diarrhea and death in young animals. Several different species of fluke including *P. cervi*, *P. microbothrium* and *P. ichikawai*, are involved. Snails act as intermediate hosts.

Diagnosis and management: see above.

Schistosomiasis (blood flukes): Bilharzia

Definition: disease caused by trematode *Schistosoma* spp. with chronic disease of hemorrhagic enteritis, anemia and emaciation in a group of cattle, many dying after months.

Clinical features: eight species of *Schistosoma* have been reported throughout Africa, the Middle East and Asia. Cercariae, released into water from the intermediate snail host, penetrate the skin or mucous membranes. **225** shows a pair of elongated flukes in a blood vessel of the stretched mesentery (A), with the female lying in a longitudinal groove of the male. Flukes may be up to 30 mm long. Pathogenic species are primarily found in mesenteric blood vessels, although one species, *S. nasale*, inhabits the nasal mucosa. The major clinical signs of hemorrhagic enteritis, anemia and emaciation are seen when the spiny eggs pass through the gut wall. In the hepatic form, granulomas form around the eggs. Lesions may also be found in the liver, lungs and bladder. *S. nasale* (**226**) produces a proliferative reaction of granulomatous masses, seen in this median section through the nasal turbinate bones. Abscesses rupture to release pus and eggs into the nasal cavity. The effect is chronic nasal obstruction and dyspnea. The parasite inhabits the veins

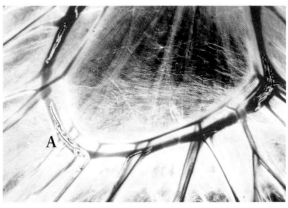

225

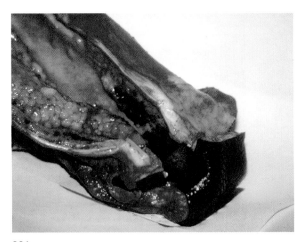

226

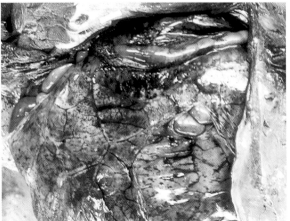

228

of the mucosa. *S. nasale* is a problem in the Indian subcontinent, Malaysia and the Caribbean.

Diagnosis: history and clinical signs are inadequate for diagnosis. Eggs must be demonstrated in feces, rectal scrapings or nasal mucus.

Management: in problem regions, e.g., China, where zoonotic spread is widespread, large-scale chemotherapy campaigns (e.g., Praziquantel), molluskicides, and habitat and management changes are effective in control.

Infectious necrotic hepatitis ('Black disease')

Definition: an acute toxemia caused by *Clostridium novyi* type B (*oedematiens*) which produces a toxin in necrotic hepatic infarcts. Most cases are seen as sudden onset incidents.

Clinical features: discrete, irregular, pale infarcts on the liver surface (**227**) are characteristic of this acute toxemia. Most frequently seen in areas of endemic fascioliasis, the larvae of *Fasciola hepatica* are the usual cause of the initial damage. The resulting lesions are then

colonized by *Clostridia*, which produce a toxin causing severe depression and rapid death from toxemia. Gross pathology may also include extensive subserosal hemorrhage, shown involving the perirenal area in **228**. The inner skin surface is dark, hence the disease pseudonym.

Differential diagnosis: other clostridial diseases and other causes of sudden death.

Management: rarely are clinical cases seen requiring treatment, but they should respond to antibiotics and NSAIDs. Vaccination is indicated if multiple cases are diagnosed.

Hepatic abscessation

Clinical features: clinical signs include nonspecific pyrexia, anorexia, abdominal pain, and depressed yield. On postmortem hepatic abscesses are usually multiple and vary in size. In this case (**229**) a large, central abscess

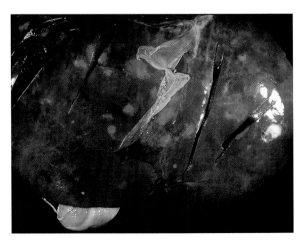

227

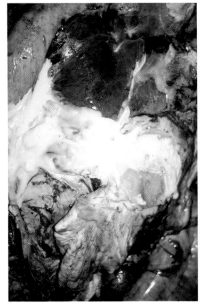

229

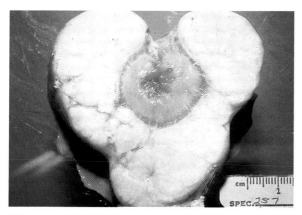

230

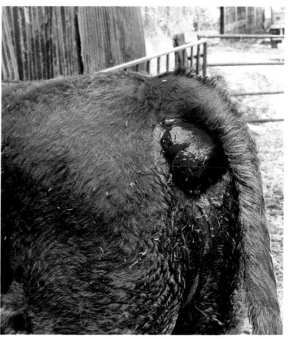

231

has ruptured to release creamy pus. Typical causes are an acute rumenitis (**193**), which is followed by hematogenous spread to the neighboring liver, or as sequelae to navel infection or traumatic reticulitis. Such abscesses usually yield *Arcanobacterium pyogenes* on culture, although the initial hepatic colonization is generally by *Fusobacterium necrophorum*. Fattening steers and high-yielding dairy cows are more susceptible owing to their relatively greater intake of concentrate feed. A specific complication of hepatic abscessation is posterior vena cava thrombosis (**262**) or pulmonary thromboembolism (**263**).

Differential diagnosis: traumatic reticulitis, abomasal ulceration and peritonitis.

Management: early cases may respond to aggressive antibiotic therapy, but as abscessation tends to become more severe, with an increasing risk of complications, early culling is advised.

Miscellaneous

Lipomatosis (abdominal fat necrosis)

Clinical features: a vertical section through the pelvic cavity of an old Angus cow (**230**) shows the rectum surrounded and severely constricted by large areas of fat necrosis, which are firm, dry and caseous. Such areas, which are also called lipomata, may occur in any part of the omental, mesenteric and retroperitoneal fat. They may cause chronic progressive bowel obstruction. However the majority cause no clinical signs and are an incidental finding during rectal examination. Although relatively rare, lipomatosis is considered more common in mature or older Channel Island breeds. Although the etiology is unclear, genetic factors, excessive intakes of soya beans and persistent pyrexia have been suggested.

Differential diagnosis: abdominal lymphosarcoma, chronic peritonitis with adhesions of abdominal viscera.

Management: lipomatosis cannot be treated.

Rectal prolapse

Clinical features: protrusion of the rectal mucosa is obvious. In **231** rectal prolapse had started 24 hours previously, primarily involving the mucosa, which is still fresh and almost undamaged. The second case (**232**) had begun 7 days previously and shows severe lacerations and edema. The only undamaged area is close to the skin–mucosal junction. Rectal prolapse occurs mainly, but not exclusively, in young animals with acute, severe or

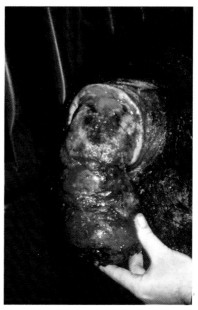

232

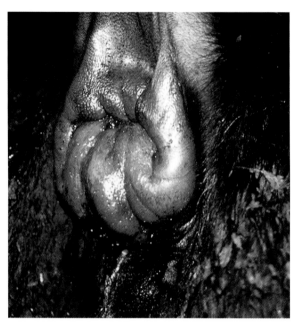

233

chronic diarrhea resulting in recurrent tenesmus. Other predisposing causes of tenesmus are coccidiosis (**59**), babesia (**684**), necrotic enteritis (**62**) and occasionally rabies (**496**).

Management: replace prolapse under epidural analgesia and keep in place with a purse-string suture. Control causes of tenesmus.

Anal edema

Anal edema (**233**) leading to protrusion of the rectoanal mucosa is an occasional consequence of rectal palpation.

Management: spontaneous recovery is seen within 12–24 hours and no treatment is required.

chapter 5

Respiratory disorders

Introduction

Although respiratory diseases have a variety of causes, infectious agents predominate e.g., infectious bovine rhinotracheitis (IBR) is caused by a herpesvirus that can affect several body systems.

A second group of important respiratory infections is caused by *Pasteurella* spp., usually following exposure of young cattle to stress (hence the alternative name for pasteurellosis, 'shipping fever'). Both *Mannheimia haemolytica* serovar 1 and *P. multocida* are normal inhabitants of the upper respiratory tract and in particular the tonsillar crypts. In order to permit colonization of the lungs, stress or a primary viral infection such as bovine virus diarrhea/mucosal disease (BVD/MD), respiratory syncytial virus (RSV) or parainfluenza type 3 (PI-3), must compromise the defense mechanisms of the body.

A third respiratory infection, termed endemic or enzootic calf pneumonia, affects groups of young calves and is of major economic importance. Both viruses (e.g., PI-3, BVD, IBR, RSV, adeno- and rhinoviruses) and mycoplasmas may be primary agents, but the etiology of many outbreaks remains uncertain, since bacterial colonization by *Pasteurella* spp. tends rapidly to supervene. Consequently, the primary virus infection may have been cleared by the time of postmortem examination. The role of *Chlamydia* is unclear.

Haemophilus somnus is of major importance as a cause of suppurative pneumonia (**491**), but, having effects on several organ systems, it is presented as infectious thromboembolic meningoencephalitis in Chapter 9.

Respiratory diseases in young cattle are of great economic importance, since their immunity to many etiological agents is poor and vaccination regimes therefore have severe limitations. Antibiotic therapy can be very costly, and recovering cattle often show poor weight gain. Contagious bovine pleuropneumonia (CBPP) is a problem in many developing countries, such as parts of Africa, India and China, where eradication through a slaughter policy and vaccination programs presents major organizational problems.

Chapter 5 is divided into infectious (viral, bacterial and other agents) and non-infectious (allergic, iatrogenic, circulatory and physiological) etiology. Where appropriate, cross-reference is made to other sections for lesions affecting

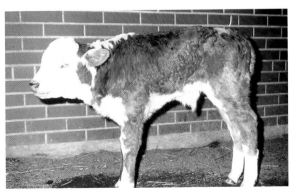

234

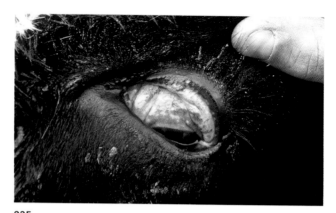

235

other systems; for example, both calf diphtheria and laryngeal abscessation (69–72) are shown in the neonatal chapter, even though they sometimes occur in older animals.

Infectious disorders

Infectious bovine rhinotracheitis (IBR) ('rednose')

Etiology and pathogenesis: IBR is caused by bovine herpesvirus 1 (BHV-1). In addition to respiratory disease, other major syndromes due to BHV-1 include abortion and genital tract infections. BHV-1.1 is the respiratory subtype, BHV-1.2 the genital subtype, and BHV-1.3 the encephalitic subtype. The last-named was recently re-classified as BHV-5, a distinct herpesvirus. *Pasteurella* spp. are common secondary invaders. BHV-1 can cause severe disease in young calves involving pyrexia, ocular and nasal discharge, respiratory distress and incoordination, leading to convulsions and death.

237

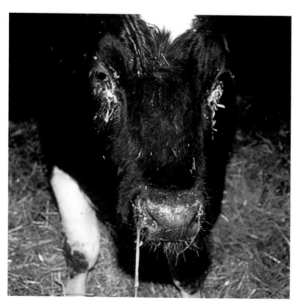

236

Clinical features: the common respiratory form of IBR has major clinical signs involving the nostrils (hence the alternative name of 'rednose') and the eyes. Feedlot cattle are at particular risk. Within a group of young cattle, several individuals may be affected simultaneously with epiphora and depression. Severely affected animals, such as the crossbred neonate in **234**, are dull, somnolent, anorexic with a tucked-up belly, and have a mucopurulent nasal discharge, nasal mucosal congestion and lympha-denopathy, and sometimes a harsh cough. The palpebral conjunctivae may be intensely injected or congested in the acute stage (**235**). Characteristic, small, raised, red plaques are visible near the lateral canthus. Secondary infection may lead to a purulent oculonasal discharge (**236**) as well as a typical purulent IBR conjunctivitis, without blepharospasm.

Postmortem examination of this animal (**237**) reveals a severe necrotizing and hemorrhagic laryngotracheitis. Another severe case is shown in **238**. In severe cases the nasal septum (**239**) sloughs its necrotic mucosa. Hemorrhage may follow the rupture of mucosal vessels.

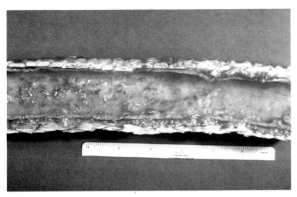

238

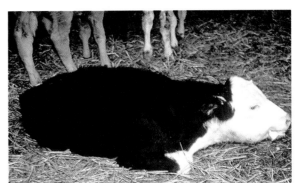

241

Balanoposthitis can occur with bovine herpesvirus 1 infection (p. 155). In **240**, the separated vulval lips reveal the multiple, discrete pustules of infectious pustular vulvo-vaginitis (IPVV). The similarity of the male and female lesions is obvious (compare **532**).

Differential diagnosis: the characteristic signs, pyrexia and eye lesions especially, make diagnosis simple in un-complicated cases. It is preferable in a field outbreak to attempt virus isolation for confirmation, or demonstration of a rising antibody titer. Bulk milk antibody tests give a simple and inexpensive indication of herd status.

Management: many cattle with eye lesions only will recover spontaneously, though there is a subsequent risk of poor fertility and an increased abortion rate. Anti-microbial therapy is needed to prevent or treat secondary infections (pasteurella). Breeding cattle, replacement

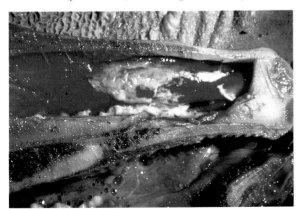

239

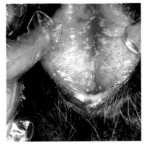

240

heifers and calves may be vaccinated from 2 months old with intramuscular or intranasal administration of modified live vaccines. Cattle entering a feedlot should be immunized 2–3 weeks before admission, but the immune response is poorer.

IBR is being successfully eradicated in some European countries by serological testing and either culling reactors or strict maintenance of a two-herd system.

Pasteurellosis ('shipping fever', 'transit fever')

Definition: pneumonic pasteurellosis is frequently caused by *Mannheimia haemolytica* serovar *1* biotype A, some-times by *P. multocida* or *Haemophilus somnus* which are all normal inhabitants of the upper respiratory tract. Often pasteurellosis is secondary to respiratory viral infections.

Etiology and pathogenesis: after stress, e.g., transport and/or viral infection, these organisms proliferate rapidly

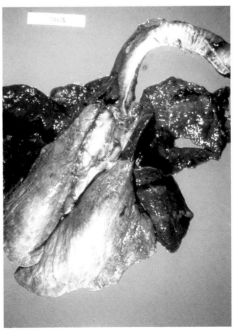

242

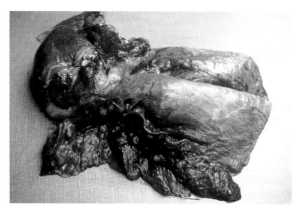

243

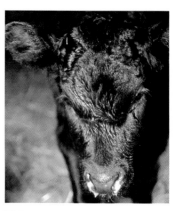

244

and extend into the trachea, bronchi and lungs. *A. pyogenes* is a frequent secondary invader.

Clinical features: severe respiratory distress (**241**), with the head and neck extended, open-mouth breathing, and froth on the lips, is obvious in this calf, which died an hour after the photograph was taken. Severe respiratory signs are evident, with dullness and anorexia, pyrexia and a moist cough. The cranioventral lung fields reveal wheezing sounds on auscultation. An expiratory grunt is possible.

At postmortem examination of another calf (**242**), in addition to froth in the major bronchi, the apical and cardiac lobes are typically dark red, slightly swollen, firm and contain microabscesses. The diaphragmatic lobes are normal. Such lungs may have fibrin deposits on the pleural surface. Lung changes tend to be symmetrical. In **243** the pneumonic areas of the apical and cardiac lobes show scattered, pale yellow abscesses. (See also *H. somnus*, **491**.)

Differential diagnosis: diagnosis depends on bacterial culture from material derived from the lower respiratory tract, or from lung tissue at postmortem. Antibiotic sensitivity testing should be done. Serology is unhelpful in diagnosis.

Management: prompt and aggressive antibiotic therapy should extend well beyond the resolution of clinical signs in affected calves to minimize the development of chronic lung abscessation. NSAIDs are important when lung congestion and respiratory signs are severe.

Pasteurella toxoid vaccines are very effective for control, but several doses may be needed in young calves where the immune response is poorer.

Hemorrhagic septicemia

Definition: a severe and frequently fatal septicemic pasteurellosis of cattle caused by *Pasteurella multocida* type B:2 or E:2.

Clinical features: the condition is characterized by sudden severe pyrexia, dyspnea, salivation, hot and painful edematous skin swellings and submucosal petechiation. It occurs primarily in Asia, Africa and occasionally parts of Southern

Europe and the Middle East. Most outbreaks are in the rainy season in river valleys and deltas.

Diagnosis is readily made on the typical postmortem features of edema, widespread hemorrhages and often hemopericardium. Pneumonic changes, except for hemorrhages, are minor.

Differential diagnosis: pneumonic pasteurellosis (**241–243**), Rinderpest (**652–657**), anthrax (**704**), and acute salmonellosis.

Management: prompt chemotherapy (sulfonamides, tetracyclines) is effective. Prevention is by vaccination twice yearly, preferably with the oil-adjuvent or alum-precipitated bacterin.

Endemic (enzootic) calf pneumonia

Definition: endemic calf pneumonia is a broad and ill-defined entity, covering infectious pulmonary disease in young cattle that is unassociated with transport stress, but frequently related to overcrowded conditions indoors or in yards.

Etiology and pathogenesis: the etiology and epidemiology involve a wide range of viral and bacterial pathogens (see Introduction).

Clinical features: the first signs are often serous ocular discharge and mild conjunctivitis. Later, a secondary

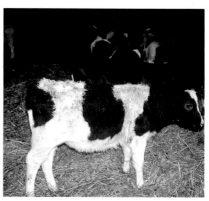

245

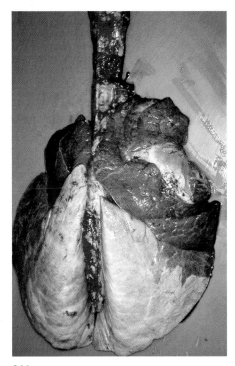

246

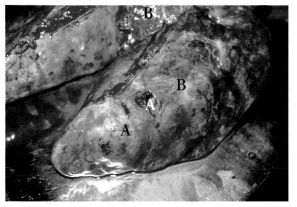

248

which, as in this calf (248), are often in the caudal (diaphragmatic) lobes, although all lung lobes may potentially be affected. Note the typical grossly distended emphysematous changes causing rounding of the lung margin.

Differential diagnosis: several viruses, as well as a secondary bacterial invader may be involved. Serology and postmortem features aid differentiation.

Management: proper housing and ventilation, adequate colostral intake as neonate, individual pens until 2–3 months old for milk-fed calves; avoid mixing multiple age groups in same air-space, as well as mixed source calves with varying immune and disease status. Provide dry, draught-free, but well-ventilated housing. Replace straw bedding frequently (e.g., 4–6 weeks). Calfhood vaccination, following identification of the causative agent is effective control. Whole group antibiotic therapy is effective in outbreaks.

Chronic suppurative pneumonia

Chronic pneumonia is often suppurative, and many organisms can be involved. Cattle of all ages can be affected. The dull beef heifer in 249 shows typical signs of chronic

infection (often *Pasteurella* spp.) can cause a bilateral mucopurulent nasal discharge (244). Some calves (245) develop a 'sweaty' coat with damp and matted hair. Similar coat changes can also be seen in some healthy, fast-growing calves on a high-concentrate feed. However coughing, with or without dyspnea, is often pronounced. Many animals in a group will be pyrexic and anorexic. Deaths may be seen within a few days of the onset of obvious clinical signs.

At postmortem the lungs contain pink-gray or purplish areas of consolidation typically in the apical and cardiac lobes and usually (246) without overlying fibrin. A cross-section of this lung (247) shows an edematous consolidated pneumonic area ventrally and normal pink lung isolated at the top. *Mycoplasma dispar.* was isolated. Secondary infection can lead to pulmonary abscessation. Respiratory syncytial virus (RSV) lungs typically show areas of emphysematous bullae (A) and patchy consolidation (B),

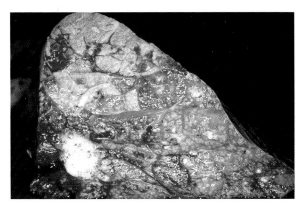

247

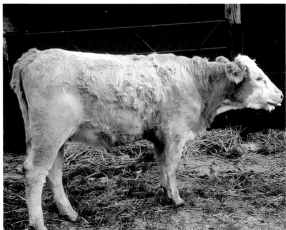

249

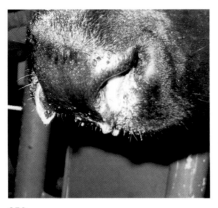

250

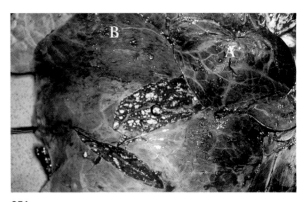

251

pneumonia, including loss of condition, an extended tongue, head and neck, and severe dyspnea, leading to froth on the lips. A profuse mucopurulent nasal discharge is also often seen in chronic suppurative pneumonia, as in a 7-year-old Holstein cow (250), together with a persistent cough. Postmortem examination (251) shows darkened areas of consolidation (A), emphysematous bullae (B), and abscessation (C). (See also 491.)

Management: prolonged aggressive antibiotic therapy (e.g., 1–2 weeks) is sometimes effective in early stages but, after this, most cases must be culled as incurable.

Contagious bovine pleuropneumonia

Definition and etiology: caused by *Mycoplasma mucoides mucoides*, contagious bovine pleuropneumonia (CBPP) is a highly contagious pulmonary disease that is often accompanied by pleurisy. It continues to be rampant in many parts of Africa, India and China, and minor outbreaks occur in the Middle East. In 1997 it occurred in Portugal.

Clinical features: CBPP infection arises predominantly from droplet inhalation in susceptible cattle, and occasionally from ingestion of infected urine or placentae. In susceptible herds the morbidity may reach 100%, the

mortality 50%, and 50% of the survivors may become carriers. The main postmortem features are a severe sero-fibrinous pleurisy (252) and fibrinonecrotic pneumonia. In 253 note the interlobular septa (A) massively distended by fibrinous exudates, creating a marbling effect. The darker areas of lung (B) are undergoing consolidation and necrosis. Chronic lung lesions include large sequestra containing viable organisms, which act as an important reservoir of infection. In 254 a large subpleural sequestrum (A) is seen to the left of a large pleuritic lesion (B). The material can be projected as an infectious aerosol by carrier cattle which may be clinically normal.

Differential diagnosis: diagnosis is readily made on clinical signs, CF test, and postmortem findings. Acute pasteurellosis (241–243) is the major differential.

Management: CBPP has been eradicated, using a compulsory slaughter policy, from North America, most of Europe (except the Iberian peninsula and parts of the Balkans), and Australia. Eradication is difficult because some infected animals become carriers and the efficacy of available vaccines is relatively poor. In most countries all outbreaks of CBPP must be notified to the central animal health authorities. Treatment is limited to endemic areas of CBPP. Elsewhere quarantine, blood testing and

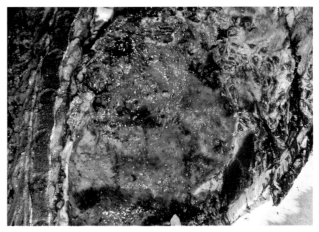

252

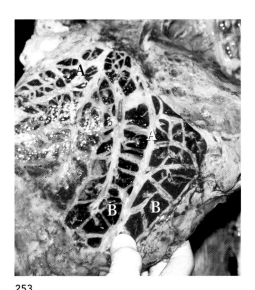

253

immunization with an attenuated vaccine can restrict disease spread.

Tuberculosis

Etiology and pathogenesis: bovine tuberculosis is caused by *Mycobacterium bovis* and is transmissible to man, usually via infected milk. Bovine organs commonly infected with tuberculosis include the alimentary tract, udder and lungs.

Clinical features: most cases of TB are identified and culled before clinical signs are seen. In advanced cases respiratory TB leads to a chronic moist cough, later dyspnea and abnormal sounds on auscultation. Lymphadenopathy, progressive emaciation and lethargy follow. Lung lesions have areas of yellow-orange pus that frequently become caseous. In **255** a section of a tuberculous lymph node shows numerous caseous granules. Gross granulomatous nodules may develop beneath the intestinal mucosa (**256**).

Diagnostic tests: TB skin test and ELISA serology.

Management: while many countries have now largely eradicated the disease, tuberculosis acquired from cattle

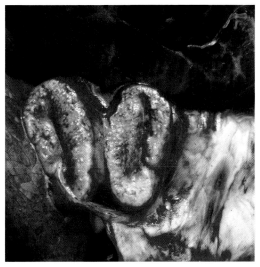

255

remains a major human health hazard in parts of Africa, the Indian subcontinent and the Far East, where the slow, chronic nature of the infection makes early clinical diagnosis difficult. Where a test and slaughter policy is not feasible, test (every 3 months) and segregation of reactors is an alternative. In some countries a wildlife reservoir (e.g., badger in UK and possum in New Zealand) has slowed down complete eradication of the disease.

Lungworm infection (verminous bronchitis, 'husk', 'hoose')

Definition: a lower respiratory tract infection caused by *Dictyocaulus viviparus*.

Pathogenesis and clinical features: the cattle lungworm causes bronchitis and pneumonia in young animals exposed to infective larvae during the first grazing season. The problem is primarily seen in the temperate areas of north-western Europe. Clinical disease does not usually occur until the late summer and autumn. Early (prepatent) infection is seen as tachypnea, partial anorexia and marked weight loss. In later stages a persistent cough develops ('husk') and the calf tends to stand with its head and

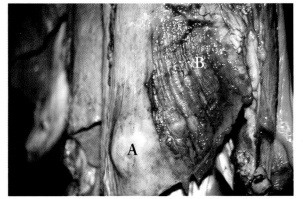

254

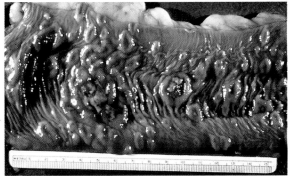

256

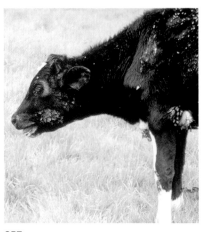

257

neck extended (257), owing to bronchial irritation from the presence of the patent forms of *D. viviparus*. A characteristic late feature is the development of a chronic, non-suppurative, eosinophilic granulomatous pneumonia, primarily in the caudal lobes of the lung. Considerable weight loss results, and clinically recovering cases still show reduced weight gain. Postmortem examination of a severe case (258) shows huge numbers of maturing larvae in the bronchi and bronchioles. Reinfection can occur in adult cattle (usually in dairy cows in the autumn) in the form of an extensive eosinophilic bronchitis. Primary infection also occurs in adult dairy cattle resulting in pronounced weight loss.

Diagnosis: larvae may be demonstrated in the feces or oronasal mucus of advanced cases, while serology can confirm exposure, but the epidemiology and clinical signs, taken together, are often characteristic.

Management: affected cattle should be given a suitable anthelmintic, and either housed or moved onto a clean pasture. Their old pasture remains infected until summer of the following year. Improve diet to restore lost weight. Strategic anthelmintic therapy (either boluses or repeated dosing) controls lungworm well at that time, but has no long-term protective effect. Optimal prophylaxis is use of an oral irradiated larval vaccine (two doses in first season,

6 and 4 weeks before turn-out). Boosted immunity derived from subsequent natural exposure can be diminished by concurrent anthelmintic therapy, which should therefore be carefully planned.

Non-infectious disorders

Atypical interstitial pneumonia (bovine pulmonary emphysema, enzootic bovine adenomatosis, 'fog fever', 'panters')

Definition: an acute hypersensitivity or allergic respiratory disease syndrome, more commonly seen in adult cattle, typically causing pulmonary edema, congestion, interstitial emphysema and alveolar changes.

Pathogenesis: it occurs predominantly in groups of heavy adult beef cattle, and, to a lesser extent, in dairy cattle and typically follows 5–10 days after a change from bare grazing onto lush pastures in the autumn, although occasional outbreaks are seen in the spring. Increased levels of nitrogenous fertilizer may be involved in some cases. The amino acid, D,L-tryptophan, the levels of which are high in lush autumn pastures, is thought to be a significant cause of this type of pneumonia, the actual toxic agent being 3-methylindole, a metabolite of D,L-tryptophan that is produced in the rumen.

Clinical features: severe respiratory distress (259) is seen, with frothing of saliva, and open-mouth breathing. Moderate exercise, such as moving off the lush pasture, can precipitate severe dyspnea and sometimes collapse and death, as in this case. In some cases subcutaneous emphysema is seen along the back from the withers. The lungs of acute cases (260) are heavy, fail to collapse, and have extensive areas of edema and emphysema (A), some of which may form large bullae.

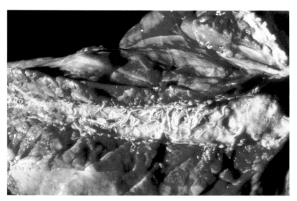

258

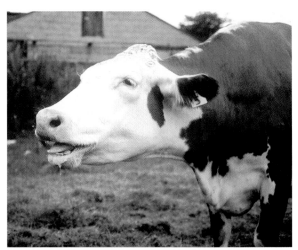

259

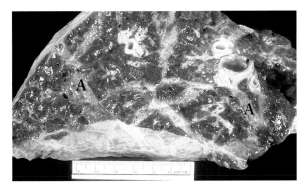

260

Management: cattle should be removed from suspect pastures as soon as possible and with extreme caution to avoid further respiratory distress. Some new cases may nevertheless occur. NSAIDs are important for treatment, and both diuretics and prophylactic antibiotics may be given. Control is by dietary management through slow introduction to lush pastures. Prophylactic feeding of monensin or lasolocid may also be effective.

Aspiration pneumonia (inhalation pneumonia)

Etiology and pathogenesis: inhalation of foreign material such as fluid drenches, or of rumen contents following bloat or occasionally during general anesthesia commonly causes a severe and often fatal pneumonia with pulmonary necrosis. Predisposing causes include abnormal head posture, struggling, bellowing, cleft palate (neonatal calves) and pharyngeal abscessation or neoplasia.

The typical pneumonia is predominantly in the anteroventral parts of the lungs. The right thoracic wall has been removed from a Holstein cow to show the effects of accidental aspiration of mineral oil (liquid paraffin) about 60 hours previously (**261**). The entire surface of the visible pleura covering the lungs appears greasy as a result

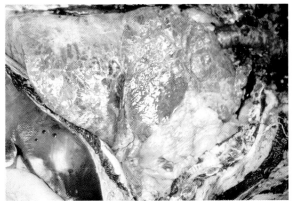

261

of oil leakage through ruptured bullae. Severe interlobular edema and emphysema are evident. Affected lobes may also reveal congestion, and early necrosis. Foreign body aspiration (drenches, rumen fluid) is frequently fatal within 48–72 hours.

Management: if aspiration has occurred, the animal should be kept quiet and given NSAIDs and broad-spectrum antibiotic prophylaxis. The prognosis is poor in all cases.

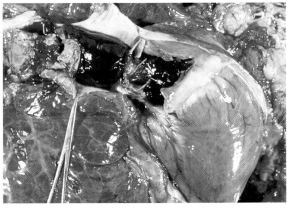

262

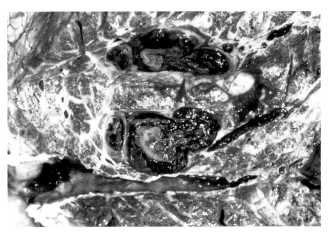

263

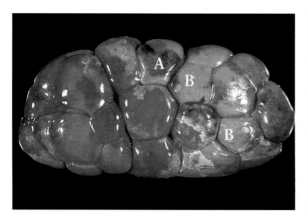

264

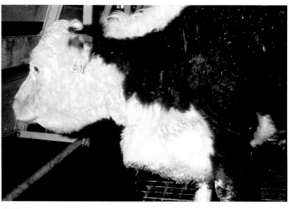

266

Pulmonary thromboembolism (caudal vena caval thrombosis)

Pathogenesis: PTE-CVC affects animals of all ages. The complex etiology of the dramatic syndrome of pulmonary thromboembolism, PTE-CVC can be a consequence of hepatic abscessation, often from navel infections or rumenitis, or can result from an earlier pulmonary disease. In some cases a localized caudal vena caval thrombosis develops (**262**). The hemostat holds the wall of the caudal vena cava. Septic emboli may seed the lungs following bacteremia and septicemia (**263**), and may result from a primary respiratory infection. Septic emboli may spread to other organs, and renal infarction (**264**) is common. The dark areas (A) in the renal cortex are recent infarcts; the paler areas (B) are older. Pulmonary arterial lesions can cause thromboembolism, aneurysm formation and

severe intrabronchial hemorrhage, hemoptysis, anemia, and melena from swallowed blood. In a fatal hemoptysis resulting from PTE-CVC (**265**), frothy arterial blood is seen on the bedding and walls of a stall.

Management: dietary control measures to prevent the development of rumenitis and acidosis. Control of respiratory disease and other bacterial infections. The acute clinical case cannot be effectively treated, but low-grade epistaxis and pyrexia may respond to antibiotic therapy.

Brisket disease (altitude sickness, high mountain disease)

Pathogenesis and clinical features: Brisket disease results from congestive cardiac failure at high altitudes (usually above 2,200 meters), where impairment of the circulatory or respiratory system overcomes the cardiac reserve capacity and causes chronic physiological hypoxia. Though individual susceptibility is great, both sexes and all ages (but predominantly <1 year) and most breeds can be affected. For unknown reasons grazing of locoweed increases the prevalence. The Hereford heifer (**266**) from Colorado, USA, shows pronounced submandibular and presternal edema, depression and dehydration.

Differential diagnosis: other causes of congestive cardiac failure.

Management: movement with due caution to a lower altitude, avoidance of locoweed.

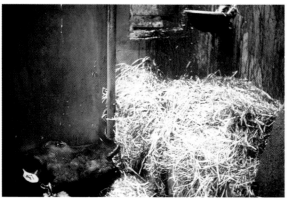

265

chapter 6

Cardiovascular disorders

Introduction

This chapter is short not because cardiovascular disorders are uncommon, but because many conditions are illustrated in other chapters. Three basic cardiac syndromes encompass most disorders: the first is congestive cardiac failure, which may result from valvular disease (270), myocardial or pericardial disease (271–273), hypertension, or congenital defects which produce shunts (27–29). Secondly, and less commonly, an acute heart failure can result from tachyarrhythmia caused by a nutritional deficiency myopathy (e.g., copper or selenium), electrocution or a lightning strike (classified under nervous disorders, 503–506), or bradycardia due to plant poisoning by *Solanum*, *Trisetum* and *Lantana* species, all of which can induce myocardial changes (731–734). Thirdly, peripheral circulatory failure can result from peripheral vasodilatation and a reduced circulating blood volume as in septic shock (e.g., acute gangrenous mastitis and acute metritis), or endotoxic shock from a peracute coliform mastitis (596–601). Peripheral circulatory failure can also be due to hematogenic failure (as a result of severe hemorrhage, see 265), or as a consequence of neonatal calf diarrhea (45–53).

Congestive cardiac failure

Definition and pathogenesis: in congestive cardiac failure reduced myocardial contractility results in reduced cardiac output and pulmonary edema when the left ventricle fails, or ascites and/or pitting edema in right-sided congestive failure, when circulatory impairment impedes venous return.

Clinical features: following right-sided failure of the heart failing to pump blood to the lungs, jugular venous distension ('jugular cording') may be marked as seen in the Friesian cow in 267. The cow was dull, pyrexic and developed a chronic cough as a result of passive venous congestion. Poor venous return in the Limousin cross bull (268) resulted in the development of a dependent edema, in the submandibular, presternal and ventral abdominal and preputial areas.

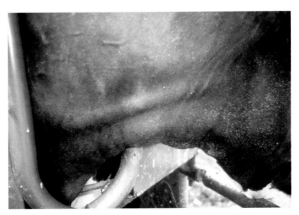

267

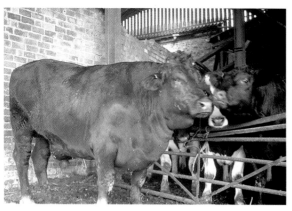

268

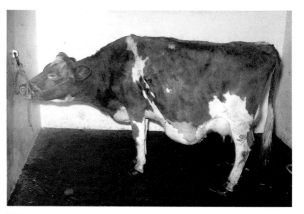

270

Differential diagnosis: ventral edema due to circulatory failure should be distinguished from a transient peripartum udder edema which is normal in dairy cows (see **642**), and from cutaneous edema (**76, 77**).

Management: largely symptomatic, including diuretics (furosemide or chlorothiazide); attempted identification of primary cause. Most cases must be culled.

Vegetative or nodular endocarditis

Pathogenesis and clinical features: another cause of congestive cardiac failure, bovine endocarditis may involve septicemia and chronic bacteremia resulting from a remote focus, such as an infected joint or the umbilicus. Characteristic signs include weight loss, drop in yield, exercise intolerance, dependent edema, tachycardia and heart murmur. Alternatively, the lesion may develop slowly in adult cattle, which remain asymptomatic, and manifest no evidence of bacterial infection (endocardiosis).

Submandibular and ventral edema are evident in a poor Friesian cow with a history of claw sepsis, which rapidly went into right heart failure. A transverse section of the heart shows massive lesions of vegetative endocarditis (**269**) in the right AV valve. In bacterial endocarditis, the tricuspid (right AV) and mitral (left AV) valves are most commonly affected.

The Guernsey cow in **270** developed a massive abscess involving the left subcutaneous abdominal vein (milk vein), which caused severe valvular endocarditis and death. Some cases that occur in young calves may have prominent valvular nodules from which *Mannheimia haemolytica* serovar *1* and α-hemolytic streptococci can be isolated, suggesting that the original infection involved the respiratory tract. Environmental streptococci, including *S. uberis*, have been isolated from clusters of cases where heifers were introduced into dairy herds under high-stress conditions.

Management: antibiotic therapy seems to stop development of lesions in early stages, and animals may well adapt to the valvular leakage. Preventive steps include control of calfhood respiratory disease, improved integration of first lactation heifers into dairy herds and reduction of the risk of septic foci.

Septic pericarditis and myocarditis

Pathogenesis: commonly follows traumatic reticuloperitonitis, less commonly from hematogenous spread.

Clinical features: septic pericarditis is usually a sequel to penetration of the pericardial sac by a wire that has migrated from the reticulum through the diaphragm (see

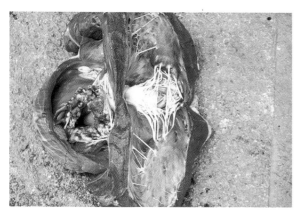

269

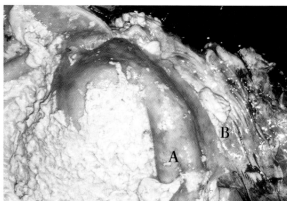

271

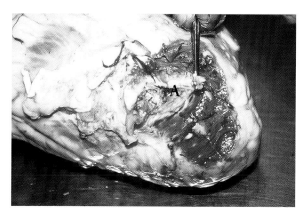

272

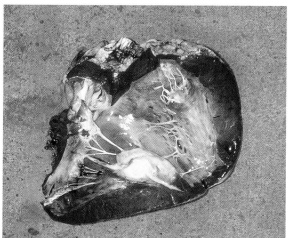

273

Traumatic reticulitis, p. 58). Congestive cardiac failure is the result of reduced contractility. In the Charolais bull in **271** a massive volume of yellow pus ('scrambled egg' appearance) fills the pericardial sac. The surface (A) below the pus is the thickened, partly fibrosed epicardium. The thickness of the pericardial wall can be judged from the depth of the sternum (B). Heart failure may result from migration of the foreign body (wire, A) into the myocardium itself (**272**). Ventral edema is often a sequel to septic pericarditis caused by traumatic reticulitis.

The absence of a septic track from the reticulum through the diaphragm to the pericardium and heart in another case (**273**) indicates that fatal myocardial abscessation can sometimes arise through hematogenous infection. In this cow (**273**), in which the original septic focus was a septic pedal arthritis, the abscess (opened) involves the papillary muscles and myocardium.

Management: treatment of individual cases is rarely successful.

Control: see Traumatic reticulitis (p. 58).

chapter 7

Locomotor disorders

Lower limb and digit

Introduction

In dairy cattle, approximately 80% of all lameness originates in the foot, particularly in the hind feet. Lameness is a major cause of economic loss, as affected animals lose weight rapidly, yields fall and, in protracted cases, fertility is affected. There is also increased culling, and considerable sums of money are spent on treatment and preventive hoof trimming. Although accurate figures are not available, lameness in beef cattle has a lower incidence and less economic importance. Many etiological factors are involved, including excessive standing, especially on hard, unyielding surfaces, feet kept continually wet in corrosive slurry, reduced horn growth at calving and high-concentrate/low-fiber feeding systems which can precipitate acidosis and subsequent laminitis. The consequences of coriosis/laminitis are an abnormal stance and hoof wear, softening of the sole horn, dropping of the distal phalanx within the hoof, and a weakening and widening of the white line, all of which predispose to digital lameness.

This chapter illustrates the common foot lesions in cattle, namely white line abscess, foreign body penetration of the sole, sole ulcer, interdigital necrobacillosis, interdigital skin hyperplasia and digital dermatitis. Complications of these primary conditions may produce deeper digital infections, involving the navicular bursa and, eventually, the pedal (distal interphalangeal) joint. Flexor tendon rupture or coronary band abscessation may result. The final section deals with vertical and horizontal claw fissures (sandcracks), claw overgrowth and laminitis. Digital lesions due to systemic disease, e.g., foot-and-mouth (650) are described in the relevant chapters.

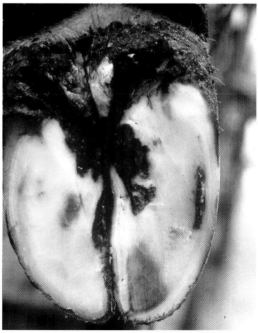

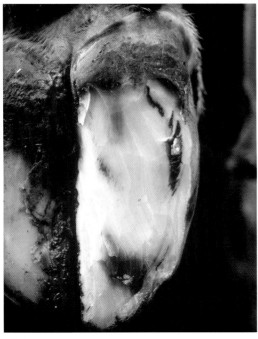

275

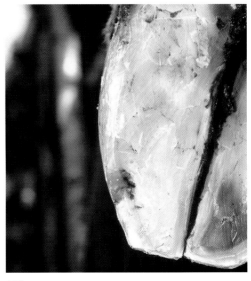

277

Disorders of the sole (bearing surface) and axial wall

White line disorders

Definition: the white line is the cemented junction between the sole horn and the hoof wall. It consists of non-tubular horn, and as a consequence it is much weaker than tubular horn of the wall and sole. Defects occur as a result of disorders in the corium leading to the production of defective white line cement. It is a point of weakness in the hoof, and the most common site for the entry of debris, dirt and infection.

Clinical features: early cases of white line disease are seen as a yellow discoloration (= serum) or reddening (= hemorrhage) of the white line cement. **274** illustrates white line hemorrhage in the right (lateral) claw; hemorrhage at the sole ulcer site (left claw) and areas of yellow discoloration in both claws. In more advanced cases (**275**) a fissure develops in the defective white line allowing the penetration of stones and other debris which then act as a wedge, producing further white line separation. Infection reaching the corium may track either across the sole, or proximally along the laminae, as in **276** to discharge at the coronary band. The abaxial white line of the hind lateral claw is most frequently involved as it represents a mechanical stress line between the rigid hoof wall and the movement of the flexible heel during locomotion.

A variety of white line abscesses are seen, depending on both the initial site of penetration of the infection, and on the direction of spread. On the left claw of **277** light grayish pus is exuding from the point of entry of infection at the white line near the toe. Pus has tracked

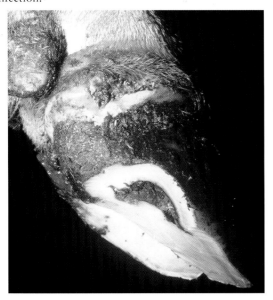

276

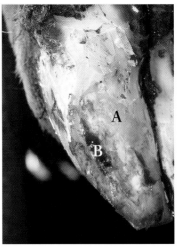

278

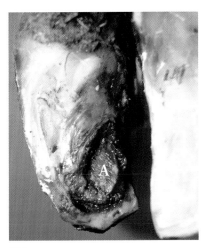

279

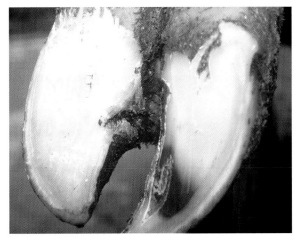

281

under the sole horn, leading to separation of the horn from the underlying corium. Lameness was pronounced. In **278** the under-run sole has been removed to expose new sole horn, developing as a layer of creamy-white tissue (A) in the center of the sole and against the edge of the trimmed horn. The hemorrhagic area (B) at the white line is the original point of entry of infection. Progressively deeper penetration of infection occurs in untreated cases. In **279**, another sole view, the corium has been eroded to expose the tip of the pedal bone (A). This resulted in severe lameness, although the cow eventually made a full recovery. Removal of the hoof wall in **280** revealed a brown necrotic line. This has permitted drainage. A wooden block has been glued onto the sound claw, to rest the affected digit. Although this cow walked soundly within 3 weeks, more than 12 months elapsed before sufficient horn had grown down from the coronet to fully repair the damaged hoof.

Differential diagnosis: punctured (FB) sole, bruised sole, sole ulcer, fracture of distal phalanx, vertical wall fissure.

Management: white line disorders are primarily a defect of the corium leading to the production of defective cement. Coriosis may be the result of a range of factors including trauma (e.g., prolonged standing due to poor

cubicle comfort, or prolonged feeding and milking times), diet (rumen acidosis leads to reduced biotin synthesis and the production of defective white line cement), and environment. An increased incidence of white line separation and abscess formation may occur when cattle walk on rough surfaces or tracks where there are small, sharp flints, or as a consequence of softening of the hoof, e.g., excessively wet conditions underfoot. Reduced horn growth at calving can lead to a thinning of the sole and this further predisposes to bruising of the corium.

Axial wall fissure and penetration

Definition: the fissure is a defect of the white line where it passes dorsally along the axial wall towards the inter-

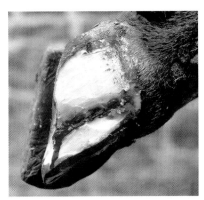

280

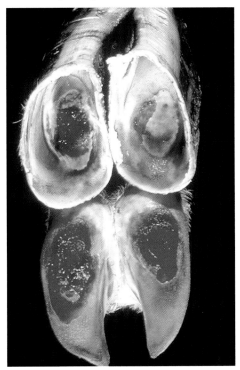

282

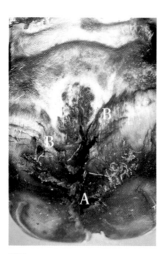

283

digital cleft. The axial groove horn is particularly thin (1–2 mm) and therefore predisposed to foreign body penetration.

Clinical features: most cases of fissure here (**281**) are seen as an impaction of the white line with black debris, often with under-running of adjacent horn. Pain and lameness are a result of the detached axial wall moving on the underlying corium. A foreign body penetrating this region resulted in a localized septic laminitis (**296**) at A, with secondary interdigital swelling and necrosis.

Differential diagnosis: interdigital FB, interdigital dermatitis.

Management: removing under-run horn treats individual cases. Predisposing factors are as in white line disorders, although wet environmental conditions are thought to be particularly important, and digital dermatitis in the interdigital space, leading to defective horn production from the coronary band may be a further cause.

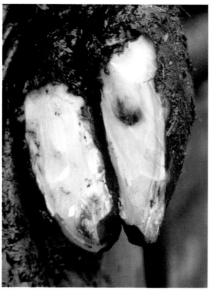

284

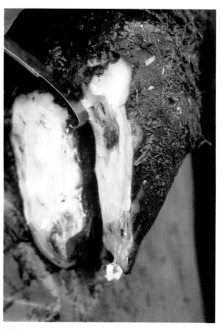

285

Sole ulcers

Definition: an ulcer is a defect in the horn exposing the underlying corium, and like white line disorders, sole ulceration originates from a damaged corium. Heel and toe ulcers are discussed in the next section. Sole ulcers are the most common and are typically found on the axial aspect of the sole in zone 4, beneath the flexor tuberosity of the pedal bone. **282** shows two exungulated claws, the left with severe hemorrhage in the corium at the sole which could develop into a sole ulcer, and the right with hemorrhage at the heel ulcer site.

Clinical features: the digit in **283** (a plantar view) has a wedge of sole horn (A) growing from the axial aspect of the right (lateral) claw towards the left claw. This wedge increasingly becomes a major weight-bearing surface and transmits excess weight to the sole corium, causing hemorrhage, bruising and eventually pressure necrosis. Note also the heel erosion (B). Another cow (**284**) shows

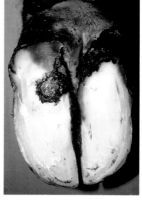

286

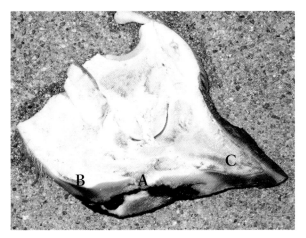

287

that when such a sole wedge is pared away, a discrete area of sole hemorrhage is exposed in the right (lateral) claw. Note the reddening of the white line in the same claw, indicative of coriosis/laminitis, and also that both claws are overgrown. Further paring and removal of the hemorrhagic horn (285) revealed under-run horn and necrosis characteristic of a sole ulcer. Some sole ulcers (286) develop a large, protruding mass of granulation tissue. The longitudinal section of another case (287) illustrates a mild, chronic ulcer in its characteristic site at the sole–heel junction. The sole horn has been perforated (A) and inflammatory changes have tracked up towards the insertion of the deep flexor tendon. The heel horn is slightly under-run (B) and there is laminitic hemorrhage (coriosis) at the toe (C). Sole ulcers are typically found on the lateral claws of hind feet and, less frequently, on the medial claws of front feet. Often the lateral digits of both hind feet are involved to a different extent. More extensive damage to the corium means that they heal more slowly than a white line abscess or an under-run sole (278).

Differential diagnosis: solar FB penetration and abscessation.

Management: coriosis is the primary defect, and hence many of the factors leading to white line disease can also produce sole ulcers, although it is not fully understood why there is sometimes a high incidence of sole ulcers and in other cases a high incidence of white line disease.

Treatment of individual cases involves paring away all under-run horn around the ulcer, and minimizing weight-bearing to allow new horn to be produced in the defective site. This can be achieved by paring the affected claw to transfer weight onto the sound claw, and/or by the application of a shoe to the sound claw.

Heel and toe ulcers

Definition: heel ulcers occur in the center of the foot at the junction of zones 4 and 6, where the heel horn joins the sole horn, and are shown as areas of hemorrhage in the exungulated right claw in 282. Toe ulcers occur at zones 1 and 2.

Clinical features: heel ulcers are seen as small black tracks penetrating the sole horn (288). Removal of overlying horn may lead to the disappearance of small lesions, but in this case there was an underlying abscess (289). In other cases the lesion discharges at the heel. Heel ulcers commonly occur in association with sole ulcers, although they are more frequently found on the medial claw of hind feet and the lateral claw of fore feet than sole ulcers. Their etiology is not understood but pinching of the corium between cartilaginous changes in the pedal suspensory apparatus above and the hoof of the sole beneath may be the cause. Toe ulcers (290) are typically larger areas of hemorrhage. They may occur when heifers and young bulls are introduced into a dairy herd without prior acclimatization to concrete. They appear to be related to trauma and excessive wear in both front and hind feet.

Differential diagnosis: as for sole ulcer.

Management: for both conditions remove all damaged horn and minimize weight bearing on the affected claw. Control by identifying initial causes of coriosis.

Toe necrosis (osteomyelitis of distal phalanx)

Definition: abscess at the toe leading to secondary infection of the apex of the pedal (distal phalangeal) bone.

Clinical features: the condition occurs in both dairy cows and in feedlot cattle, and may be associated with

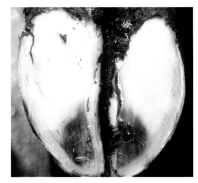

288

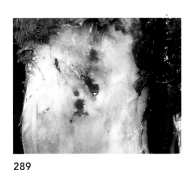

289

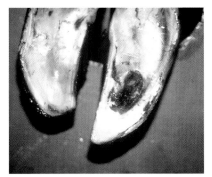

290

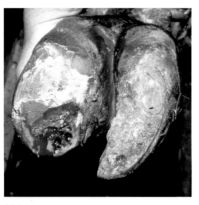

291

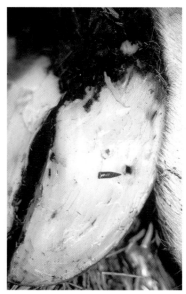

293

excess wear leading to thinning of the horn at the toe. In **291** the under-run sole at the toe has largely been removed to reveal a black necrotic area tracking up under the dorsal wall. The lesion commonly has a pronounced putrid smell, rarely present in other hoof disorders. The necrotic tip of the pedal bone can be palpated at the site of hemorrhage at the toe. Many of these lesions fail to heal and recur a few months later. In a cross-section of another affected digit (**292**), the apex of the pedal bone has clearly been eroded, dry fecal debris is impacted into the residual cavity at the toe and gray areas of necrotic pedal bone are visible on its ventral and dorsal surfaces.

Management: thorough removal of under-run horn, debridement and cleaning will result in recovery of a few cases, but many need more radical treatment such as amputation of the osteomyelitic and necrotic tip of the pedal bone, or of the whole claw.

Foreign body penetration of the sole

Definition: penetration of the sole by a foreign body allowing access of infection to the corium and subsequent abscess formation.

Clinical features: the most common foreign bodies are nails, stones and cast teeth. In **293** a metal staple is firmly impacted in the sole, towards the heel. Unless the foreign body penetrates the sole horn, leading to infection and under-run corium, lameness is relatively mild. In **294** a portion of nail has penetrated the sole horn on the axial aspect of the white line, carrying infection into the corium. In **295** superficial horn has been removed to provide drainage and to expose the new sole (A) developing beneath. In the center (B) is the sensitive corium. Foreign body penetration can also occur near the axial groove (**296**) as the wall horn is thinnest here, leading to secondary interdigital swelling and necrosis and a septic laminitis. Sole puncture at the toe can cause osteomyelitis of the distal phalanx or pedal bone (**291**, **292**).

Management: removal of foreign body and paring of surrounding under-run horn to permit optimal drainage.

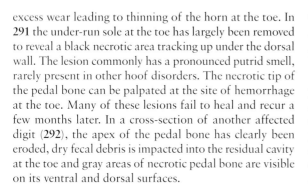

292

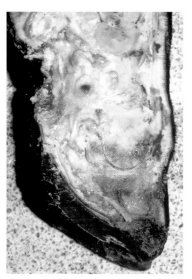

294

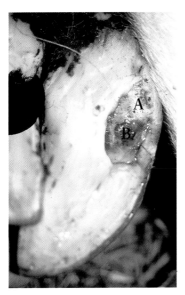

295

False sole

Clinical features: removal of the under-run sole in **295** reveals a thin layer of epidermal horn covering the corium. The detached horn is often called a 'false sole'. In another example (**285**) the point of the hoof knife is lifting the false sole. In other cases acute coriosis may lead to a total but temporary cessation of horn production, and the production of a secondary or false sole, with no external signs of penetration or white line disease.

Management: the under-run false sole horn is trimmed off to stimulate regrowth.

Complications of digital hoof disorders

Introduction

Superficial under-running of the corium is easily treated by removal of separated horn and allowing regrowth of new hoof. Infection of deeper tissues leads to further

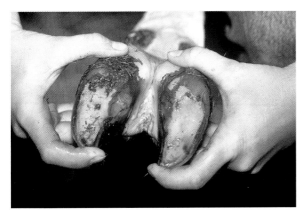

296

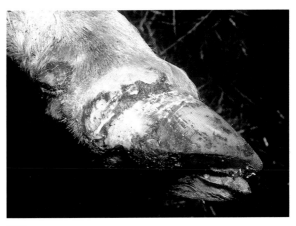

297

clinical signs and usually a more severe and protracted lameness. A range of conditions may be seen including abscesses at the coronary band or the heel, rupture of the deep flexor tendon, and deeper sepsis.

Abscess at the coronary band

Infection originating at the white line has passed proximally under the hoof wall to the coronet in **297**, where it has penetrated the deeper tissues of the collateral digital ligaments to produce a septic cellulitis, with pronounced swelling around the coronary band. As well as highlighting the overgrowth of the sole horn, this chronic lesion shows that the horn wall is detached from the coronet beneath the abscess. The affected toe has deviated dorsally, suggesting partial rupture of the flexor tendon, and leading to relative horn overgrowth from lack of wear.

Abscess at heel (retroarticular abscess; septic navicular bursitis)

Clinical features: neglected ulcers may penetrate deeper structures: in a longitudinal section of a claw (**298**), purulent infection can be seen in the digital cushion (A) adjacent to the navicular bone, the deep digital flexor tendon (B) and the pedal joint (C). This is sometimes referred to as a retroarticular abscess, and needs surgical drainage.

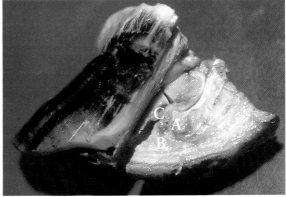

298

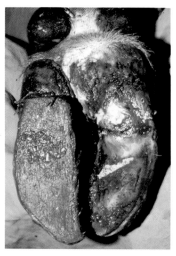

299

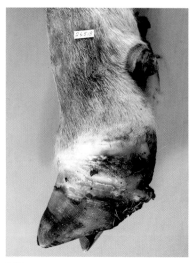

301

Similarly **299** shows heel enlargement, and a purulent exudate, probably from an infected navicular bursa or a retroarticular abscess discharging through the original ulcer site. A wooden block has been applied to the sound claw. Flexor tendon rupture (**300**) may result from complicated cases (see below).

Management of pedal abscesses and deep sepsis: removal of all under-run horn, drainage of abscesses by curettage and flushing, and aggressive antibiotic therapy. Distal joint sepsis requires amputation or joint fusion, but many cases are best culled on welfare and economic grounds.

Rupture of the deep flexor tendon

Clinical features: complications from severe white line abscess, a sole ulcer, or, as in **301**, a retroarticular heel abscess, can lead to infection and the subsequent rupture of the deep flexor tendon. In **301** the coronary band is severely distorted, the heel is swollen and the toe deviates upwards (plantigrade), leading to continual overgrowth and lack of wear of the affected claw. A longitudinal section of a septic digit (**300**) reveals the site of the ulcer

that perforated the sole horn (A), and the point of rupture of the deep flexor tendon (B). Note the horn overgrowth at the toe. At this stage the joint is not affected and recovery is possible with prompt treatment.

Septic pedal arthritis (distal interphalangeal sepsis)

Definition: infection of the distal interphalangeal joint (pedal joint).

Clinical features: pedal arthritis typically results from a neglected white line abscess, sole ulcer or interdigital necrobacillosis infection. Note the marked unilateral enlargement of the left heel in **302**, with inflammation tracking up towards the fetlock and causing distortion of the claw. The navicular bursa and pedal joint are also

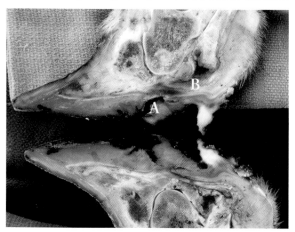

300

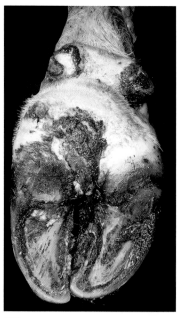

302

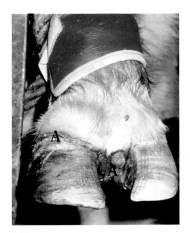

303

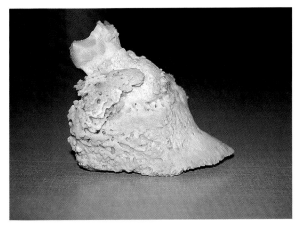

306

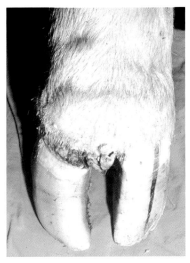

304

infected, producing a septic pedal arthritis. Gross enlargement can result in lifting of digital sole and heel horn, especially at the heel and towards the interdigital space. The Hereford cow in **303** had been lame for 8 weeks. The affected lateral claw is grossly enlarged and inflamed, there is swelling of the coronet and separation

of horn at the coronary band (A), and granulation tissue protrudes into the interdigital space at the point where pus discharges from the infected joint. Despite a less severe degree of swelling in the more chronic case in **304**, the hoof on the affected lateral claw is being evulsed by pressure and necrosis from a septic coronitis.

Long-standing digital infections may lead to an osteitis and a proliferation of new bone, as in **306**, which is a boiled-out specimen of a chronically infected sole ulcer in a Holstein cow. A deep cavity was present at the ulcer site, with extensive new bone proliferation in the navicular, digital cushion and coronary areas. When P2 and P3 became ankylosed, the severity of lameness decreased. In **305**, which is a sagittal section following digital amputation, necrosis in the navicular bone has extended to cause severe sepsis in the distal joint (A). Infection at the coronary band (B) has produced swelling above the coronet.

Management of pedal abscesses and deep sepsis: as with all abscesses, drainage and flushing are of paramount importance. Removal of all under-run horn, deep pedal curettage, flushing, and aggressive antibiotic therapy may prove effective. Insertion of a drainage tube along the track of the original discharging fistula to exit above the coronary band is easily achieved and improves drainage. Cases involving a marked bony swelling above the coronary band from extensive and longer-term periostitis require amputation. Joint sepsis requires amputation or joint ankylosis, but many cases are best culled on welfare and economic grounds.

Disorders of the digital skin and heels

Whereas hoof disorders arise from the corium and are largely managemental in origin, diseases of the interdigital skin have a large infectious component.

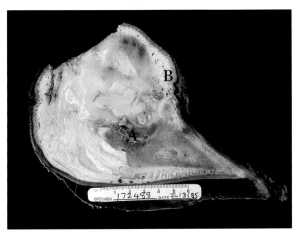

305

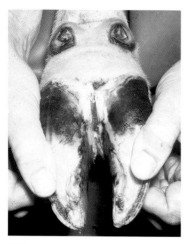

307

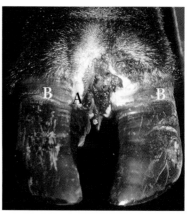

310

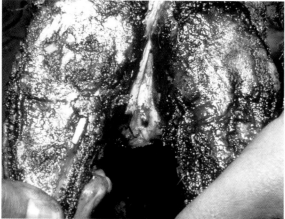

308

Interdigital necrobacillosis (phlegmona interdigitalis, 'foul', 'footrot')

Definition: a common cause of lameness, interdigital necrobacillosis is an infection of the dermal layers of interdigital skin associated with *Fusobacterium necrophorum*

and other bacteria such as *Porphyromonas assacharolytica* and *Prevotella* spp. Infection starts in the dermis.

Clinical features: early cases have an obvious lameness and show a symmetrical, bilateral, hyperemic swelling of the heel bulbs that may extend to the accessory digits. At this stage, the interdigital skin is swollen but intact, and the claws appear to be pushed apart when the animal stands. After 24–48 hours the interdigital skin splits (**307**) (some sloughed epidermis has been removed), and in later cases, the dermis is exposed (**308**). There may be a foul-smelling, caseous exudate, as seen in **309**. **310** is a dorsal view of a neglected case after cleansing, with sloughed necrotic debris in the interdigital space. The depth of the necrotic process has caused proliferation of granulation tissue. Early separation of the axial wall of the left claw (A) and swelling of the coronet suggest early inflammatory changes in the pedal joint. The horizontal groove (B) distal to the coronary band indicates that the problem has existed for about 1 month.

A peracute form of interdigital necrobacillosis exists known as 'Super Foul' (**311**), where severe necrosis extends

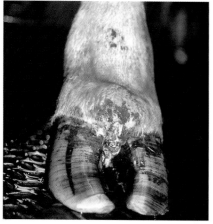

309

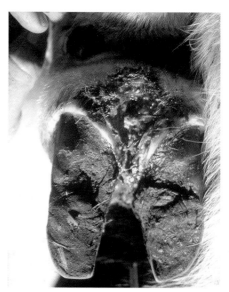

311

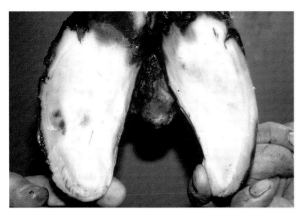

312

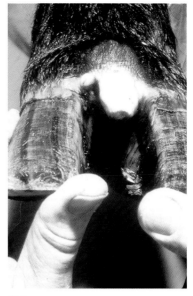

314

from the interdigital cleft onto the heel skin. The dermal necrosis is savage in onset and there may be joint involvement within 48 hours of initial clinical signs. The same causative organisms are involved, although the antibiotic sensitivity pattern may differ. Prompt and aggressive therapy is vital.

Differential diagnosis: interdigital dermatitis (321), interdigital foreign body (325), digital dermatitis (315–317).

Management: improved foot hygiene by cleaner floor areas and regular foot bathing can dramatically reduce the incidence. Avoid rough gateways and other surfaces that can traumatize the interdigital cleft. Treatment by parenteral and topical antibiotics.

Interdigital skin hyperplasia (fibroma, 'corn')

Definition: hyperplasia in the interdigital space develops from skin folds adjacent to the axial hoof wall, as shown in 312.

Clinical features: the lesion, which may be inherited and is then usually bilateral, is a problem in heavier breeds of beef and dairy cows as well as mature beef bulls. Lameness is produced either when the claws pinch the interdigital skin during walking, or following secondary (necrobacillary) infection in areas of pressure necrosis (313) and commonly as a result of secondary infection with digital dermatitis. Note the superficial but severe slough of necrotic material.

In a few cases, hyperplasia is restricted more to the dorsal interdigital space (314), when lameness is less likely.

Differential diagnosis: interdigital necrobacillosis (307), digital dermatitis (315–317).

Management: irritation to the interdigital skin from trauma, excess stretching when walking over rough surfaces, and chronic irritation from digital dermatitis and interdigital necrobacillosis are all predisposing factors and should be avoided in the control of the condition. Small lesions can be treated by removing overgrowth of the axial wall to minimize pinching, or by regular foot bathing through astringents such as formalin or copper sulfate solutions. Larger lesions require amputation.

Digital dermatitis ('hairy warts')

Definition: a bacterial infection of the epidermis of the hoof skin involving *Treponeme* species.

Clinical features: the lesion is typically seen on the skin above the heel bulbs, proximal to the interdigital space.

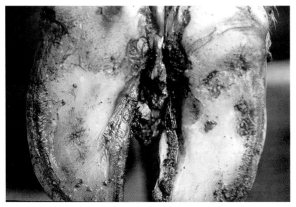

313

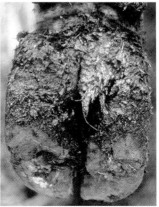

315

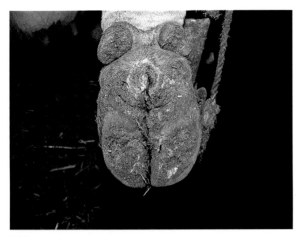

316

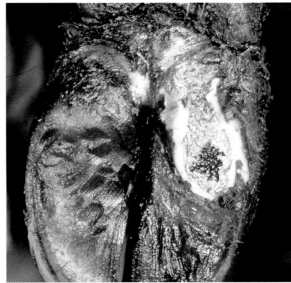

319

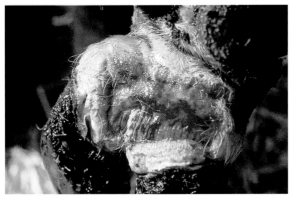

317

lesions, involving perioplic horn of the coronary band, may produce complications such as vertical fissure and pedal osteitis, and a much more protracted lameness. Another complication involves an under-run sole from an initial heel lesion (319). Chronic infection produces 'hairy warts', seen typically as tufts of proliferating skin at the back of the heel (320).

Differential diagnosis: interdigital necrobacillosis (307), interdigital dermatitis (321), mud fever (322), and heel erosion or slurry heel (323).

Management: digital dermatitis is associated with repeated exposure to slurry, especially to the mixture of urine and feces which is typically associated with automated slurry scrapers. Low-grade lesions present in dry cows often rapidly progress to produce raw open lesions in early lactation animals. This explains why disease is most commonly seen at peak lactation. Control is based on meticulous foot bathing to prevent lesions developing, and improved environmental foot hygiene. More advanced lesions causing lameness can be treated individually by topical antibiotics

On initial inspection, early cases (315) show hairs that are erect and matted with a serous exudate. Cleaning off superficial debris (316) in a similar case reveals a circular area of epidermitis, 1–2 cm in diameter. Affected animals are acutely lame, even though dermal tissues are not significantly involved (compare interdigital necrobacillosis, 307). In advanced lesions (317) the heel horn becomes eroded and under-run, with an extensive raw area of epidermitis extending up towards the accessory digits. Although the majority of cases occur at the plantar aspect, ulcerating dorsal lesions, as seen in 318, are not uncommon. Such

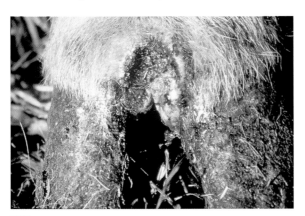

318

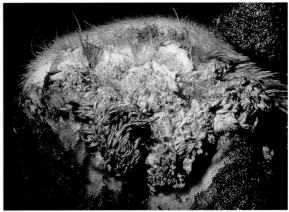

320

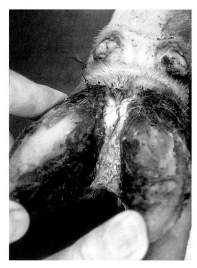

321

or by surgical removal of 'hairy warts'. Herd outbreaks can be controlled by foot bathing in antibiotic or formalin, but this may not be permitted in some countries.

Interdigital dermatitis

Interdigital dermatitis is a superficial, moist inflammation of the interdigital epidermis (321) not involving the deeper tissues, and hence differs from necrobacillosis (307). *Dichelobacter nodosus* has occasionally been recovered from lesions. Several cattle may be affected at one time. Despite the superficial nature of the lesion, lameness is sometimes pronounced. Many consider that this lesion is related to digital dermatitis.

Differential diagnosis: interdigital necrobacillosis (307), digital dermatitis (315–317).

Management: topical antibiotic aerosol.

'Mud fever'

Clinical features: mud fever occurs following exposure to cold, wet, muddy conditions and may involve secondary *Dermatophilus* infection (see 106). In 322 the leg is swollen, especially around the pastern. The cleansed skin is thickened with a dry eczema and there is some hair loss from the coronet, extending to above the fetlock. Lameness was pronounced. All four limbs may be affected.

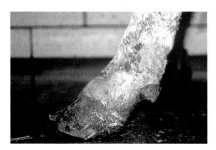

322

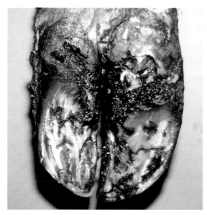

323

Differential diagnosis: digital dermatitis (315).

Management: affected areas should be thoroughly washed and a greasy antiseptic ointment rubbed onto the area, alternatively the skin may be sprayed with emollient teat dip. Severe cases benefit from a 3-day course of systemic penicillin.

Heel erosion ('slurry heel')

Definition: erosion of the heel horn. The heel is an important weight-bearing surface. Its normal structure has been demonstrated in preceding illustrations, e.g., 313.

Clinical features: erosion is commonly seen in housed dairy cows that stand in slurry. Loss of the heel horn destabilizes the hoof, alters weight-bearing, increases concussion, and may predispose to sole ulcers. Slurry heel may be related to digital and interdigital dermatitis. *Bacteroides nodosus* has occasionally been isolated from both lesions. In 323 the original smooth horn has been eroded, producing a deep fissure in the left heel. More severe erosion of the right (lateral) heel horn has led to the appearance of granulation tissue from the sole. In the advanced case of 324 both heels are almost completely eroded. Digital

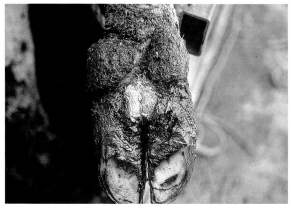

324

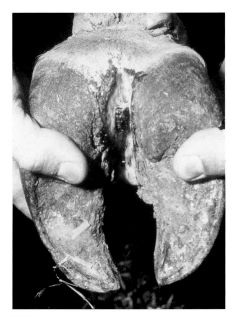

325

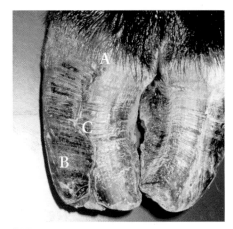

326

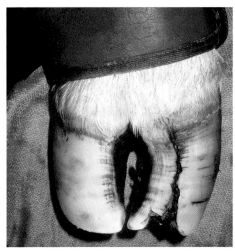

327

dermatitis and slurry heel often occur together, as in **324**, as poor environmental hygiene predisposes to both conditions.

Differential diagnosis: digital dermatitis (**315**).

Management: spontaneous recovery is seen when cattle are kept at pasture. Some housed cases require horn trimming.

Interdigital foreign body

Clinical features: in **325** a stone is impacted in the interdigital space, ulcerating the axial skin of the left claw. Small pieces of twig, especially thorns, can lie longitudinally in the cleft, damaging the interdigital skin and leading to secondary necrobacillosis (see also **296**).

Differential diagnosis: interdigital necrobacillosis.

Management: removal and careful examination of depth and extent of interdigital trauma. Topical antibiotic.

Disorders of the hoof wall

Vertical fissure (vertical sandcrack)

Definition: a split, of varying depth, in the hoof wall running from the coronary band to the weight-bearing surface at the sole, more common in heavy beef breeds.

Clinical features: vertical fissures occur as a result of damage to the superficial periople, and underlying coronary band, for example following hot, dry weather, or damage to the coronary band from trauma or a digital dermatitis infection at the coronary band. Both claws of the overgrown left forefoot in **326** are affected, although the major fissure appears only on the medial claw. Note its irregular

course and its origin at the coronary band (A). Note also the section (B), which is slightly loose due to an oblique crack at (C). In **327** only the right claw is affected, where the fissure is much deeper and the toe is broken off. An extensive, wide, vertical horn crack is shown, in which the laminae are very liable to become exposed, resulting in severe lameness, even though little pus may be present. In advanced cases (**328**), granulation tissue with blood may protrude from the fissure.

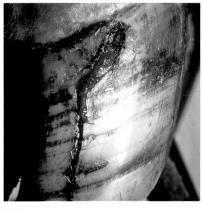

328

Management: distal weight-bearing horn on each side of the crack should be removed, as should any hinged portion of horn, to reduce movement of the fissure. If granulation tissue is protruding from the fissure, as in **328**, it is likely that there is also an osteomyelitis of the pedal bone. Digit amputation is then the only treatment. Supplementary biotin has been shown to decrease the prevalence in beef cattle. Control in dairy herds necessitates lowering the incidence of digital dermatitis.

Horizontal fissure (horizontal sandcrack)

Definition: horizontal fissures result from a temporary cessation of horn formation, often as a result of a metabolic disturbance. If the cessation was marked, the fissure may extend down to the corium. Less severe disruptions cause simple lines of interrupted horn growth, sometimes known as 'hardship lines'. Unlike vertical fissures, these are usually evident in all eight claws.

Clinical features: in **329** both claws are affected: the hand-held, cracked, medial hoof wall resulted from a temporary cessation of horn formation 4 months previously, due to an abrupt dietary change. Because the length of the anterior wall is greater than the height of the heel, the 'thimble' of horn eventually loses its support from the heel, but remains attached at the toe. Lameness results from the pressure of the hinged portion of horn on the underlying laminae, or from exposure of the sensitive laminae when the thimble becomes detached (broken toe). In **329** a smaller fissure of the lateral claw has been partially trimmed off, without exposing sensitive laminae, to reduce movement of the thimble. Sometimes both claws of all four feet may be affected as a result of a severe systemic insult, for example following acute mastitis, foot-and-mouth disease or acute metritis.

Management: herds with a high incidence of horizontal fissures must be suffering periodic bouts of coriosis/laminitis, the cause of which needs to be identified and rectified. Dietary factors or disease could be involved, especially in the periparturient cow. Investigation of a

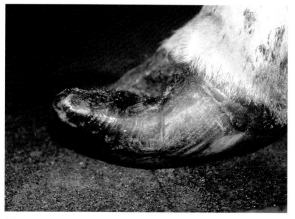

330

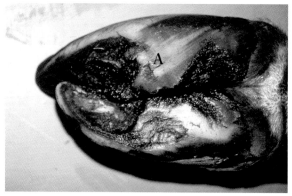

331

herd problem begins with a detailed examination of the history of the transition cow.

Corkscrew claw

Definition: the claw, usually the lateral claw of both hind legs, is twisted spirally throughout its length.

Clinical features: the lateral claw of the front or the hind feet can be affected by this partially heritable growth defect. The overgrown lateral toe in **330** deviates upwards, and in the same digit, the abaxial wall curls under the sole (**331**), inevitably altering the weight-bearing surfaces. The axial sole overgrowth (**331**, A) consequently becomes a major weight-bearing surface and lameness can result from sole ulcers and/or pedal bone compression (see also **334**). In the pedal bone specimen in **332**, osteolysis secondary to corkscrew claw compression is seen near the toe, at A. The left pedal bone and the cavitation are normal. **331** also shows early bilateral heel erosion (see also **323**), and cavitation of the sole of the medial claw due to impaction by debris.

Scissor claw

Definition: scissor claw differs from corkscrew claw in that one toe grows across the other, there is less wall involvement, and rotation along a longitudinal axis is absent.

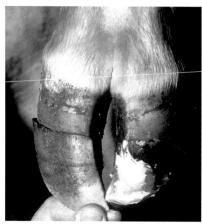

329

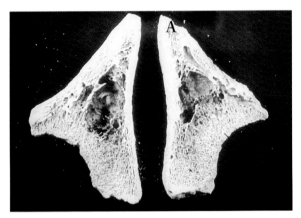

332

Clinical features: in 333 the wall of the left claw curls slightly axially at the point of contact with the ground, and may form a false sole. Slight mechanical lameness can result from the pressure of one toe on top of the other during walking.

Management: both corkscrew claw and scissor claw require repeated radical trimming. Intensive farming practice usually necessitates early culling for economic reasons.

Sole overgrowth

Definition: the central sole area, *viz.* zone 4 beneath the flexor tuberosity of the pedal bone, should be non-weight-bearing. However, it is not uncommon for a wedge of sole to grow out from zone 4 to become the major weight-bearing area of the sole. Sole ulcers may then develop beneath this wedge.

Clinical features: the lateral (left) claw in 334 is much larger than the medial claw, and the outer wall is over-grown, curling axially towards the sole. A wedge of sole horn (A) is growing across towards the medial claw. This wedge predisposes the animal to sole bruising and/or sole ulcers (see also 283, 314, 331). The black areas on the heels

are early heel erosions (323). In front feet sole overgrowth is most commonly seen in the medial claw.

Management: thought to be a consequence of coriosis/laminitis, sole overgrowth is seen especially in heifers 6–12 weeks after calving. Heifers that have been reared in straw yards prior to calving have a less well-developed sole thickness which is more prone to bruising when they move onto concrete postpartum. The problem is exacerbated by other causes of coriosis such as poor cubicle/free stall comfort and an inappropriate diet. Corrective trimming to restore normal weight distribution is required.

Fracture of distal phalanx

Definition: occurring primarily in the front feet, distal phalangeal fracture is usually traumatic and intra-articular, although it may be pathologically associated with fluorosis (749) or osteomyelitis.

Clinical features: the medial claw is often involved, forcing the animal to adopt a cross-legged stance, and hence transferring weight to the lateral claw (335). The fracture line (A) in 336 runs vertically from the distal interphalangeal joint, and the two fragments of pedal bone are separated. This type of fracture leads to a sudden onset of severe lameness, often with no initial visible signs of heat or swelling. Later, the affected claw may be palpably hotter, but in the early stages, diagnosis without radiography is difficult. The most common cause of a crossed foreleg stance is bilateral sole ulceration.

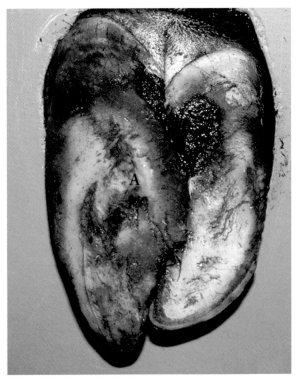

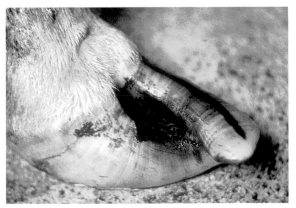

333   334

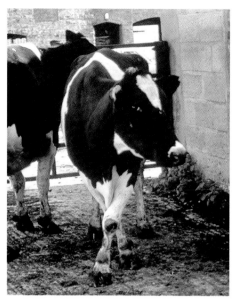

335

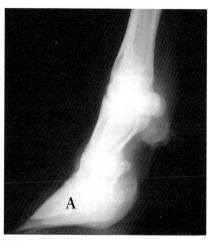

336

Differential diagnosis: bilateral ulcers of medial claws of forefeet; foreign body perforation of the interdigital space or the sole.

Management: as the bone is 'self-splinted' by the hoof casing, most cases recover with limited intervention. A surgical block put on the sound claw minimizes weight-bearing on the affected claw, improving the welfare of the cow by abolition of pain, and speeding the healing process.

Laminitis

Definition: although 'laminitis' remains a widely used term, rarely are changes limited to the laminar area of the corium. In most instances inflammation of the entire corium is involved, and hence the term 'coriosis' is more appropriate. Recent research into the pathogenesis of sole ulcers and white line disease has suggested that the laminar corium remains normal when the distal phalanx sinks,

and hence use of the term laminitis may not be justified in cattle. The primary changes are microvascular, the causes being multifactorial and including trauma, infections and metabolic disease and dietary disturbances.

Acute laminitis

Clinical features: the Friesian cow in 337 has a typical acute laminitic stance: the front legs are abducted, the hind legs are placed forward under the abdomen, the back is arched, the neck is extended, and the tail is slightly raised. Hoof changes following laminitis are shown in 338. Hemorrhage can be seen over the heel bulb and along the white line. Note the black debris impacted into the widened white line towards the heel, which could result in white line infection (277). Intense congestion of the blood vessels in the corium is the most probable cause of the blood clot in the sole horn at the toe. The heifer had calved 2 months previously and the coriosis/laminitis was probably the result of depressed horn synthesis around the time of calving, leading to a thin sole susceptible to bruising, and a change from a fibrous to a high-concentrate diet (producing acidosis), combined with excessive

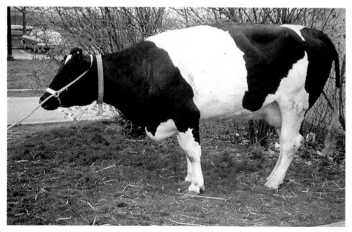

337

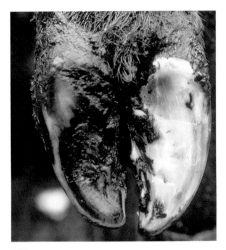

338

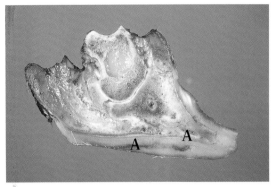

341

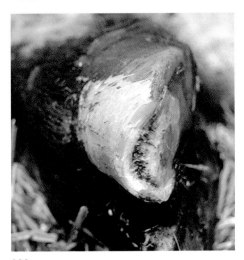

339

standing on concrete. The condition is frequently seen when heifers that have been reared in yards or on pasture are introduced postpartum into cubicles for the first time.

The gross widening and hemorrhage of the white line in the 3-year-old Simmental bull (339) was the result of excessive exercise in a cubicle-housed dairy herd over several months, at the beginning of which acute laminitis developed. These changes caused softening of the white

line, permitted penetration of dirt, and resulted in acute lameness due to the under-run sole. White line abscesses (277–280) and sole ulcers (284–287) are the common sequel to acute coriosis.

Chronic laminitis

Clinical features: in this longitudinal section (340) through the foot of a 6-year-old Shorthorn bull with early chronic coriosis/laminitis, the sole laminae are thickened and hemorrhagic, and pink striations indicate that there is blood in the sole horn, particularly at the toe. The pedal bone is displaced downwards, away from the overlying hoof wall. At a later stage (341), the line of hemorrhage (A) in the sole horn beneath the pedal bone is easily recognizable. The inflammatory insult responsible for this line would have occurred about 5 weeks previously. Note the thickening and the dorsal deviation of the toe. These changes lead to growth irregularities of the

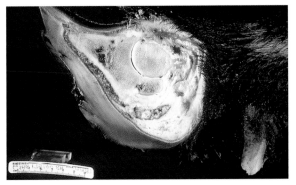

340

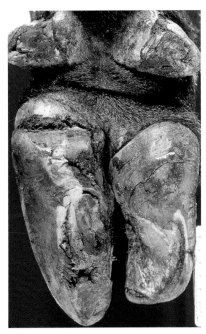

342

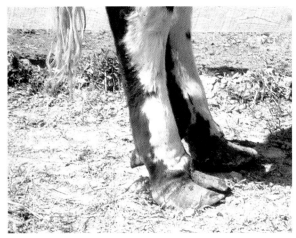

343

type seen in **342** and **343**. In **342** the wall of the outer claw (left) is curling axially. A deep heel fissure and an obvious false sole are developing. The medial claw (right) has an expanded white line. Both hind claws in **343** are elongated and the heels are sunken. The toe angle is small, there are prominent horizontal lines, and the periople at the coronary band is flaky.

Management: the causes and control of coriosis have been discussed under sections on white line disorders, sole ulcers and horizontal fissures.

Upper limb and spine

Introduction

The illustrations in this section have been grouped primarily by affected area and type of damage. Although the 'downer cow' syndrome is not a physical injury, it is included here because many of the conditions subsequently illustrated can be a consequence of the 'downer cow'. This is followed by spinal conditions, and trauma affecting joints and long bones (e.g., fractures). Paralyses, excluding those illustrated in the downer cow section, form another small group. Infectious causes are pictured in the septic arthritides section. Finally, a miscellaneous group includes vitamin and mineral deficiencies and metabolic disorders that can result in lameness.

Downer cow

Definition: animals that fail to rise after treatment for hypocalcemia, (p. 137, see **473, 474**) and where no obvious cause of recumbency can be diagnosed, are commonly referred to as 'downer' cows. The reason often remains obscure.

Clinical features: metabolic disease, and specifically a non-responsive milk fever or hypocalcemia (see **473, 474**), is the major cause of the downer cow syndrome. Such cows

fail to rise after treatment for hypocalcemia. The etiology is often puzzling. Lying on hard concrete or on the edge of the gutter in a standing or cubicle for as little as 6 hours can cause permanent nerve damage in the hind leg. Struggling may cause dislocation of the hip joint, muscle rupture, femoral fracture or other trauma that prevent the animal from rising, despite being normocalcemic. Other more insidious conditions, such as metritis, mastitis and toxicities, can also cause a cow or a bull to become a downer. Blood changes include a rapid elevation of muscle enzymes, such as serum glutamic-oxaloacetic transaminase (SGOT) and creatine phosphokinase (CPK), as a result of ischemic muscle necrosis.

Management: care of the downer cow is very important. Good nursing on a soft surface, e.g., straw on top of sand, which provides an adequate grip when the animal attempts to rise, is the prime requirement. Several times daily the animal should be turned from one side to the other. Loss of appetite and progressive signs of dullness and toxicity suggest a poor prognosis, but some alert downers have been known to rise spontaneously after several weeks. Hip clamps, slings and inflatable bags have a role in temporarily elevating the hindquarters.

Compartment syndrome

Definition: ischemic muscle degeneration of the hind limb leading to intense pain, limb dysfunction and eventual toxemia from by-products of muscle breakdown.

Clinical features: the cow in **344** had been recumbent on her right side for 24 hours, and was turned over to help examination of the right leg. There was pronounced swelling and thickening of the gluteal region and further swelling around the tibia. On palpation the enlargement was hard and painful. The prognosis for such cases is poor. The animal is disinclined to move and the resulting toxemia leads to anorexia.

Differential diagnosis: primary nerve paralysis (**398–400**), pelvic fracture (**367, 368**), femoral fracture (**352**).

Management: put on soft bedding, turn from side to side several times daily and ensure access to feed and water.

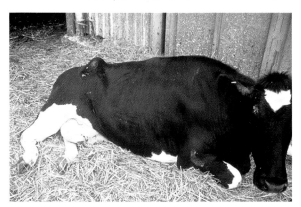

344

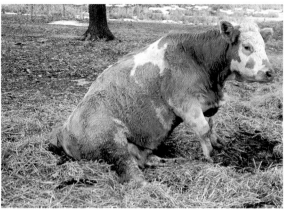

345

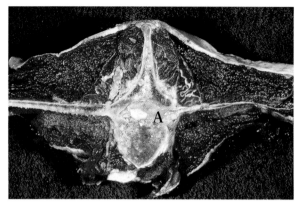

347

Spinal or pelvic damage

Clinical features: suddenly, after dystocia, the mature Simmental female in **345** adopted this 'dog-sitting' position, which is suggestive of lumbar or pelvic canal trauma. The posterior paresis resolved after 3 weeks, and the cow recovered completely. Occasionally, this odd position is habitual as a result of spondylarthrosis. Progressively severe posterior paresis with 'knuckling' of the hind fetlocks (**346**) developed in this mature Holstein cow as a result of vertebral lymphoma. Necropsy of a similar case (**347**)

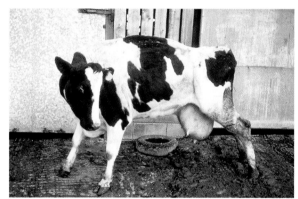

348

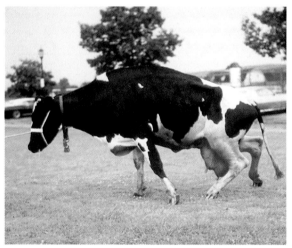

346

shows a transverse section of the caudal lumbar vertebral area with yellow-brown lymphomatous tissue (A) and normal, white, epidural fat within the spinal canal. The lymphoma caused marked compression of the spinal nerves, including the sciatic supply. The Friesian cow in **348** had lumbar spondylosis and stood and walked only with great difficulty. Body condition is very poor and the thoracolumbar spine is convex and prominent owing to muscle atrophy. The position of the hind legs relieves pain on spinal nerves. A lateral radiograph of a similar case (**349**) shows lumbar degenerative arthropathy, with ventral osteophyte proliferation (A). Progressive ankylosis brings a risk of fracture of the newly deposited bone of the spinal body, leading to the downer syndrome.

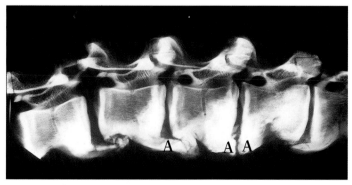

349

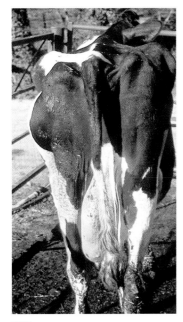

350

Differential diagnosis: metabolic disease or toxic infection, hind limb trauma (350–356).

Management: some cases (345) respond to good nursing in a deeply bedded loose box. Any deterioration necessitates an immediate full clinical re-examination.

Dislocated hip

Clinical features: although hip dislocation can be a cause of a 'downer cow', it is more commonly a consequence of injury from falling, for example during estrus activity. Craniodorsal dislocations are more frequent (80% of hip dislocations), as in the cow in 350, which shows an abnormal posture and silhouette of the left leg. In the Friesian heifer in 351 the left femoral head is dislocated upwards and forwards (craniodorsally). The bony landmarks of the hindquarters are incongruent. The left gluteal musculature is prominent owing to dorsal dis-

placement of the greater femoral trochanter (A). Crepitus can occasionally be detected on circumrotation of the femur. Ventral and caudal dislocation of the femoral head into the obturator foramen may also occur, when damage may be caused to the obturator nerve (354).

Differential diagnosis: pelvic fracture, proximal femoral fracture (352, 353, 370), obturator paralysis (354, 355), spinal fracture (357, 358).

Management: early cases may be reduced by manipulation, especially in younger cattle with craniodorsal luxation. Dislocations incurred over 24 hours previously must usually be culled as untreatable.

Fractured femur

Clinical features: most femoral fractures in periparturient animals occur close to the femoral head and are diagnosed on the basis of abnormal limb position and the detection of crepitus on limb movement. The downer cow in 352 has a right femoral midshaft fracture and related soft-tissue swelling. The lower part of the right limb is deviated laterally owing to outward movement of the lower femoral shaft. The area is very painful. Such fractures do not always result in recumbency. Another femoral fracture (353) shows extensive soft tissue swelling and the forwards and outwards position of the leg. After one or two attempts, cattle usually abandon further efforts to stand. The underlying, nonfractured hind leg is liable to develop severe ischemic muscle necrosis (see p. 101). Femoral fracture in calves is discussed and shown in 370.

Differential diagnosis: dislocated hip (350, 351), pelvic fracture (367, 368).

Management: usually untreatable except for mid- or distal shaft fractures in immature cattle where internal fixation (plate, pins) may be attempted in valuable stock.

Obturator paralysis

Definition: the obturator nerve supplies the adductor muscles of the hind limb. Dystocia from fetal oversize

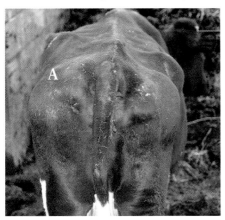

351

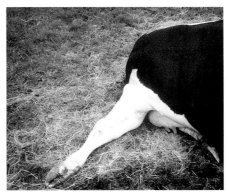

352

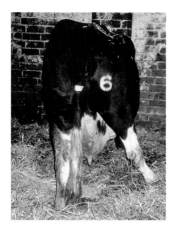

353

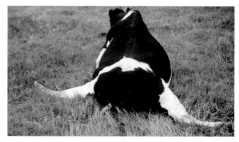

355

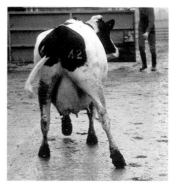

356

may produce unilateral or bilateral nerve paralysis, with subsequent limb abduction.

Clinical features: in 354 the abducted and symmetrical position of the hind legs is characteristic of bilateral obturator paralysis. Less severe cases will simply walk with limb abduction, but if allowed onto slippery concrete (as happened in 354), may slip ('do the splits'), and a dislocated hip or femoral fracture may result as a secondary feature. Compare the degree of limb adduction in 354 with that in 355, where there is secondary hip or femoral damage. This cow will not recover. Another cow (356), partially recovered from an obturator paralysis incurred 9 months previously, still abducts the right leg when walking; the left leg is normal and weight-bearing.

Differential diagnosis: dislocated hip (350, 351), femoral fracture (352, 353).

Management: confinement to well-bedded straw box. If obturator paralysis is suspected the animal should be retained on a soft surface where grip is optimal until locomotion has improved. Hobbles applied to the fetlocks or hocks will help to prevent excessive abduction and may permit the cow safely to walk for milking, etc. Regular brief attempts may be made with a hip clamp to raise the cow to a standing position to assess development and to aid the circulation to the hind limbs.

Spinal conditions
Spinal compression fracture

Clinical features: spinal cord compression (A) (357) can be caused by a vertebral fracture (B). Posterior paresis had developed suddenly in this 8-month-old Holstein heifer and was probably associated with clinical rickets of several months' duration. A compression fracture had resulted in the vertebral body being slowly forced dorsally, causing kyphosis (arched back). The spinal canal became progressively stenosed and another fracture of the rachitic bone then compressed the spinal cord. Both compression

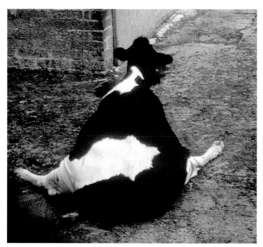

354

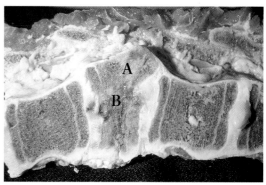

357

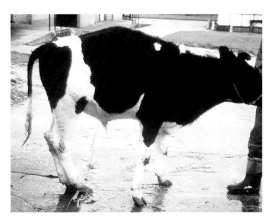

358

fractures and septic foci in vertebral growth plates usually occur in younger cattle.

In a Friesian steer that suddenly developed kyphosis, with a discretely localized convexity of the caudal thoracic spine (358), its rapid deterioration necessitated slaughter. Postmortem examination revealed a collapsed and infected intervertebral disc space (359) between the first (A) and second (B) lumbar vertebrae, resulting from a septic physitis. Deviation of the spinal canal and some spinal cord compression were evident (C). Kyphosis can also be congenital, and is progressive with increasing age. Many affected calves eventually become recumbent.

Differential diagnosis: other types of spinal trauma, e.g., infiltrating lymphosarcomatous masses, pelvic or sacral fracture, osteomyelitis.

Management: early identification and where possible correction of the primary cause is clearly essential. Most affected animals require slaughter, but it may be possible to prevent further cases by dietary management. High-concentrate maize-based diets with no supplementary minerals are commonly involved, and may also lead to spontaneous limb fractures.

Spinal (vertebral) spondylopathy

Definition: any vertebral disease including osteomyelitis, spinal abscessation and ankylosis (spondylosis).

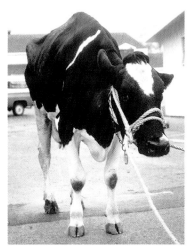

360

Clinical features: osteomyelitis of the spinal vertebrae is a painful progressive disease, seen in both young and mature animals as a result of hematogenous spread. The cow in 360 had a pained expression due to vertebral abscessation, walked stiffly and was soon reluctant to stand.

Specimen 361 is a longitudinal section of the thoracolumbar spine of a 6-month-old Holstein calf. Osteomyelitis affects the whole depth of a lumbar vertebral physis (growth plate). The intervertebral disc has been destroyed and the vertebral canal is stenosed. Hemorrhage is evident beneath the meninges over the stenosed cord. The infection was probably hematogenous (*Arcanobacterium pyogenes* was isolated).

The cow in 362 has an arched thoracolumbar spine and the hind feet are placed further to the rear than normal. The right hind foot is lifted in an attempt to relieve spinal pain. Such cows often 'paddle' with the hind legs and may have difficulty in rising. The condition (compare lumbar spondylosis (348) and spinal osteomyelitis (360), is a slowly progressive, aseptic process. Proliferating bone on the spinal bodies may eventually produce ankylosis (349).

Differential diagnosis: spinal osteomyelitis (360, 361), spinal compression fractures (357–359).

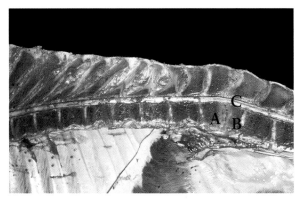

359

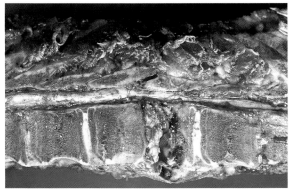

361

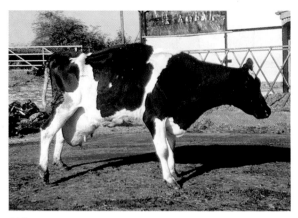

362

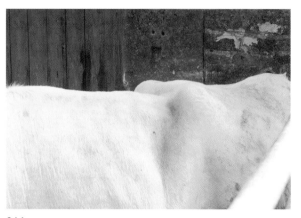

364

Management: most causes are slowly or rapidly progressive and should be culled on welfare grounds, especially when rapidly becoming recumbent.

Cervical spinal fracture

A fracture of the fifth and sixth cervical vertebrae made the 2-year-old Friesian heifer in **363** unable to lift the head and neck. A prominent dip is apparent in the dorsal cervical spine, in front of the scapula. In another similar case, the cow grazed on her knees as she was unable to bend her neck sufficiently to reach the pasture.

Sacroiliac subluxation and luxation

Definition: the ligamentous attachment at the junction of the pelvis and the sacrum relaxes in the periparturient animal to allow passage of the fetus through the birth canal. Rotation of the sacrum on the spine can result when severe traction is applied to an oversized fetus. A partial loss of integrity of the fibrous union of the sacroiliac joint (subluxation) occasionally results, as can complete loss of contact of the two articular surfaces (luxation).

Clinical features: subluxation can cause temporary recumbency, the downer cow syndrome (p. 101). The wings

of the ilium in the Friesian cow (**364**) are raised relative to the lumbar spine. Rectal palpation revealed the sacral promontory to be pushed backwards and depressed, resulting in a reduced dorsoventral diameter of the pelvic inlet. In contrast, a cow with a complete luxation (with no persisting contact of the sacrum with the ilial wings) is unlikely to recover to a normal stance and gait.

Differential diagnosis: pelvic fracture (367–369), lumbar spinal fracture, spinal spondylopathy (360, 361), downer cow syndrome.

Management: cases of subluxation often improve over a few days to survive the lactation, but cases with complete luxation should be culled as soon as possible. Cows with subluxation should not be retained for breeding as the reduced pelvic inlet could predispose to dystocia.

Sacrococcygeal fracture and tail paralysis

Clinical features: the Hereford bull (**365**) could not raise his tail to defecate. The prominent swelling at the tailhead (A) is an old sacrococcygeal fracture. It resulted from a fall during attempted service of a cow, and led to compression of the coccygeal nerve supply. However, sacrococcygeal fracture does not invariably lead to nerve dysfunction, but sometimes to minor disfigurement, as in

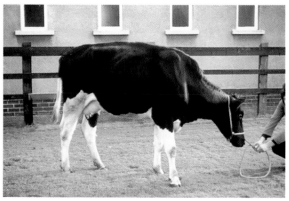

363

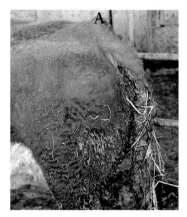

365

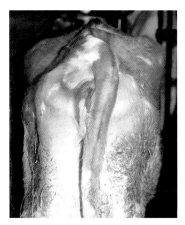

366

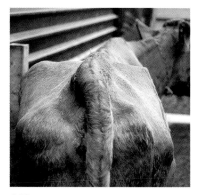

368

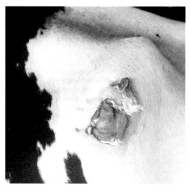

369

the 2-year-old Guernsey heifer in **366**. The growing animal is especially susceptible to compression fractures of the spine and to localization of metastatic septic foci in the growth plates of vertebral bodies (compare **360** and **361**).

Management: in dairy cows tail paralysis results in gross fecal contamination of the back of the udder and teats. Such cows should be culled, though tail amputation is a theoretical but ethically dubious alternative.

Trauma of joints and long bones

Pelvic fracture

Definition: most pelvic fractures involve the ilial wing and are of minor significance. Iliac shaft and pubic fractures are much less common but cause severe lameness and sometimes recumbency, as in the downer cow.

Clinical features: an open fracture of the left ilial wing of the cow in **367** is grossly contaminated, and as drainage is poor, lesions in this area are slow to heal. Such fractures arise from trauma incurred with rough handling or overcrowding, when cows are rushed through doorways, or from a sudden fall onto a hard surface. Most fractures of the ilial wing are closed, the fragment of bone being pulled downwards by the fascia lata, as in the Guernsey cow

(**368**), where the bony prominence is absent ('dropped hip') on the right side. In other cases, the skin over the bone becomes gangrenous and sloughs (**369**). Most ilial wing fractures are nothing more than cosmetic blemishes.

Management: routine wound treatment is needed in open cases, after removal of any bone fragments.

Femoral fracture

Clinical features: the soft tissue swelling in this Simmental bull calf (**370**) overlies a femoral shaft fracture of 2 days' duration. The stance could be confused with femoral paralysis or a hip injury such as coxofemoral luxation or

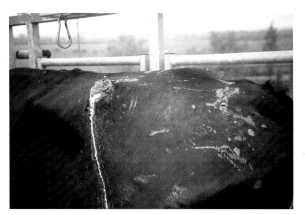

367

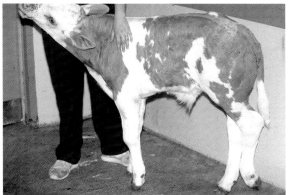

370

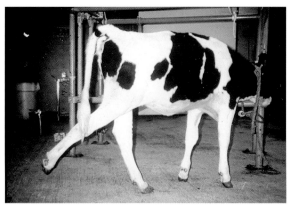

371

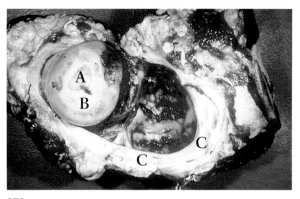

373

femoral neck fracture. Other femoral fractures are shown in 352 and 353.

Patellar luxation

Definition: upward or lateral, intermittent or permanent displacement of the patella, of uncertain etiology.

Clinical features: the respective clinical signs differ markedly (compare 371 and 372). The right hind leg of the Holstein heifer in 371 was held in maximal extension for a few seconds and was then jerked forward. The patella was temporarily fixed above the femoral trochlea. Diagnosis of upward patellar fixation, made on palpation during locomotion, is confirmed by the response to medial patellar desmotomy. One specific form of upward luxation and fixation occurs in growing and mature cattle, and is also common among draught animals in the Indian subcontinent. Some forms are inherited.

In contrast, the young Holstein calf (372) had a flexed stifle. The patella was easily palpable, and luxated lateral to the femoral trochlea, increasing the total width of the joint. Note the accompanying gross quadriceps femoris atrophy and left hind plantigrade stance. Lateral patellar luxation is generally encountered in calves less than 1 month old.

Differential diagnosis: in upward patellar fixation spastic paresis (404); in lateral patellar luxation femoral paralysis (399).

Management: medial patellar desmotomy in the upward luxation or fixation; medial overlap procedure in lateral luxation though prognosis in later surgery is guarded. Some cases of intermittent upward luxation resolve spontaneously.

Degenerative joint disease (DJD)

Definition: a chronic degeneration of the articular cartilage with thickening of the joint capsule and peripheral osteophyte formation in one or more major joints in older cows and bulls, which may be unable to mount for natural service.

Clinical features: degenerative joint disease (DJD) affects the hip and stifle more frequently than other weight-bearing joints. This hip joint of an old Hereford cow (373) shows the classical features of DJD: extensive erosion of articular cartilage (A), eburnation of the underlying bone (B), and

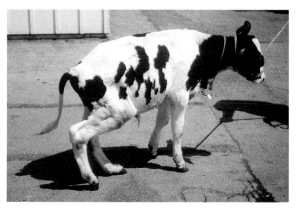

372

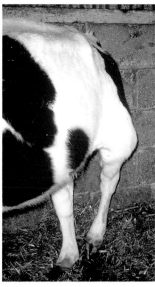

374

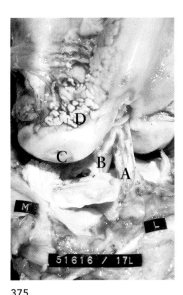

375

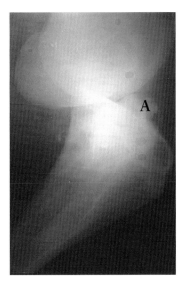

376

a thickened joint capsule (C). The presence of blood suggests that a more recent traumatic incident had occurred after the chronic changes became established.

Differential diagnosis: DJD of stifle (see aseptic gonitis (374–376)), pelvic fracture (367–369).

Management: rest, confinement, analgesics and NSAIDs.

Aseptic gonitis (stifle osteoarthritis)

Definition: degenerative joint disease (see hip arthritis above) of one or both stifle joints, often in older cattle.

Clinical features: aseptic or noninfectious gonitis results from trauma, and animals experience a severe and chronic lameness. Some cows have a slow progressive enlargement of the stifle and move the limb without flexing the joint. Muscle atrophy of the limb rapidly develops. The swelling in the yearling Friesian (374) comprises fibrosis and in-flammatory fluid around the joint with secondary bone proliferation. Typically, young cattle may have a partial rupture of a collateral ligament. Some such cases remain slightly lame owing to a secondary degenerative osteo-arthritis. In mature cattle (375) cranial cruciate ligament rupture (CrCL) is a common cause of severe stifle lameness (ruptured ligament (A)). A lateral radiograph (376) of the stifle joint of a similar, old, beef cow shows considerable cranial movement of the tibial articular surface on the femoral condyles (about 3 cm). A small chip is evident near the tibial eminence (A). The cranial view into the opened stifle joint in 375 shows a mere fragment of the CrCL (A), although the caudal cruciate ligament is intact (B). The medial meniscus is torn and fragmented. The medial femoral condyle shows bone loss from erosion (C), and the margin of the condyle has extensive osteophyte prolifer-ation (D). The palpably thickened joint capsule and bony enlargement are prominent clinical signs of CrCL rupture.

Differential diagnosis: septic gonitis, distal femoral fracture, periarticular abscess.

Management: few cases will recover. NSAIDs and analgesic drugs may help locomotion, but lactating cows are best confined to yards and loose boxes.

Metacarpal/metatarsal fractures

Definition: fractures of metacarpal/metatarsal shaft may be closed or open. The age range is wide and includes sporadic cases in both young calves and adult cattle.

Clinical features in calves: the Friesian calf in 377 had severe angulation following a recent distal metacarpal shaft fracture. The fracture had not been reduced and immobilized. The small amount of overlying soft tissue makes such fractures liable to perforate through the skin and become infected, hence producing osteomyelitis. Such fractures, or separation of the metacarpal physis, are very

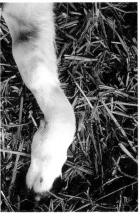

377

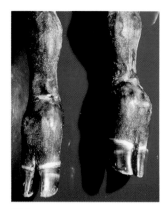

378

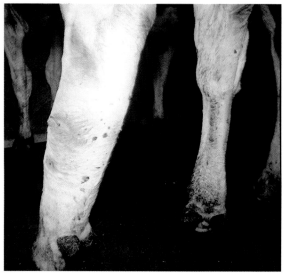

380

likely to occur following excessive traction in dystocia. The bilateral metacarpal shaft fractures in the Angus heifer in **378** were caused by traction on obstetrical chains placed just above the fetlocks. Note the residual scar. In this view, healing was taking place 2 weeks after external splintage, but note the 10–20° malalignment.

Metacarpal fracture may occur with epiphyseal separation, as seen in the radiograph (**379**). This shows a partial separation and displacement of the distal metacarpal growth plate (A), and fracture of the metaphysis (B) (Salter type II) in a neonatal calf.

Differential diagnosis: careful manipulation should reveal whether the shaft is fractured or the distal physis separated. Radiography can confirm the precise conformation.

Management: the prognosis is good with careful management. Check carefully whether the fracture is open and therefore infected. Such cases, carrying a more guarded prognosis, need debridement and irrigation before external fixation is applied, and an optional 'porthole' may be left

for catheter and further irrigation. External support (e.g., resin) should extend proximal to the carpus and distal to the coronet. Systemic antibiotics should be given for 5–7 days.

Clinical features in adult cattle: most cases present as sudden onset lameness. Typical metatarsal/metacarpal shaft fractures are very common and account for 50% of all long bone fractures in adults.

A second type (chip fracture), involving a sequestrum chipped from the cortex, is also occasionally seen (**380**) although changes in the metacarpal/metatarsal shafts may be difficult to detect in the early stages. As the condition progresses, a pronounced hard swelling develops, as in **380**, where two discharging sinuses are visible on the lateral aspect of the left metatarsus. This animal injured her leg as a heifer when transported to the farm several months previously. On X-ray a large saucer-shaped sequestrum of bone cortex was visible on the lateral aspect of the mid-shaft region of the metatarsus. Most cases are traumatic in origin and the discharge is a foreign body reaction, although bacterial infection may also occur.

Management: the common fracture type should be managed as for calves though the risk of an open fracture is greater. In chip fractures surgical removal of the sequestrum is possible but not easy. In many cases lameness will resolve if exercise is limited for 2–3 months, and although the leg swelling persists this does not cause a problem.

Infectious arthritis: septic arthritis and epiphysitis

Clinical features: this section excludes joint ill and polyarthritis of calfhood (see **73** in the neonatal chapter). Most forms of septic or infectious arthritis are bacterial in origin. They originate from penetrating wounds, extension from adjacent tissues (both forms being common in digital

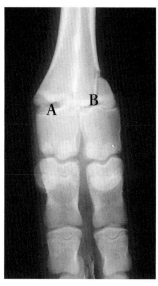

379

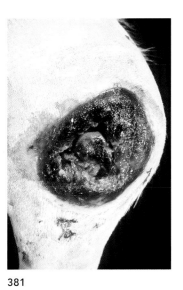

381

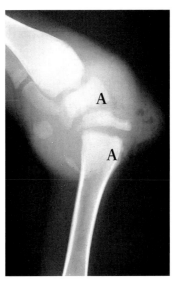

382

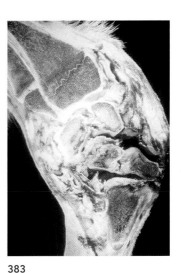

383

sepsis, see p. 90), or by the hematogenous route. Some examples are given.

In a case of septic carpitis, pressure necrosis of the skin over the carpus (knee) in a 4-month-old Holstein heifer (381) has exposed the carpal bones. Note the peripheral epithelialization and necrosis. A lateral radiograph of the flexed carpus (382) shows soft tissue swelling, bone destruction of the middle and distal rows of carpal bones, and an extensive osseous proliferative reaction (A). A sagittal section through the limb (383) confirms the massive tissue destruction. Infection also extends along the tendon sheaths. Detected some weeks earlier such an infection could have been successfully managed.

The 4-month-old calf in 384 has a wound (not visible in this view) on the medial surface of the fetlock, severe septic cellulitis, tenosynovitis and arthritis leading to massive joint swelling.

The fetlock joint of the Friesian cow in 385 (with flexor tendons reflected) contains inspissated pus (*Arcanobacterium pyogenes*), but has minimal damage to the articular cartilage. In such cases, joint infection often results from ascending digital sepsis. *Erysipelas* is also commonly isolated.

The longitudinal section of the metacarpus of a 7-week-old Angus heifer (386) shows skin necrosis, and infection has led to sepsis of the metacarpophalangeal (fetlock) joint. The skin necrosis had developed from overlong application of splints and a plaster cast (4 weeks) for the immobilization of a midshaft metacarpal fracture (A), which is seen to have healed.

In a case of septic arthritis of the elbow in the 14-month-old Holstein heifer in 387, brownish pus adheres to the joint surfaces. The articular surfaces, especially of the distal humerus, are severely eroded (A). Periarticular fibrosis is present. The usual age range for septic arthritis in calves is 1–3 months.

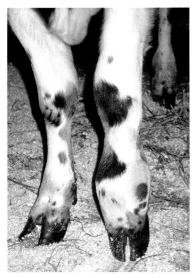

384

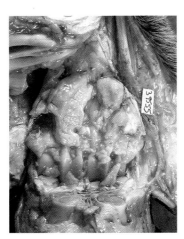

385

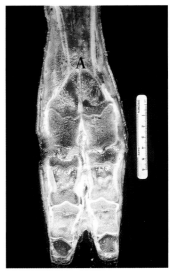

386

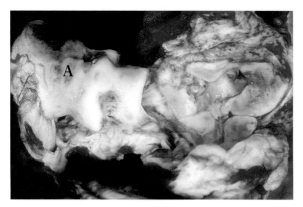

387

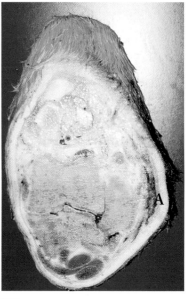

390

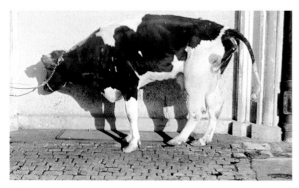

388

Some cases of infection of major joints occur in adult cows and develop insidiously. This old cow from Czechoslovakia with chronic infectious gonitis (388) had lost a lot of weight and was in obvious pain. Longstanding degenerative and proliferative changes had caused considerable enlargement of the stifle joint. *Brucella abortus* was recovered from the synovial fluid. Such cows with an infectious, albeit non-septic, arthritis should be culled.

Conditions of the hock region

Introduction

Hock trauma is commonly seen in confinement housing systems with inadequate bedding, and especially when the cubicle/free-stall size and design are deficient. Solid, horizontal, wooden dividing rails and vertical uprights often cause injuries, although lack of bedding and a slippery

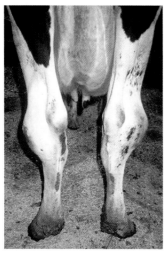

389

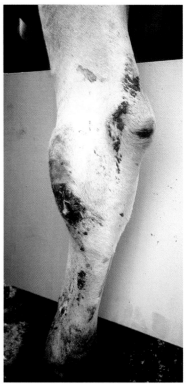

391

surface, leading to abrasive trauma as the weight-bearing limb moves over the floor surface during rising and sitting, are the major causes. Trauma may also develop secondary to digital lameness, when cows are recumbent for long periods and have difficulty in rising. Many forms of hock swelling and injury nevertheless cause little or no lameness.

Tarsal bursitis and cellulitis

Clinical features: lateral swellings over the subcutaneous bursae of both hocks (also called cellulitis) are common in cattle housed on concrete (**389**). Carpal hygroma (**403**) causes a similar foreleg problem. The hair loss results from chronic abrasion. A horizontal section through an affected hock (**390**) shows a discrete discolored cavity (A) lined with granulation tissue. The synovia-like fluid is sterile. The majority of cases are not infected. An outward deviation of the digits (cow-hocked) often contributes to the development of tarsal bursitis.

Cellulitis develops when the skin barrier is broken and the wound becomes infected and discharges pus (**391**). The swelling then tends to be more diffuse than in aseptic bursitis, the joint capsule may become involved, and marked pain and lameness result. In another cow the right hock and adjacent limb are very swollen with an extensive cellulitis (**392**). The injury resulted from a puncture wound which introduced infection into the subcutaneous tissues. Although such animals do become very lame, this cow recovered after antibiotic therapy.

Differential diagnosis: infectious (septic) tarsitis, tarsal fracture.

Management: unless very large, non-infected lesions are best treated conservatively by simply removing the animal

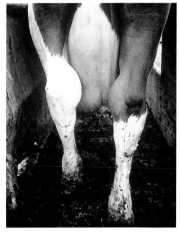

393

from the traumatic environment and allowing natural resolution, which commonly occurs when cows go out to pasture at the end of the winter. If winter-housed, cows should be put onto straw bedding for several weeks. Larger lesions can be drained by sterile aspiration, although the puncture wound produced can lead to secondary infection. If a sterile bursitis is lanced, secondary infection is a common sequel. Cellulitis lesions require prolonged and aggressive antibiotic therapy.

Medial tarsal hygroma

Clinical features: the bilateral synovial swelling in **393** is fluctuating, painless, and its size results in slight mechanical lameness. The condition is sporadic and may result from trauma on the edge of the cubicle kerb.

Tenosynovitis of the tarsal sheath ('capped hock')

Clinical features: a firm swelling surrounds the point of the hock of this 3-year-old Holstein cow (**394**) and extends distally towards the tibiotarsal joint. Six months previously, the cow had fallen through a metal grid,

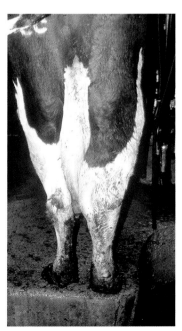

392

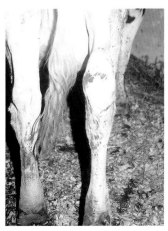

394

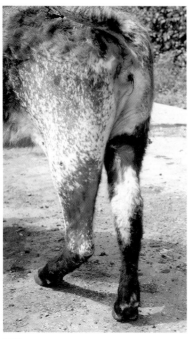

395

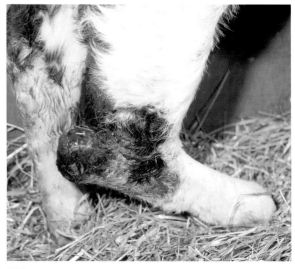

397

sustaining an open wound involving the medial aspect of the tarsal sheath. Sepsis resulted, but the wound eventually healed with fibrosis.

Gastrocnemius trauma

Clinical features: trauma to the gastrocnemius muscle-tendon group arises sporadically from struggling, as when a cow with hypocalcemia (milk fever) attempts to stand following a period of recumbency. Rare cases are associated with vitamin D deficiency and aphosphorosis. The prognosis is generally hopeless, except in young animals, where external support may permit slow healing by fibrosis. Two manifestations of gastrocnemius rupture are shown. The first (395) shows a dropped hock and swelling of the gastrocnemius muscle belly in a Shorthorn heifer.

The cross-bred beef steer in 396 has a complete bilateral rupture, cannot stand, and bears weight on the plantar surfaces of the hock. The appearance is similar to avulsion of the epiphyses of the os calcis, whereby the gastrocnemius muscle-tendon is intact. Another form of gastrocnemius injury is traumatic transection, as shown in the 2-year-old Friesian heifer in 397. This injury arises from a slicing action and can be very severe. The wound is invariably infected. Since both gastrocnemius and superficial flexor tendons are involved, weight-bearing is made impossible.

Differential diagnosis: fracture of the os calcis, rupture of the gastrocnemius muscle belly.

Management: most cases of complete rupture or gastrocnemius transection fail to heal as a result of continuing attempts at weight-bearing. In smaller growing stock splintage in non-infected cases may permit recovery in some weeks.

Peripheral paralyses

One form of peripheral paralysis (obturator) has already been illustrated (354–355). Other types of nerve damage are illustrated in the following section.

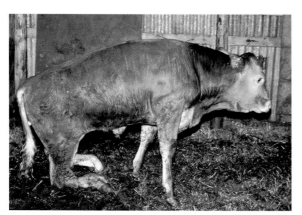

396

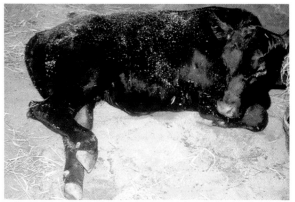

398

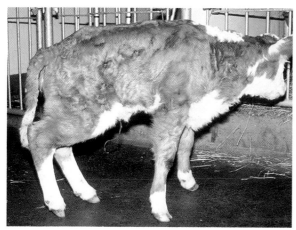

399

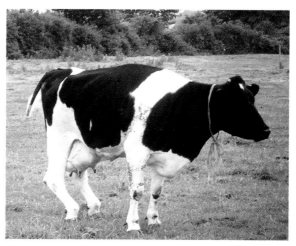

400

Sciatic paralysis (L$_6$, S$_{1-2}$ nerve roots)

Left sciatic paralysis resulted from the accidental (iatrogenic) perineural injection of an antibiotic solution into the deep gluteal region of this Angus heifer (398). Longacting antibiotic preparations are commonly implicated. Sciatic paralysis occasionally develops following prolonged recumbency resulting from parturient paresis. Severe ischemic muscle necrosis is evident around the damaged nerve (see downer cow, p. 101).

Femoral paralysis (L$_{4-6}$ nerve roots)

The flexed stifle cannot be extended to allow weight-bearing, owing to dysfunction of the quadriceps group in this 4-day-old Simmental calf (399). Skin sensation was absent over part of the medial aspect of the thigh. A secondary lateral patellar luxation is sometimes present (372). A hollowed-out appearance of the quadriceps muscle (atrophy) is seen after about 7–10 days. Neonatal cases are the most common and their pathogenesis is often unclear. Fetal hyperextension caused by excessive traction during delivery, muscular compression and ischemic anoxia may account for the clinical signs.

Differential diagnosis: lateral patellar luxation.

Peroneal paralysis (cranial division of sciatic nerve roots)

Peroneal paralysis is a common postpartum injury, as in the 6-year-old Holstein in 400. The stance resulted from paralysis of the hock flexors and digital extensors. Paresis or paralysis may persist for days or weeks or occasionally indefinitely. The peroneal nerve is most susceptible to damage over the lateral surface of the stifle joint, and injury with subsequent paralysis is therefore seen following recumbency on a hard surface. Most are unilateral. Knuckling may be so pronounced as to cause abrasion of the dorsal aspect of the fetlock leading to joint damage.

Differential diagnosis: tibial paralysis (not shown), sciatic paralysis or paresis.

Management: avoid hard and slippery surfaces which could result in further injury.

Radial paralysis (C$_{7-8}$, T$_1$ nerve roots)

This mature Holstein cow (401) shows a dropped elbow, a flexed carpus and fetlock, and an inability to bear weight. The cow had been maintained under general anesthesia, in right lateral recumbency on a padded table for $2\frac{1}{2}$ hours. Paralysis was immediately evident on standing but the gait was normal 2 days later.

Differential diagnosis: humeral fracture.

Brachial plexus injury (C$_6$–T$_1$ nerve roots)

The elbow of the Friesian cow in 402 was dropped, but the forelimb could be advanced for some limited weight-bearing. This injury can result from severe abduction of the forelimb, for example when falling after mounting a cow in estrus. Some radial paralysis (the radial nerve being one component of the plexus) was present.

Management: if weather conditions permit, keep the cow at pasture to promote exercise and avoid further

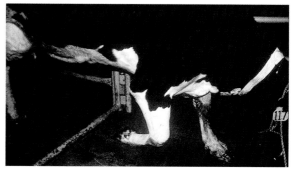

401

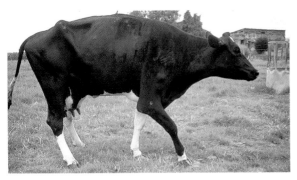

402

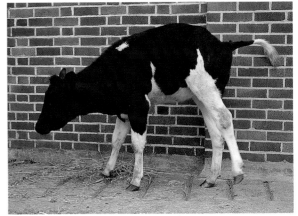

404

injuries, otherwise place into bedded loose box. Avoid self-trauma from struggling to rise (sciatic), or abrasion to dorsal aspect of fetlock (radial). NSAIDs reduce discomfort.

Miscellaneous locomotor conditions

Carpal hygroma

Definition: large fluid-filled sac on the front of the carpus.

Clinical features: carpal hygromata rarely reach the size seen in the forelegs of this old Friesian cow (403). They are usually bilateral, contain thin serum-like material, and cause little or no lameness. Like tarsal bursitis (see 389), carpal hygromata result from repeated contusions on hard surfaces (concrete) in poorly designed housing, or, rarely, from brucellosis.

Management: transfer to straw yard or pasture for slow resolution.

Spastic paresis ('Elso heel')

Definition: uncommon progressive hind limb extensor spasms of unknown etiology.

Clinical features: in this 6-month-old Friesian heifer (404) the left hock is overextended, and the gastrocnemius

tendon and muscle were tense on palpation. This inherited condition, sporadically seen in both dairy and beef breeds, affects one or both hind limbs, producing a progressive disability that starts at 2–9 months old. Surgical correction can be performed, but is not recommended in breeding animals.

Differential diagnosis: dorsal patellar luxation, joint ill, gonitis, localized spinal trauma or space-occupying lesion.

Management: surgery to permit animal to be fattened, otherwise early culling.

Hip dysplasia

Definition: a progressive and probably inherited, bilateral, degenerative joint disease, seen in several beef breeds including the Aberdeen Angus and the Hereford.

Clinical features: the yearling Hereford bull in 405 has severe atrophy of the hindquarters. The forefeet are placed caudally and the hindfeet cranially to increase the proportion of weight borne by the forequarters. The acetabulum of another Hereford bull (406) shows the extensive cartilaginous erosion and areas of bone loss that result from this degenerative process. The clinical signs start at 2–18 months old. Hip dysplasia is generally progressive.

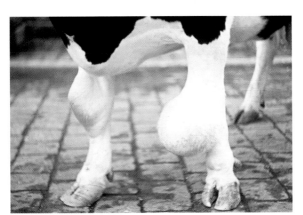

403

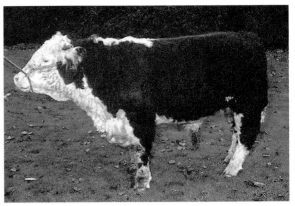

405

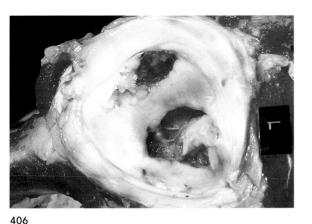

406

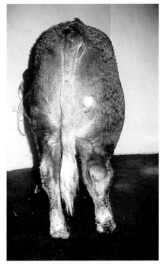

408

Differential diagnosis: osteochondrosis dissecans of stifle.

Osteochondrosis dissecans (OCD)

OCD occasionally causes a degenerative and aseptic joint problem of unknown etiology in groups of young, fast-growing beef cattle. The opened joints of a yearling Angus crossbred steer (**407**) that had chronic, bilaterally enlarged shoulder joints, leading to lameness and poor growth, show loss of cartilage and subchondral bone (A), and periarticular fibrosis (B). Joints commonly involved are stifles, hocks and shoulder.

Differential diagnosis: septic polyarthritis, hip dysplasia, muscle dystrophy.

Management: the development of OCD is poorly understood, but it has been associated with rapid growth rates on high-concentrate diets in the young animal, insufficient exercise, inadequate mineralization of the diet and suboptimal floor surfaces. Several such factors need thorough investigation for management advice on prevention.

Septic myositis (popliteal abscess)

Clinical features: the massive swelling seen in the right thigh of this 2-year-old Simmental bull (**408**) caused a moderate lameness. The lighter area had been clipped for exploratory puncture. The swelling contained 12 liters of pus (isolate: *Arcanobacterium pyogenes*). For a further discussion, see popliteal abscess (**129**).

Management: ensure adequate drainage following a long incision and initially irrigation and gentle curettage of the focus.

Rupture of the ventral serrate muscle

The right scapula of the mature Flemish Maas-Rijn-Ijssel cow in **409** projects above the thoracic spine owing to the rupture of the ventral serrate and subscapularis muscles. The scapula returns to its normal anatomical position when the leg is not bearing weight. In mature cattle the etiology is probably chronic muscle degeneration and atrophy.

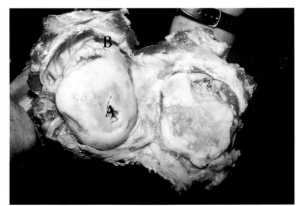

407

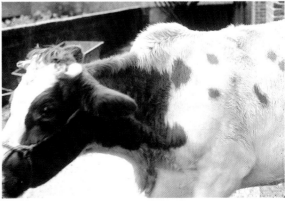

409

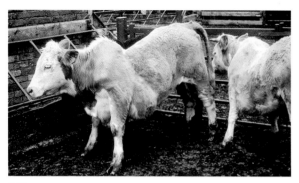

410

Management: although a cosmetic blemish, such cows can easily be retained to the end of a lactation.

White muscle disease (enzootic muscle dystrophy, 'flying scapula')

Definition: muscle degeneration caused by vitamin E and/or selenium deficiency in which an accumulation of free peroxide radicals leads to muscle degeneration and a calcium deposition necrosis.

Clinical features: clinical signs are often seen following spring turn-out when a sudden increase in exercise and general muscle stress is combined with a dramatic intake of FFA in lush springtime grazing. This is particularly the case if poor winter feeding had induced a vitamin E/selenium deficiency. Affected cattle may show lameness, general locomotor impairment, dyspnea if the diaphragm is affected, and sudden death from cardiac degeneration. In 410 ventral serrate and subscapular muscle function has been lost allowing the scapula to rise above the thoracic spine in the two beef steers. Note the wide-based foreleg stance to accommodate the abnormal support mechanism. The heart of a calf with white muscle disease (411) has extensive pale grayish areas (A) on the epicardium, typically extending into the myocardium. There may also be endothelial plaques. The cardiac shape is globular following chronic hypertrophy (411). White muscle lesions, usually bilateral, are also seen at postmortem in skeletal muscle and diaphragm.

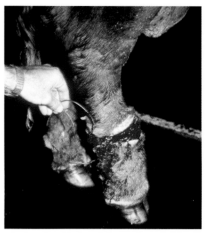

412

Management: provision of a balanced diet and where necessary supplementation with vitamin E and/or selenium. Requirements increase with rapid growth rates and high oil diets, especially high PUFAs (polyunsaturated fatty acids). Individual affected animals respond well to parenteral therapy with vitamin E and selenium.

Foreign body around the metatarsus

In 412 a piece of wire is being removed from a characteristic, deep, circumferential, granulating wound of the metatarsal soft tissues. The 2-year-old Limousin bull was moderately lame and recovered rapidly.

Differential diagnosis: other forms of wounds.

Management: adequate restraint and deep exploration with forceps down to metatarsus to detect and remove metal wire.

Distal limb gangrene: traumatic origin

In 413 a clear line demarcates the dead from the healthy skin. The Holstein cow had caught her leg at the metacarpal

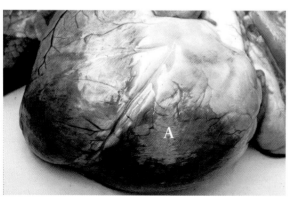

411

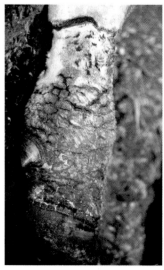

413

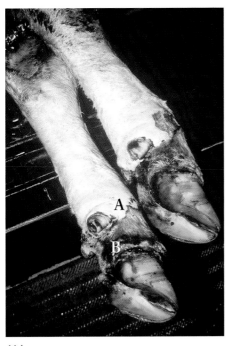

414

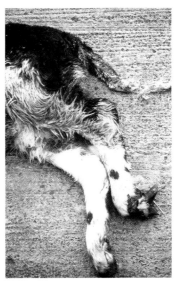

416

level in a stanchion chain, and was found recumbent the following morning, with the chain still in place. A few days later the skin was dry and painless. It sloughed 3 weeks later, together with the distal soft tissues and hoof horn capsule, necessitating euthanasia. Compare skin changes in **412**.

Management: early culling.

Fescue foot gangrene

Definition: fescue foot is caused by an ergot-like toxin, consumed by cattle grazing certain endophyte-infested strains of tall fescue grasses in many states of the USA, as well as in New Zealand, Italy, Australia and Orkney (UK).

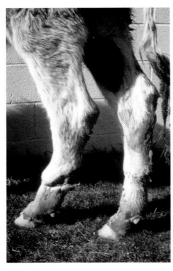

415

Clinical features: in the 11-month-old Hereford steer in **414**, the dark areas of skin on the hind pasterns are dry gangrene. A sharply defined oblique line (A) extending over the fetlock, separates the dead from the normal skin. Skin has also separated from the coronary band to expose infected subcutis (B). The upper (right) limb shows a pink area where the gangrenous skin has sloughed. The ear tips and tail may also become gangrenous. The problem affects several younger cattle in a group, all of which are at risk.

Differential diagnosis: ergotism (**415**), frostbite (**133**), trauma (**413**) and salmonellosis (**55**).

Management: change of pasture if practical, or confinement and feeding of endophyte-free hay. The individual case cannot be cured.

Ergot gangrene

Definition: ergotism results from ingestion of the parasitic fungus *Claviceps purpurea* on hay, grain or seeded pastures.

Clinical features: gangrene of the extremities resulting from the ingestion of ergot-infested cereals and other feeds is a worldwide problem. The clinical features resemble fescue foot' (**414**). The lower limb and tail tip are affected in the yearling heifer in **415**. Gangrenous skin is sloughing from the left metatarsal region, and a similar line of demarcation is seen in the right leg. The distal 25 cm of the tail is twisted, moist and gangrenous. More advanced changes in the feet are shown in **416**. The left foot has almost sloughed at the pastern, and the distal third of the tail is detached.

Differential diagnosis: fescue foot (**414**), frostbite (**133**), trauma (**413**), and salmonellosis (**55**).

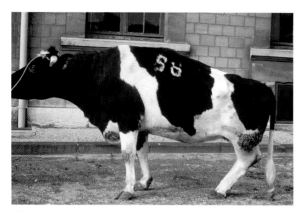

417

Hyaena disease

Definition: a rare chondrodystrophy of the hindlimb bones and lumbar vertebrae of unknown etiology, often accompanied by aggressive behavior.

Clinical features: this severely affected, $3\frac{1}{2}$-year-old French Friesian cow (**417**) has a hyaena-like silhouette, with underdevelopment of the hindquarters. Calves are normal at birth, and manifest the initial signs of the disease at 6–10 months. Compared with a normal tibia of a 2-year-old animal (**418**, left), the tibia of an affected individual (22 months) is considerably shortened, although the width and articular surface area are comparable. The condition is thought to result from a bone dysplasia.

Management: incurable.

Deficiency diseases

Rickets

Definition: caused by a calcium, phosphorus or vitamin D deficiency, rickets involves a failure of calcification of osteoid and cartilage.

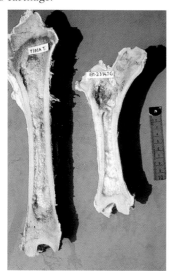

418

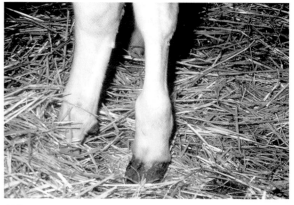

419

Clinical features: swelling and pain generally involve all the major limb joints. In the 6-month-old Holstein heifer in **419** the fetlock is enlarged due to widening of the distal metatarsal physis. The articular surfaces are normal. The calf is lame. Poorly mineralized high-concentrate diets that promote rumen acidosis can lead to a type of rickets producing spontaneous fractures in rapidly growing cattle.

Differential diagnosis: copper deficiency (**426**) and epiphysitis. See also spinal compression fracture (**357**).

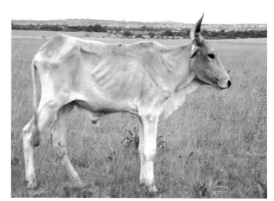

420

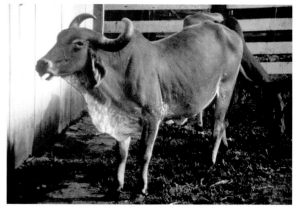

421

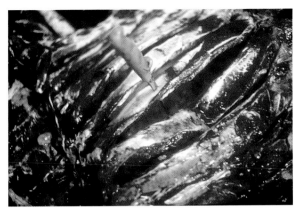

422

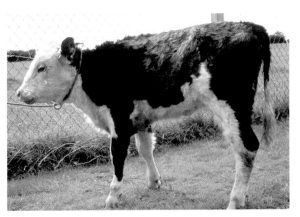

423

Phosphorus deficiency (osteomalacia, 'peg-leg')

Definition: impaired mineralization of bones of adult cattle, with excess osteoid accumulation, caused by phosphorus and/or vitamin D deficiency. Phosphorus deficiency is the most common mineral deficiency worldwide.

Clinical features: affected cattle are unthrifty, have a poor appetite and walk stiffly. The Brazilian steer in **420** is stunted, extremely emaciated, and walked with great difficulty. The local term for this severe aphosphorosis is 'entreva'. The Brazilian Zebu (Gir) cow (**421**) is eating a bone, demonstrating pica; other bones litter the ground. This habit may result in botulism (**709**). A carcass of a phosphorus-deficient animal from the Australian outback has multiple fractured ribs that are so soft they can easily be cut with a knife (**422**). A phosphorus deficiency in young cattle causes rickets (**419**) with slow growth and joint deformities.

Differential diagnosis: other mineral deficiencies, e.g., calcium, copper and cobalt, and starvation.

Management: the easiest and cheapest prophylaxis is the supply of a phosphatic mineral supplement in troughs or boxes protected from the rain. In Australian beef cattle, due to low soil P levels, a phosphorus concentrate may be needed all the time. Problem of supply of supplements is common in range conditions.

Copper deficiency (hypocuprosis, 'pine')

Definition: abnormally low blood and tissue copper levels.

Clinical features: the crossbred Hereford heifer in **423** is unthrifty and has enlarged fetlocks and a characteristic brownish tinge to the hair coat. (The Hereford also has lice.) The loss of hair and hair pigment may produce a 'spectacled' appearance, as seen in the crossbred Holstein/Friesian calf in **424**, which also shows coarse hair typical of copper deficiency. Bone fragility and anemia are other clinical features. The Brazilian cows in **425** show poor growth, poor hair coat and loss of pigment. The fetlock joint enlargement (**426**) is due to widening and irregularity of the distal metacarpal physes, as seen in the radiographs (**427**) of an affected animal (left) compared with a normal animal (right). Similar radiographic changes are seen in the digits. Other cattle may become stunted, developing bowed legs, contracted tendons and kyphosis. Excluding phosphorus deficiency, a deficiency of copper may be the most severe mineral limitation to grazing livestock in extensive tropical regions.

Differential diagnosis: aphosphorosis (**420**), rickets (**419**), and cobalt deficiency (**429**).

Management: copper supplements.

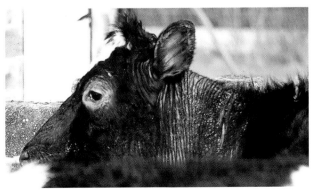

424

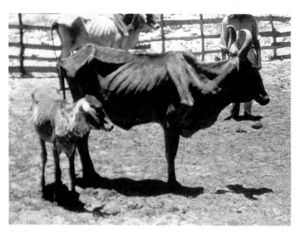

425

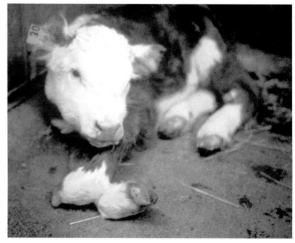

428

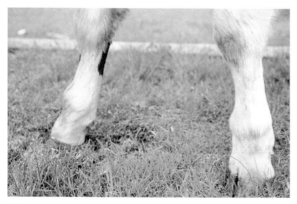

426

Manganese deficiency

Definition: abnormally low blood manganese levels in dam or offspring leading to various skeletal deformities and infertility.

Clinical features: this Hereford neonate (**428**) cannot stand owing to a congenital twisting and flexion of the enlarged fetlock joints. Various other skeletal abnormalities are also present. These changes resulted from a severe manganese deficiency in the dam during gestation. In a 100-head Hereford herd in Canada, of the 5–10% of calves

that were born with abnormalities, this calf was among the most severely affected. Following external splintage, many calves recovered from tendon contracture.

Management: supplementary manganese to pregnant beef cattle at risk, limb splintage where needed in young calves. Good nursing.

Cobalt deficiency ('pine', enzootic marasmus)

Definition: inadequate intake of cobalt over prolonged period, causing poor weight gain and anorexia.

Clinical features: the Brazilian Zebu cattle are depressed, emaciated, eat little and have a poor hair coat (**429**). They are also anemic. Visual evidence of cobalt deficiency is nonspecific, resembling the signs of semistarvation. Young animals are more susceptible. Diagnosis may ultimately rest on the response to cobalt supplementation.

Differential diagnosis: aphosphorosis (osteomalacia) (**420**), hypocuprosis (**423**), parasitism and low feed intake.

Management: confirmation of deficiency by biochemical analysis of blood and other tissues, also feed, followed by adequate access to mineral supplements.

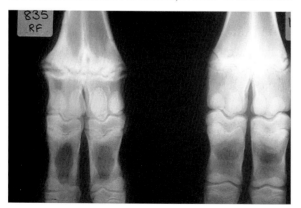

427

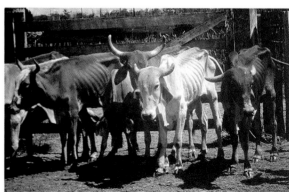

429

chapter 8

Ocular disorders

Introduction

Disorders of the eye are relatively easily seen and photographed. The disorders may be congenital, nutritional, infectious, traumatic or neoplastic in origin. Examples of each are illustrated. Some conditions, for example infectious bovine keratoconjunctivitis (IBK), occur worldwide, and may be a significant cause of economic loss. Pain associated with the active phase of disease restricts feeding and leads to weight loss. If sight is lost, affected animals are less able to forage, particularly under extensive ranch conditions, and they are more susceptible to predators.

Congenital disorders

Although by definition congenital abnormalities are present at birth, some may not be recognized until the calf is much older. Strabismus (squint) is a typical example. Congenital disorders may be genetic, and therefore inherited, or they may be caused by environmental factors. Some abnormalities have more than one cause. For example, congenital cataract may be inherited, or it may have been caused by maternal BVD infection during pregnancy. The cause of many abnormalities is unknown. Congenital disorders in organs other than the eye are described in Chapter 1.

BVD/MD, discussed under Alimentary disorders (p. 43) can give rise to congenital or acquired ocular changes. Congenital BVD/MD can cause retinal dysplasia and

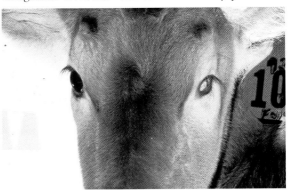

430

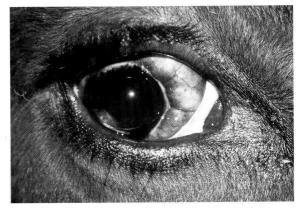

431

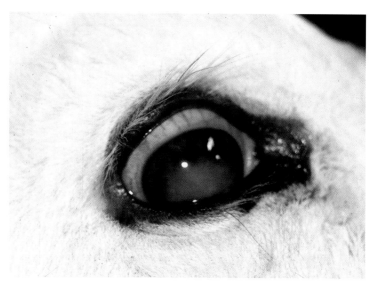

432

degeneration, focal capsular cataract as well as optic nerve gliosis, microphthalmos (see below) and optic neuritis.

Anophthalmos (anophthalmia); microphthalmos (microphthalmia)

Definition: anophthalmos is a developmental absence of the eye; microphthalmos is an abnormal smallness of one or both eyes.

Clinical features: the two examples illustrate both abnormalities. The left eye of the Guernsey heifer in **430** has a small orbit and there is no evidence of the globe. Note that the entire orbit appears collapsed and smaller, compared with the normal right eye. This condition can be inherited. A Jersey cow with microphthalmos (**431**) and prolapse of orbital fat had possibly had an insult to the eye in calfhood, leading to this shrunken globe (*phthisis bulbi*).

Cataract

Definition: opacity of the lens or its capsule or both, present at birth or acquired from trauma or systemic disease.

Clinical features: both eyes of the 4-day-old Hereford crossbred calf in **432** were affected and the animal was totally blind. In other animals, only one eye may be affected, or the cataract may not cause total loss of vision. Congenital cataract is not normally progressive. Cattle cope with blindness remarkably well and can be reared in confinement systems. They quickly learn to remain within the group, although handling can be difficult. Blind dairy cows will learn to follow the herd to and from pasture. Congenital cataract may be inherited, or may result from the teratogenic effects of maternal BVD infection during

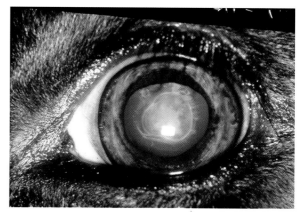

433

early/mid pregnancy. **433** shows a congenital nuclear cataract in a young Friesian calf.

Note in acquired cataract the two large synechiae (adhesions of the iris to the cornea), and the opacity and wrinkling of the lens in the Guernsey cow in **434**. Cataracts may be secondary to inflammatory processes within the eye, when they can be progressive. In contrast, congenital cataracts (**432**) are rarely progressive.

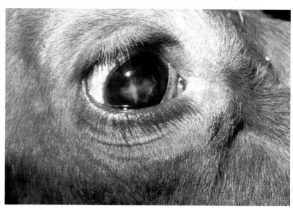

434

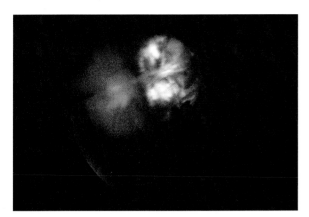

435

Coloboma

Definition: a coloboma is a congenital cleft caused by failure of the embryonic optic fissure to close.

Clinical features: it can occur in the eyelids, iris, lens, or, as shown in **435**, the retina. Note the pale area devoid of functional retinal cells. The condition is inherited in certain breeds of cattle (e.g., Charolais), but vision is not normally impaired.

Dermoid

Definition: an uncommon tumor of developmental origin containing various tissues such as hair follicles, various glandular structures and nerve elements, located often on the cornea, conjunctiva and eyelids.

Clinical features: a typical dermoid is seen in a 4-month-old Friesian heifer (**436**). The tumor is attached to the conjunctiva of the lower lid and presents long hairs which led to the presenting sign of unilateral epiphora.

Management: most ocular dermoids can be resected surgically. Recurrence is unlikely.

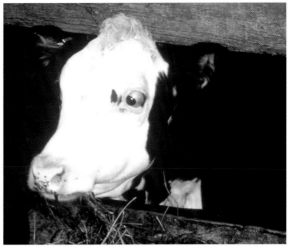

437

Strabismus ('squint')

Definition: involuntary deviation of the eye.

Clinical features: strabismus may be convergent (esotopia), when the visual axes of the eyes converge more than is required for normal vision, or divergent. It may involve one or both eyes. The globe is deviated from its proper axis due to excessive tension in opposing extra-ocular muscles. **437** shows convergent strabismus in the left eye of a Hereford cross heifer. Exophthalmos with strabismus may be inherited, although it is often unnoticed until 6–9 months old, and it is often progressive. Some animals may become so badly affected that total impairment of vision results.

Neonatal corneal opacity

A reduction in intraocular pressure in stillborn calves leads to cloudiness in the cornea and indicates that the

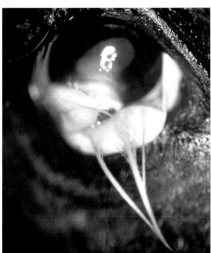

436

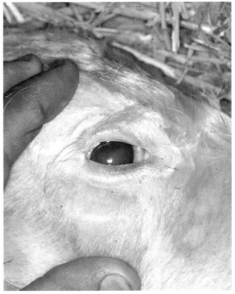

438

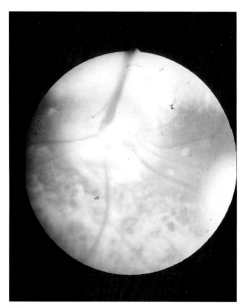

439

calf has died at least 12 hours before birth. In the stillborn Charolais calf in **438** the eyeball is also slightly sunken in the socket.

Acquired disorders

Vitamin A deficiency

In young growing animals, vitamin A deficiency blindness is associated with stenosis of the optic foramen and consequent pressure on the optic nerve. The pupil becomes dilated and degenerative changes may be seen on the retina (**439**). For comparison, **440** shows a normal fundus. The optic disc is pale and enlarged, with indistinct margins (papilloedema). White mottling of the nontapetal area suggests chorioretinal degeneration. The steer was blind. The diet had been barley straw, rolled barley and, occasionally, poor-quality hay.

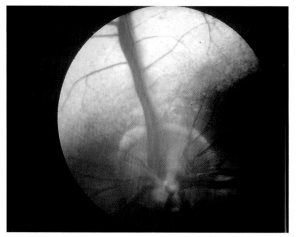

440

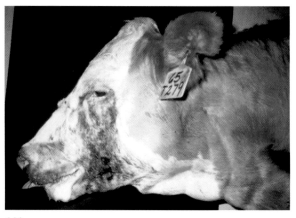

441

Management: ensure diets of cereals, straw and similar feeds are adequately supplemented with vitamin A, especially for rapidly growing stock.

Conjunctivitis

Mild conjunctivitis is seen clinically as epiphora. Typically, a wet, black-stained facial area radiates from the medial canthus. More advanced cases (**441**) show a degree of photophobia. Purulent conjunctivitis (**442**) may also be seen. Caused by a variety of infections and irritants, conjunctivitis and epiphora commonly occur in association with other diseases, for example, calf pneumonia, IBR (**235**), IBK (**443**), and ocular foreign body (**453**).

Infectious bovine keratoconjunctivitis (IBK, infectious ophthalmia, 'New Forest disease' or 'pinkeye')

Definition and pathogenesis: a bacterial infection caused by *Moraxella bovis*, IBK produces blepharospasm, conjunctivitis, keratitis and corneal ulceration.

Clinical features: in mild cases, corneal ulceration may not be apparent and the only clinical signs are epiphora and partial bletharospasm. Typically the ulcer is in the center of the cornea and may be superficial or erode deeply

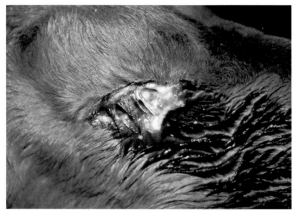

442

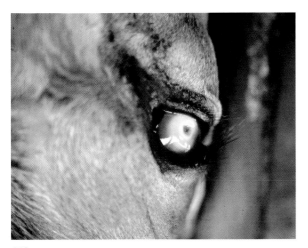

443

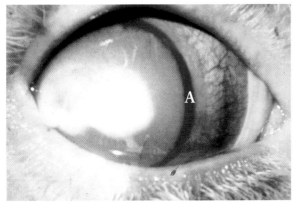

444

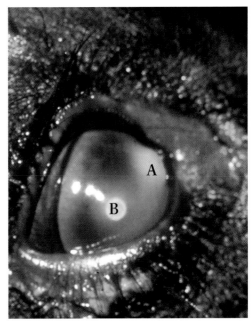

446

ulcer, is clearly evident. The pannus will regress when healing is complete.

into the stroma as shown in a more advanced case (443). Conjunctivitis is always present. The condition is very painful, leading to photophobia, blepharospasm and epiphora. Early (adventitious) corneal vascularization has developed into pannus formation in 443. Later stages (444) develop corneal opacity due to increased intra-ocular pressure. The bright red rim of pannus (A), progressing from the corneoscleral junction to fill the

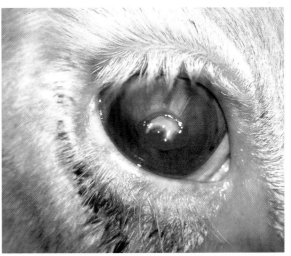

447

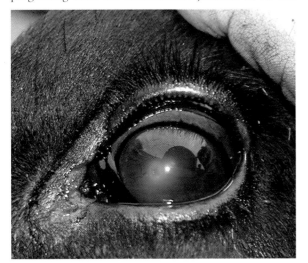

445

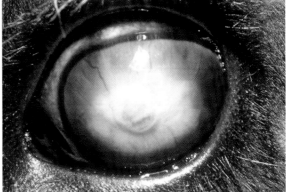

448

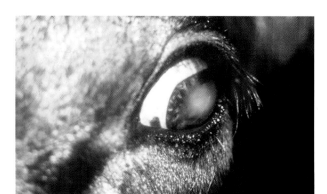

449

Pannus formation does not occur with shallow, superficial lesions, where the ulcer is seen in a localized area of corneal opacity (445). If corneal rupture does not occur, healing may be complete, or may leave a small corneal scar (A), as seen towards the medial canthus in 446. Partial sight has been regained. The circular plaque (B) on the cornea is an artefact caused by flash photography.

Deep ulcers may perforate through to the aqueous. In 447, tissue from the iris plugs the ruptured ulcer and can be seen as a red ring protruding from the surface of the cornea. This is a staphyloma. More advanced cases lose

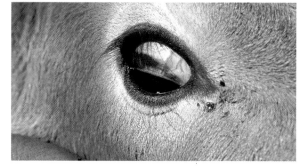

452

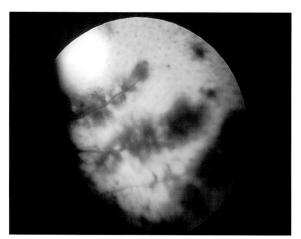

450

their red appearance and some may eventually heal, but they leave an opaque, scarred cornea (448) and glaucoma from impaired drainage of the aqueous humor.

Differential diagnosis: diagnosis is easily made on ocular signs especially if several cattle are affected. Differentials include bovine iritis, and foreign bodies (usually peripheral, see 453), parasites (455) and IBR. *M. bovis* infection can be confirmed on culture in doubtful cases. Note that IBK and IBR eye lesions can rarely be present in the same animal.

Management: bright sunlight, dry, dusty and irritant conditions, flies, and a tight stocking density are all predisposing factors. Separation of affected animals is advisable, preferably in the shade. *M. bovis* is susceptible

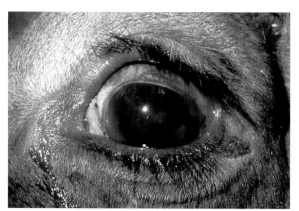

451

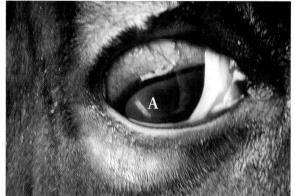

453

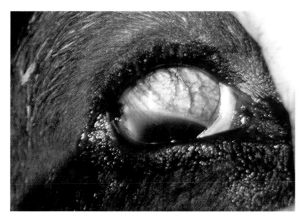

454

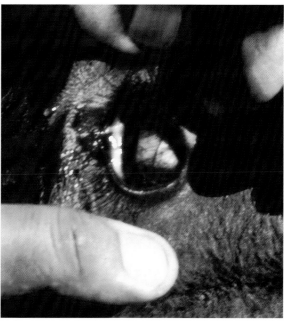

455

to various antibiotics which may be administered sub-conjunctivally, topically or parenterally. Surgery (third eyelid flap) may help severely affected individuals. The efficacy of *M. bovis* bacterins is still disputed.

Hypopyon

Definition: pus in the anterior chamber.

Clinical features: this 4-week-old calf (**449**) was dull, pyrexic and anorexic due to calfhood septicemia resulting from colostrum deficiency. Note the white blood cells in the anterior chamber. This calf recovered following antibiotics and NSAIDs. *Haemophilus somnus* septicemia can produce blindness from retinal hemorrhages and edema (**450**).

Ocular trauma

Clinical features: although the eye is well protected within the bony orbit and by the rapid reflex closure of the lids to approaching foreign bodies, traumatic eye lesions are common, particularly those due to incoming objects. Irritation due to dust or ultraviolet light may produce keratitis and conjunctivitis. The Guernsey cow in **451** has a congested scleral conjunctiva (seen below the upper eyelid), an indistinct pupil, and mild corneal opacity at the medial canthus, probably the result of a blow. The 4-day-old Jersey calf in **452** shows marked scleral hemorrhage resulting from dystocia.

Management: many cases resolve completely within a few days. If persistent, a further check for a FB should be made before starting topical therapy.

Ocular foreign body

Clinical features: grass seeds or other plant material may become lodged in the conjunctiva and, as the eyeball

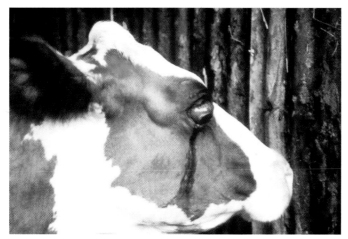

456

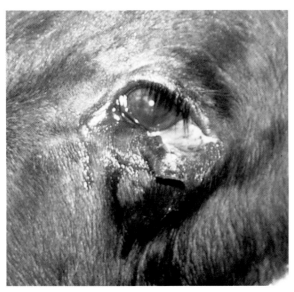

457

moves, repeatedly traumatize the area to produce erosion and ulceration. Cattle reaching up to feed from overhead hay racks are particularly at risk. In **453** a small fragment of plant material (A) is embedded in the corneal surface near the lateral canthus. Note the surrounding early peripheral keratitis and corneal opacity. Keratitis with early corneal ulceration is seen in the more advanced case in **454**. Most of the foreign body is lodged in the lateral canthus, with one small fragment protruding across the cornea.

Management: following good restraint and possibly use of a topical local anesthetic, the foreign body can be removed manually or with fine blunt-tipped forceps. Topical therapy should be given for several days

Thelazia ('eyeworm')

Definition: spiruroid worm (e.g., *T. rhodesii*) of family *Thelazidae* which parasitizes the lacrimal duct and conjunctival sac of cattle, being deposited in the sac by flies as the intermediate host (*Musca* spp.).

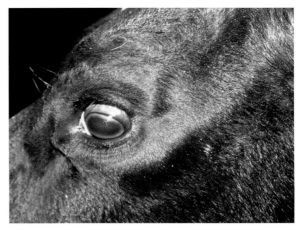

459

Clinical features: infection causes chronic conjunctivitis, lacrimation, blepharospasm and keratitis. This example shows white *Thelazia* larvae floating in tear secretion in the lower conjunctival sac (**455**). Diagnosis is made on inspection.

Differential diagnosis: IBK (**443**), bovine iritis (**460**), ocular trauma (**453, 454**).

Management: mechanical removal with forceps after instilling a local anesthetic solution. Prevention is by levamisole and ivermectin with doramectin, along with control measures against face flies.

Prolapse of the eyeball (proptosis)

Definition: forward displacement or bulging of the eye.

Clinical features: it is an infrequent condition caused by trauma to the head. In the Ayrshire cow in **456**, note the congested and edematous sclera and the eyeball protruding beyond the lids.

Management: under sedation and local anesthesia the eyeball can be returned to its socket. If held in place for

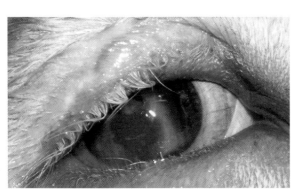

458

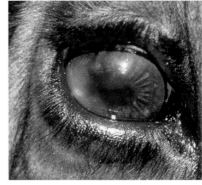

460

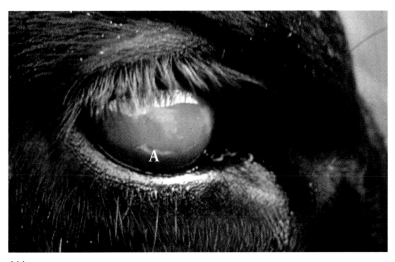

461

4–5 days by suturing the lids together, most cases (as in 456) resolve well.

Eyelid laceration

Clinical features: lacerations of the lower eyelids are fairly common. They are often caused by an animal rubbing the head and catching an eyelid on projections from troughs, buildings or fragments of wire. In the Angus heifer in 457, the lower lid injury near the lateral canthus was sustained several days previously and was healing well.

Management: sometimes the resultant rough eyelid edge leads to incomplete lid closure with persistent low-grade corneal ulceration and lacrimation. More severe cases should therefore benefit from suturing.

Entropion

Definition: inversion of the margin of an eyelid, a congenital or acquired condition.

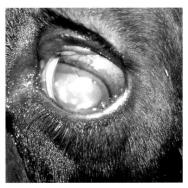

462

Clinical features: a Simmental bull, following uveitis (see Bovine iritis, p. 132) developed entropion of the right lower lid (458) where secondary corneal pannus formation is also evident. The entropion was of the spastic type and resolved following topical treatment.

Hyphema

Definition: hyphema is blood in the anterior chamber, with many possible causes such as trauma, clotting disorders and sepsis.

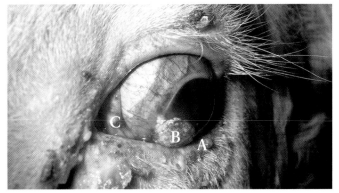

463

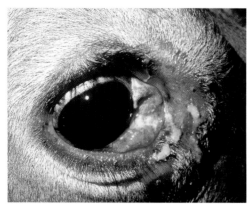

464

Clinical features: in **459** note the fresh blood which has settled at the bottom of the anterior chamber. (See also bracken poisoning, **720**.)

Management: many traumatic cases are bilateral and the animal has total but temporary loss of sight. Most cases resolve spontaneously over 2–3 weeks without treatment.

Bovine iritis (uveitis, iridocyclitis, 'silage eye')

Definition: inflammation of the anterior uveal tract (iris and ciliary body) is iridocyclitis, while posterior uveitis is inflammation of the ciliary body and choroid.

Clinical features: several neonatal (e.g., navel ill) as well as systemic diseases of growing and adult cattle may be associated with uveitis, such as malignant catarrhal fever, tuberculosis and IBR. Bovine iritis has been more recently associated with *Listeria monocytogenes* infection and is possibly caused by the feeding of big-bale silage. One or both eyes are affected. Early cases (**460**) show an enlarged and wrinkled iris, leading to a central miotic pupil. Near the lateral canthus is a white endothelial plaque on the inner surface of the cornea (Descemet's membrane), with corneal opacity and early pannus formation. As the condition progresses (**461**), pannus develops circumferentially (A), with increasing corneal discoloration and opacity. In severe cases (**462**) the endothelial plaques produce a very irregular surface on the cornea and cause complete blindness.

Diagnosis: the association of close contact with big-bale silage and ocular disease in a group is characteristic. Other differentials include IBK (**443–448**) and ocular foreign body (**453**).

Management: even advanced cases (**461, 462**) recover following subconjunctival anti-inflammatory and antibiotic treatment. Major outbreaks occur when silage was cut at a fairly mature stage of grass growth. Feeding from round feeders and along windy troughs, both of which increase eye contact with silage, increases disease risk.

Neoplastic conditions

Malignancy of the third eyelid (membrana nictitans) and the globe is common in cattle worldwide. Lymphosarcomas may occur within the globe itself or in the orbit, leading to prolapse of the globe. Papillomas have been occasionally reported.

Squamous cell carcinoma

Pathogenesis: squamous cell carcinoma (SCC) is the most common ocular neoplasm of cattle, and is seen particularly in mature white-headed beef cattle, such as the Hereford, and other breeds with little pigmentation around the eye (e.g., Simmental). The disease is associated with sunlight (ultraviolet light).

Clinical features: common sites for SCC include the lower lid, the third eyelid and the corneoscleral junction of the globe. Often both eyes are affected to a varying degree. Small benign precursor lesions will often regress. The Hereford bull in **463** has SCC at several points along the eyelids (A), a grayish plaque, 10 mm in diameter, extending over the cornea from the corneoscleral junction (B), and early SCC in the third eyelid (C). In the Guernsey cow in **464**, pink, neoplastic tissue protrudes from the third eyelid (membrana nictitans) at the medial canthus. There is a secondary superficial purulent infection. If neglected, about 10% will eventually metastasize to the regional lymph nodes, (resulting in slaughterhouse condemnation) and a small proportion to the lungs, as in **465**. The multiple irregular pale areas are tumor tissue.

Differential diagnosis: IBK (**443–448**), periorbital lymphosarcoma (**466**).

Management: early third eyelid lesions are easily removed under sedation and local anesthesia using forceps and

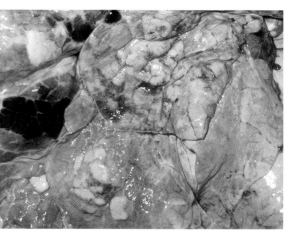

465

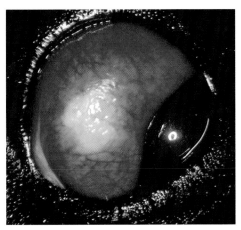

466

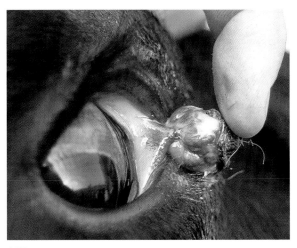

467

scissors. More advanced cases require cryotherapy or total removal of the eyeball to avoid regional spread.

Lymphosarcoma (malignant lymphoma)

Definition: a malignant neoplasm of lymphatic tissue, lymphosarcoma can develop at several sites (abomasum, uterus). When in the eye it usually presents as a retrobulbar mass with progressive expansion and spread.

Clinical features: in **466** a large neoplastic mass has produced a smooth, red, bulbous enlargement of the conjunctiva, compressing the eyeball towards the medial canthus (right). Ocular lymphosarcoma causes progressive exophthalmos.

Diagnosis: the tumor is almost invariably present in other sites, as clinical examination often reveals superficial, abdominal and pelvic lymphadenopathy and other lymphosarcomatous foci. Biopsy and histopathology of the mass or enlarged lymph node can confirm diagnosis.

Management: affected cattle should therefore be culled. Secondary spread results in carcass condemnation.

Papilloma of the third eyelid

In **467** the papilloma is attached to the third eyelid by a 'stalk' and has a very irregular keratinized surface. It is much less common than a SCC, and is easy to remove surgically.

chapter 9

Nervous disorders

Introduction

The nervous diseases discussed in this chapter are those in which nervous signs comprise the major part of the clinical syndrome. Consequently, a wide etiological range is covered including nutritional conditions (e.g., cerebrocortical necrosis), metabolic disorders (e.g., hypomagnesemia), bacterial and viral infections (e.g., listeriosis and rabies), parasites (e.g., *Coenurus cerebralis*), physical and traumatic incidents (lightning stroke and electrocution) and miscellaneous conditions of uncertain etiology (e.g., bovine spongiform encephalopathy). However, other diseases with significant clinical nervous signs may be featured elsewhere and include tetanus (707), botulism (709) and lead poisoning (747).

Nervous conditions may be difficult to appreciate in 'still' photographs, since their clinical assessment is based on changes in behavior, movement, gait and stance. An understanding of the normal animal is therefore extremely important. Where problems of recognition occur, the text has been expanded in an attempt to describe those changes that cannot be photographed.

Cerebrocortical necrosis (polioencephalomalacia)

Etiology: cerebrocortical necrosis (CCN) is an induced thiamine deficiency caused by products of abnormal ruminal fermentation (thiaminases). Concentrate feeding leading to excessive growth of specific thiaminase 1 enzyme-secreting rumen bacteria is the most likely cause. The syndrome can also be induced by feeding high levels of certain ammonium sulfate mixtures used as dietary urinary acidifiers for the prevention of urolithiasis (511–515).

Clinical features: CCN is seen most commonly in calves that are 2–6 months old, often following a dietary change when on high-concentrate rations. In the Friesian calf in **468**, note the pronounced opisthotonos, the rotation of the eye to expose the sclera, and the extensor spasm of the front legs. Other signs include depression, ataxia, head-pressing (**469**) and cortical blindness. Postmortem lesions (**470**) are normally symmetrical and occur in the frontal, occipital and parietal lobes. Congestion and yellow degener-

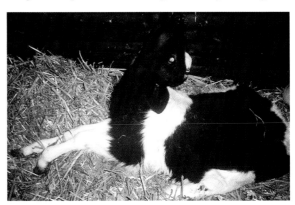

468

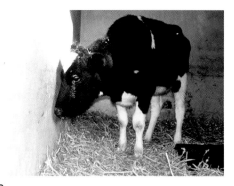

469

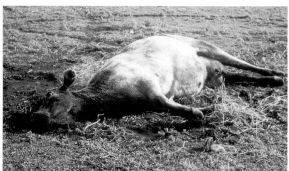

471

ation of the cortical gray matter (A) is seen, typically at the junction of the white and gray matter, particularly on the left and right extremities. Affected brains will fluoresce blue-green under ultraviolet light.

Differential diagnosis: acute lead poisoning, hypomagnesemia, brain abscess, vitamin A deficiency. Diagnosis is based on the clinical signs and response to thiamine therapy.

Management: multiple injections of thiamine HCl, the first i.v., within a few hours of onset of signs, possibly also diuretics and/or dexamethasone, can lead to a marked improvement. Mortality in untreated animals can exceed 50%. Prevention involves avoidance of possible risk factors.

Metabolic diseases

Metabolic diseases are included in this chapter, since many of their presenting clinical signs are behavioral or nervous. Typically, such signs occur when homeostasis has been extended beyond physiological limits. Four conditions are illustrated: hypomagnesemia, hypocalcemia, acetonemia and fatty liver syndrome.

Hypomagnesemia ('grass staggers', 'grass tetany')

Definition: hypomagnesemia is a complex metabolic disturbance involving lowered blood and CSF Mg leading

to hyperexcitability, muscle spasms, convulsions and death, usually in adult lactating dairy or beef cows. Death in severe cases can occur within a few hours.

Clinical features: the Friesian cow in **471** fell and developed extensor spasm when being brought in for milking. Note the 'staring' eye, dilated pupil, frothing at the mouth and sweaty coat. In **472** the crossbred cow from Queensland, Australia, shows similar eye changes. The head and the hind legs are in extensor spasm. Violent paddling movements of the forelegs and head have resulted in loss of foliage, exposing the bare earth. Less severely affected cows may walk stiffly, are hypersensitive to touch and sound, and urinate often. Precipitated by stress and seen especially in temperate climates, the condition is induced by grazing magnesium-deficient or high-potassium pastures, and other pastures where magnesium uptake is poor. Concurrent hypocalcemia may be an exacerbating factor.

Differential diagnosis: hypocalcemia (**473**, **474**), BSE (**498–500**), encephalitis, listeriosis (**477**, **478**), ketosis (**475**).

Management: individual treatment involves sedation to control spasms and to prevent cardiac arrest, and subcutaneous injection of 25% solution of magnesium sulfate, possibly with calcium borogluconate. Small amounts of MgSO$_4$ can be given slowly i.v.

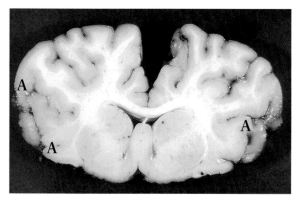

470

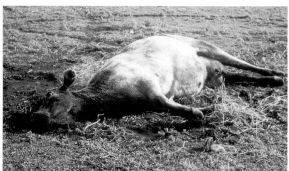

472

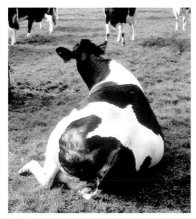

473

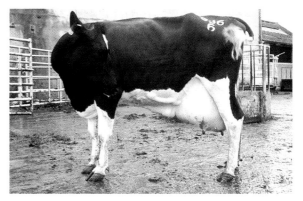

475

Prevention: maintain adequate intake of Mg, either by sward management, buffer feeding, or by addition of Mg salts to diet or drinking water.

Hypocalcemia ('milk fever', post-parturient paresis)

Clinical features: hypocalcemia (**473**) occurs typically in older cows immediately pre- or post-calving. Early signs include hypersensitivity and increased excitability. Later, affected animals are unable to rise owing to lack of muscle power and poor nerve function. Note also the protruding anal sphincter (due to accumulation of feces in the rectum, and increased intra-abdominal pressure), slight ruminal bloat (ruminal atony) and the typical 'S-bend' in the neck (**473**). This is thought to be a self-righting response, as the animal attempts to avoid full lateral recumbency. Some affected cows lie with their head resting on their flank (**474**).

Differential diagnosis: toxic mastitis or metritis, periparturient hemorrhage, severe hindlimb trauma, or bilateral obturator paralysis.

Management: slow i.v. injection of 400 ml of 40% Ca borogluconate, possibly with additional magnesium and

phosphorus. Calcium may also be given by s.c. injection. Prevention includes avoidance of over-fat cows at calving, and dietary management during the transition period. Avoid lush high-K^+ and high-Ca^+ rations such as grazing, and feed long fiber and diets which have an appropriate cation : anion balance.

Nervous acetonemia (ketosis, 'slow fever')

Nervous acetonemia is an intoxication by circulating ketone bodies and is associated with an energy deficit in early lactation. Typical clinical signs are anorexia and lethargy (hence 'slow fever'), depressed yields and constipation, although some cases develop nervous signs such as compulsive licking, salivation, biting flanks (as seen in

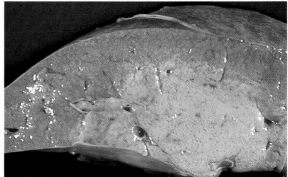

476

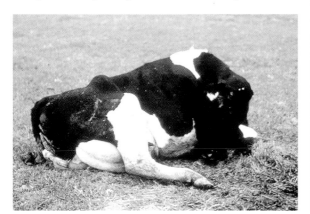

474

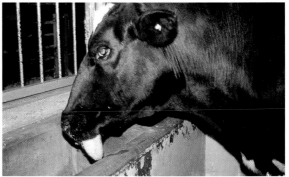

477

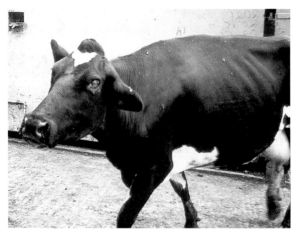

478

this 5-year-old Holstein in **475**) or even maniacal behavior. This cow was difficult to get in the parlor for milking. Six hours later her frantic licking of udder and forelegs resulted in bleeding. The cow rapidly responded to dextrose and corticosteroids.

Differential diagnosis: hypomagnesemia (**471, 472**), BSE (**498–500**), listeriosis (**477, 478**).

Management: avoid over-fat cows at calving. Provide suitable transition rations (see Hypocalcemia), and palatable high-energy feed in early lactation.

Fatty liver syndrome (fat cow syndrome)

Definition: a condition of anorexia, ketonuria and hepatic dysfunction in over-fat cows at parturition, precipitated by other peripartum diseases and disturbed feed intake, especially in cows that are fed an energy-deficient diet after calving.

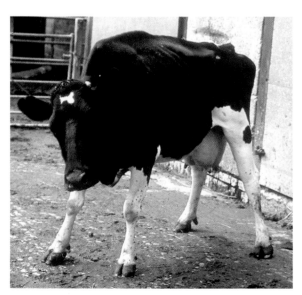

479

Clinical features: many cows show no precise clinical signs. More advanced cases develop anorexia and 'stargazing', progressing to toxemia and terminal recumbency. Massive fatty infiltration of the friable liver is seen in **476**.

Differential diagnosis: hypocalcemia (**473, 474**), mastitis, metritis and other forms of toxemia.

Management: early cases may respond to i.v. glucose solutions, parenteral glucocorticoids and bovine somatotrophin (if licensed). Advanced recumbent cases should be culled. Prevention as for ketosis (p. 137).

Bacterial infections
Listeriosis ('circling disease')

Definition: infectious disease caused by *Listeria monocytogenes*, resulting in either a meningoencephalitic syndrome, neonatal septicemia or abortion.

Clinical features: the meningoencephalitic form produces pyrexia, dullness, blindness, headpressing and a unilateral facial nerve paralysis, leading to prolapse of the tongue (**477**) and drooping of the ears. Compulsive circling towards the affected side (**478**) is also often seen, and abortions may occur, but they are usually not concurrent with nervous signs. Note the typical paralysed eyelids and resulting development of keratitis sicca in both **477** and **478**. In 2–4-day-old calves septicemia leads to sudden death. *Listeria* can be isolated from many organs at postmortem. The organism is ubiquitous, being found in the environment and in most wildlife. Disease may be associated with cold weather and silage feeding.

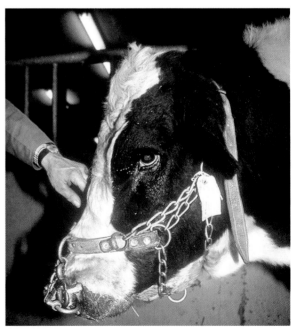

480

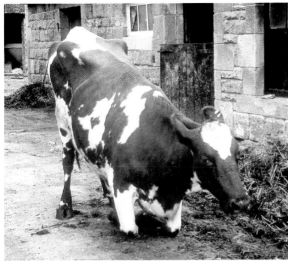

481

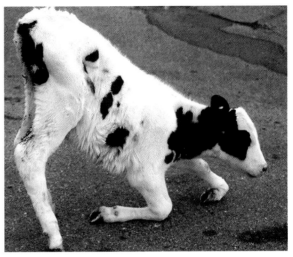

483

Differential diagnosis: rabies (**495**), acute lead poisoning (**747**), CCN (**468**), BSE (**498**), botulism (**709**), bacterial meningitis (**484**), viral encephalitis and pituitary abscess (**482**).

Management: early cases may respond to aggressive penicillin therapy with NSAIDs in initial stages. *Listeria* is more prevalent in high-pH silage, and in moldy silage, so prevention is based on silage management. Preventive parenteral penicillin at birth may reduce deaths from neonatal septicemia.

Middle ear infection (otitis media)

Clinical features: in middle ear infections, the head is typically held to one side, as in the Friesian cow in **479**. However, she remained alert, continued feeding and was not pyrexic. Note the base-wide stance to maintain balance. *Pasteurella* spp. and other respiratory bacterial pathogens are often involved.

Differential diagnosis: listeriosis (**477**) and meningitis (**484**).

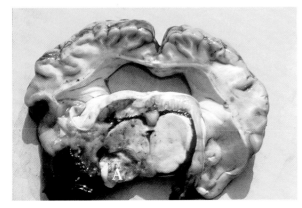

482

Management: some improvement is seen with parenteral antibiotics, but many cases continue to thrive, apparently unaffected by the head tilt. Prevention involves control of respiratory infections.

Facial nerve paralysis

Clinical features: in **480** the ear, upper eyelid and muzzle are drooping. In this bull the cause was unknown, but possible etiology includes trauma, middle ear disease, listeriosis and other brain infections.

Differential diagnosis: includes botulism (**709**), rabies (**495**) and listeriosis (**477**).

Brain abscess

Clinical features: the Ayrshire cow in **481** looks apprehensive, holds her head to one side and is unable to stand on her front legs. An abscess (A) was seen in the base of the brain on postmortem (**482**). A common location for such abscesses is the pituitary fossa.

Differential diagnosis: as for listeriosis.

Management: individual treatment is usually unsuccessful. Prevention depends on control of foci of bacteremia such as lameness, mastitis and respiratory infections.

Meningitis/meningoencephalitis

Definition: a pathological inflammation of the meninges of variable etiology.

Clinical features: meningitis produces a range of clinical signs. Some calves have difficulty in standing and walking, as in this 4-week-old Holstein heifer (**483**), which collapsed in the forequarters, and shortly afterwards went into

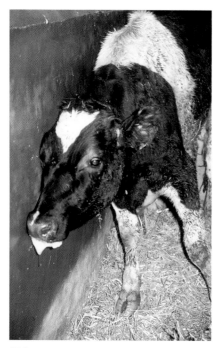

484

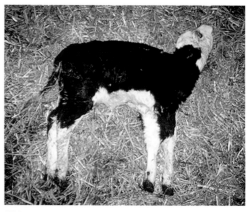

486

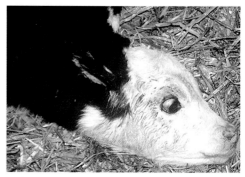

487

extensor rigidity. The calf in **484** is leaning and pushing its head against the wall, its pupils are dilated and it is frothing at the mouth. Some calves (**485**) are recumbent and dull, with drooping ears and eyelids, giving the appearance of an intense headache. The calf in **485** exhibited a hypopyon (see p. 129) which resolved surprisingly rapidly following treatment. Hypopyon is also just evident in **484**. A more extreme case developed extensor spasm (**486**) and opisthotonos (**487**), but recovered. Adult cattle can also be affected with similar signs. **488** shows a congested brain at postmortem. A range of organisms may be involved including *Streptococci*, *Haemophilus*, *Pasteurella* and *Listeria*.

Differential diagnosis: rabies (**495**, **496**), brain abscess (**481**), acute lead poisoning (**747**) and infectious thromboembolic meningoencephalitis (**489**).

Haemophilus somnus disease complex (TEME, ITEME), thrombotic meningoencephalitis (TME), (hemophilosis)

Definition: an acute often fatal septicemic disease involving one or multiple body systems, caused by *Haemophilus somnus*.

Clinical features: it is seen primarily in North American feedlot cattle but has also been reported in Europe and Israel. The correct terminology is disputed. TME (TEME, ITEME) is sudden in onset, occurring initially with marked pyrexia. Affected animals are dull and severely depressed, as in the Charolais bull in **489**. Note the salivation, drooping

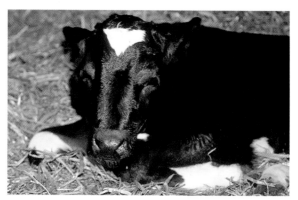

485

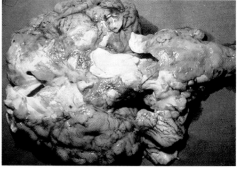

488

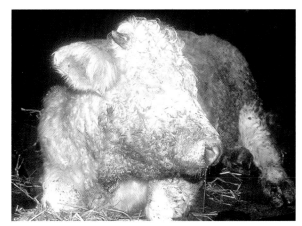

489

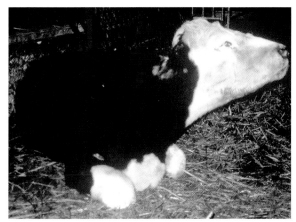

492

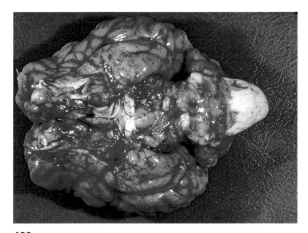

490

ears and eyelids. Recumbency and death may follow within a few hours. Blindness from retinal hemorrhages with gray foci of retinal necrosis and edema are early features. Marked cerebral edema, congestion and hemorrhage are seen in a ventral view of the brain (490) at postmortem, with congestion of the gray matter, cerebral hemorrhages (in the lateral ventricles), meningitis and discolored cerebrospinal fluid (CSF). *H. somnus* alone can cause a suppurative bronchopneumonia with severe cranioventral

changes (491), or it may be involved in shipping fever or pasteurellosis. The pathogen can be cultured from many organs including synovia, CSF, pleural cavity and myocardium.

Differential diagnosis: cerebrocortical necrosis (468, 470), hypovitaminosis A, acute lead poisoning (747), listeriosis (477, 478), pasteurellosis and rabies (495, 496).

Management: sick animals should be isolated and immediately given antibiotic therapy. Cattle which become recumbent with TME infection rarely recover, despite intensive care. Attempts to develop an effective preventive program with bacterins of *H. somnus* have generally been unsuccessful in North America. Mass medication with longacting tetracycline on arrival in feedlots did not reduce mortality from *H. somnus*, but has reduced the incidence of subsequent respiratory disease.

Coenurus cerebralis (coenurosis, 'gid')

Etiology: *Coenurus cerebralis* is the intermediate stage (metacestode) of the canine tapeworm, *Taenia multiceps*. Although common in sheep, it occasionally encysts in cattle brains, producing a slow, progressive nervous disease.

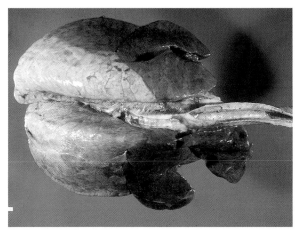

491

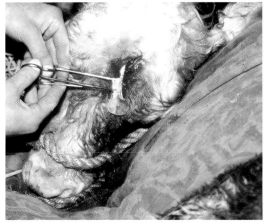

493

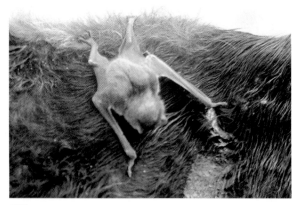

494

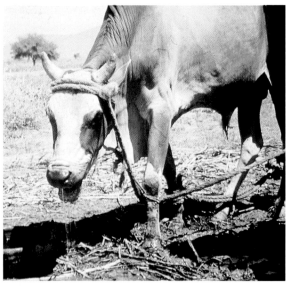

495

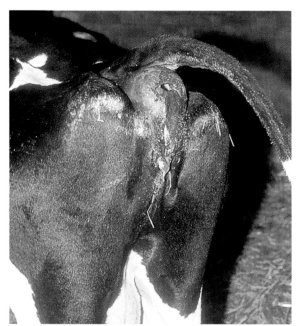

496

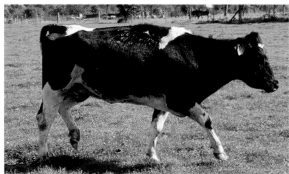

497

Clinical features: starting with blindness, head-pressing, sleepiness and aimless wandering, affected animals eventually become recumbent over a period of 1–4 months. The Hereford cross heifer (**492**), unable to stand, has its eyes closed and head extended, typical of a headache. The cyst often lies immediately beneath the frontal bone, from where it can be removed from the external surface of the cerebral hemispheres (**493**). This animal made a full recovery.

Management: correct carcass disposal to avoid dogs becoming infected with tapeworms. Regular 3-monthly treatment of all farm dogs and others in contact with livestock.

Viral infections

Rabies

Definition: rabies is a rhabdoviral infection that produces a fatal encephalomyelitis in all warm-blooded animal species, including man.

498

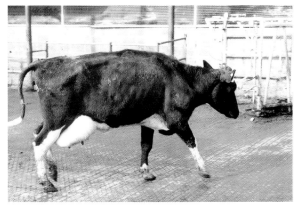

499

Clinical features: dogs, cats and wild carnivores (e.g., foxes, racoons, coyotes) are primarily affected. Carrier animals transmit infective saliva to cattle by biting, e.g., the vampire bat shown feeding from a cow in Brazil in **494**, was later found to harbor the rabies virus. The virus then passes to the brain via peripheral nerves (ascending paralysis), hence the variation in incubation period depending on the site of injury. Initially seen simply as a change in behavior, early cases progress to show salivation, apprehension, bellowing (**495**) and knuckling of the hind fetlocks. Some cattle show marked tenesmus (**496**). This may lead directly to paralysis and death, although in the more classic 'furious' form of rabies, with characteristic bellowing, aggression sometimes occurs in cattle. Pending euthanasia in the tropics a steer may be shackled for restraint (**495**) due to the lack of isolation facilities.

Differential diagnosis: bacterial meningitis (**484**), brain abscess (**481**), listeriosis (**477**), botulism (**710**), Aujeszky's disease (**497**), hypomagnesemia (**471, 472**) and nervous ketosis (**475**).

Management: countries free of rabies maintain strict quarantine measures for dogs and cats entering from abroad. Many other countries have active eradication campaigns and a compulsory vaccination policy for certain domestic species.

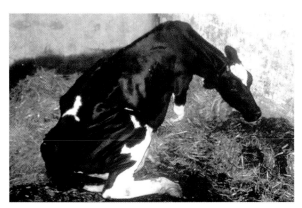

500

Aujeszky's disease (pseudorabies, 'mad itch')

Definition: caused by porcine herpesvirus 1, infection is occasionally acquired from pigs to cause a progressive and fatal disease with a characteristic frenzied scratching and marked excitement.

Clinical features: although primarily a herpes infection of pigs, other species, including cattle, can sporadically develop a meningoencephalitis that is usually fatal within 48 hours. Apprehension, licking, trembling and salivation (**497**) are early signs, typically followed by an intense pruritis, marked excitement, convulsions and death. The grossly swollen eyelids in **497** are the result of intense rubbing to relieve the pruritis.

Differential diagnosis: nervous acetonemia (**475**), rabies (**495, 496**), PPH (**501**), and acute lead poisoning.

Management: this disease is notifiable. Some countries practise vaccination of cattle which are in close contact with potentially infected pigs.

Bovine spongiform encephalopathy (BSE)

Definition: BSE is a progressive non-febrile, fatal brain degenerative condition. The full etiology is not yet understood, but the current theory is that it is an infectious disease caused by ingestion of an agent ('prion'), present in ruminant-derived concentrate feed which is similar to,

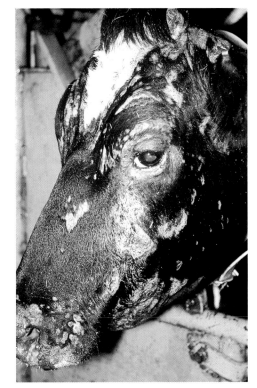

501

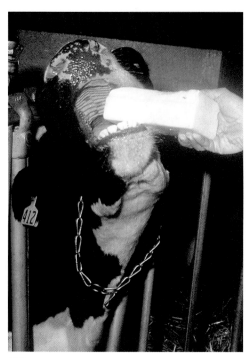

502

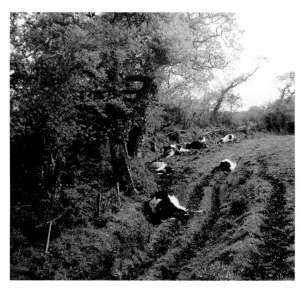

503

but not necessarily identical to, the scrapie agent in sheep. The political and economic effects of BSE, worldwide, have been enormous.

Clinical features: cows that are between 3 and 6 years old are primarily affected by bovine spongiform encephalopathy. Occasional cases occur in bulls, and cases are more common in dairy than beef cows, because the former are more likely to have been given concentrates as calves. Clinical signs include weight loss (**498**), an unsteady, stiff-legged gait, especially in the hind legs, and behavioral changes such as teeth grinding, excessive licking of the muzzle, muscle twitching, nervousness, over-reaction to stimuli such as a hand-clap, and occasionally aggression. Severe posterior ataxia and, eventually, recumbency develop after a period of days to months. The change in gait is

difficult to visualize in a photograph. The Friesian cow in **499** is typically in poor bodily condition, with arched back, raised tail, stiffness of hind legs, and her base-wide stance is an attempt to maintain balance in walking. She was difficult, indeed almost dangerous to handle. Recumbent cases (**500**) often adopt a characteristic dog-sitting posture. Typical microscopic spongiform changes were seen in the brain at postmortem.

First seen in 1986, BSE was originally largely confined to the UK, with many fewer cases seen in Eire and Switzerland. Recently several hundred cases have been diagnosed in Portugal, France, Germany and other European countries. Susceptibility to infection is possibly inherited and maternal transmission via placenta or colostrum may occur. The disease is notifiable worldwide due to its possible association with the human form of new variant Creutzfeld-Jacob Disease (nvCJD).

Differential diagnosis: rabies (**495, 496**), Aujeszky's disease (**497**), listeriosis (**477, 478**), meningitis (**484–488**), brain abscess (**481, 482**) and hypomagnesemia (**471, 472**).

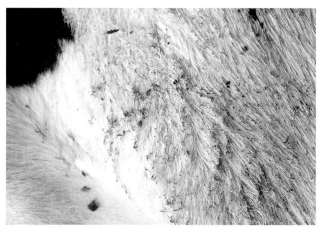

504

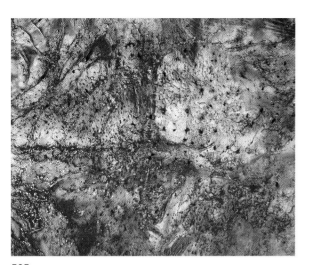

505

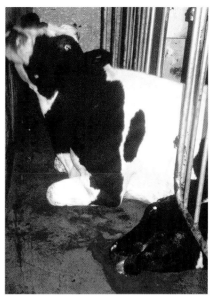

506

Management: following notification, suspect cases are euthanased on the farm, and the brain is examined for diagnostic changes. Antemortem tests are currently under trial. In the UK only about 85% of clinically suspect animals prove to be positive. Control is based on the destruction of all potentially infected and suspect cases, and by the total elimination of mammalian protein from ruminant feeds.

Miscellaneous disorders
Pruritis-pyrexia-hemorrhagica (PPH)

Definition: a rare, non-infectious disorder of adult cattle of uncertain etiology, causing an intense pruritis and variable other systemic signs.

Clinical features: in PPH, raised plaques of skin on the head (501), neck, tail and udder may initially resemble ringworm (97, 98), but are intensely pruritic. More severe cases are pyrexic, anorexic and pass blood from the mouth, nose and rectum. The cause is unknown, but a fungal toxin, citronin, produced by *Penicillium* and *Aspergillus* molds and sweet vernal grass have both been implicated. On post-mortem intense hemorrhage is seen throughout the carcass including the heart, and also white, necrotic renal foci.

Differential diagnosis: Aujeszky's disease (497), mange (85), nervous ketosis (475), winter dysentery, especially the hemorrhagic form (159), and ringworm (97).

Salt-craving pica

Prolonged, deficient diets lead to an intense craving for salt. Affected animals will often lick and bite any object (pica), and may avidly attack salt blocks (502). Milk production, food intake, growth and fertility may be depressed.

Lightning stroke

Clinical features: animals that have been struck by lightning are typically found beside a hedge, a wire fence (503), or under a tree. The tree may show evidence of lightning damage. Trees that have shallow-spreading root systems are particularly dangerous, especially if the ground is damp or has underground drains. Dead animals may be found with fresh food in the mouth and scorch marks of burned hair on the coat, especially the legs (504). Removal of the hide reveals extensive bleeding due to rupture of the subcutaneous blood vessels (505). Mildly affected animals may recover after a variable period of time.

Differential diagnosis (of sudden death): hypomagnesemia (471), bloat (197), pulmonary thrombo-embolism (262–265), cardiac failure (see Chapter 6), anthrax (704).

Electrocution

Clinical features: electrocution is quite commonly seen in cattle, partly owing to an inherent susceptibility, but also because they are more often exposed in milking parlors (506). Clinical signs vary from being stunned, with resulting nasal, oral and ocular bleeding, to death (as in the cows in 506), also with profuse bleeding. Death is due to ventricular fibrillation and respiratory arrest. Exposure to lower levels of high-amperage electric current produces a variety of nervous and behavioral changes, depending on the voltage intensity. 'Stray electricity', due to poor earthing, can be a problem in milking parlors, leading to poor milk let-down, and/or nervous cows liable frequently to kick off the cluster.

chapter 10

Urinogenital disorders

Urinary tract

Introduction

The main infectious and bacterial diseases of the bovine urinary tract are pyelonephritis and leptospirosis. Urolithiasis is a multifactorial urinary problem resulting from metabolic and nutritional disorders. Finally, amyloidosis, although an uncommon sporadic disease of adult cattle, requires differentiation from pyelonephritis.

Conditions with secondary renal pathology include pruritis-pyrexia-hemorrhagica (PPH) (501), oak (acorn) poisoning (724, 725), renal infarction secondary to caudal vena caval thrombosis (264), babesiosis (redwater, 679), and the many causes of bacteremia and septicemia.

Pyelonephritis

Definition: a bacterial infection (usually *Corynebacterium renale*) of the kidney and renal pelvis, pyelonephritis usually ascends from the vagina and vulva.

Clinical features: it is worldwide in distribution, sporadic and most often seen in the first 3 months postpartum. It may result from contact with infected urine or from a genital tract infection. Most infections start in the winter housing period when cow-to-cow contact increases. Affected cows are pyrexic, lose weight, show polyuria, hematuria or pyuria, and may develop a dry, brownish discoloration of the coat, often with urine staining over the tail and perineum which resembles cystitis (519). Rectal palpation may reveal a thickened ureter or enlarged (left) kidney. 507, an 18-month-old Limousin heifer, ill for several days, showed at postmortem a granular renal cortex with areas of recent hemorrhage. In addition, several small discrete renal abscesses are evident, one of which has burst.

Severe chronic pyelonephritis is illustrated in 508 where the left kidney is contracted and pale, and the right kidney is enlarged and appears granular. Both ureters, particularly the left, are thickened as they contain pus and cellular debris (pyoureter).

Other cases of pyelonephritis have multiple caseous and purulent centers, primarily in the renal medulla which may be appreciated on rectal palpation.

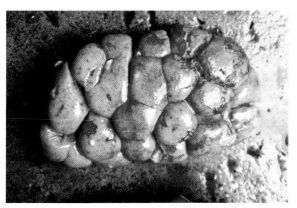

507

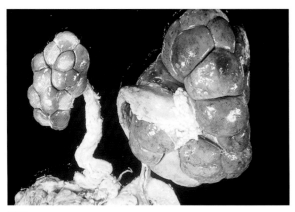

508

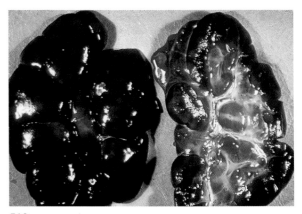

510

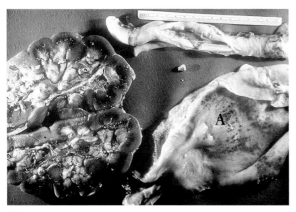

509

In a case of chronic pyelonephritis (509) calculi are present in the renal calyces, further calculi are in a thickened fibrotic ureter, and the bladder mucosa contains multiple petechiae (A).

Differential diagnosis: urolithiasis, acute intestinal obstruction (in acute pyelonephritis) and cystitis. Diagnosis is usually made on gross appearance of a urine sample, urine staining of the tail and perineum, and rectal palpation of the bladder and kidneys. Pyelonephritis and cystitis may co-exist.

Management: early cases may respond to aggressive parenteral antibiotics for 7–10 days (e.g., amoxycillin, potentiated sulfonamides). Affected animals are best isolated. Advanced cases are best culled.

Leptospirosis

Definition: infectious disease of both adult and young cattle with different clinical syndromes caused by the spirochete *Leptospira*.

Clinical features: the main effects of *Leptospira interrogans* serovar. *pomona* or *hardjo* infection are abortion (see 587 for a fetus from a possible leptospiral abortion), stillbirths, loss of milk production and reduced fertility. *L. pomona* causes an acute septicemia, with hemoglobinuria,

jaundice, anemia and possibly death, in calves. Dark swollen kidneys (510) are usually indicative of a hemolytic crisis. Recovered cattle show little more than ill-defined, grayish, cortical spots, indicative of a focal interstitial nephritis. The spirochaete may be seen under dark field microscopy of urine, but confirmation of diagnosis otherwise depends on serology or histopathology.

Differential diagnosis: babesiosis (679–684), anaplasmosis (685–688), rape and kale poisoning (728), postparturient hemoglobinuria, and bacillary hemoglobinuria (227). Note the completely different appearances of the kidney in pyelonephritis (508) and amyloidosis (518).

Management: early clinical cases of *L. pomona* in adults with a hemolytic crisis may respond to tetracyclines. Blood transfusions may be additionally useful in acute syndromes in the calf. In early stages of a herd outbreak, further abortions may be avoided by prompt vaccination and antibiotic therapy of the entire herd.

Prevention: annual vaccination and rearing in confinement. *L. hardjo* control is difficult except in herds where only sporadic cases (abortion) are seen, when infected cows and seropositive young stock may be culled. All new purchased cattle should be tested and only negative cattle retained. Whole herd vaccination has the risk of persistent renal *hardjo* carriers.

Urolithiasis

Definition: formation of calculi within the urinary tract.

Etiology: urolithiasis has a multifactorial etiology including a relatively reduced fluid intake, mineral imbalance, high-concentrate intake and castration. The condition begins with microcalculus formation in the kidneys (509), and clinical problems arise when the calculi grow to a sufficient size to obstruct the urethra. The clinical syndrome is confined to the male (castrate or entire) where the urethral diameter is smaller.

Clinical features: early cases are dull, anorexic and walk stiffly. If grown sufficiently, rectal examination may reveal an enlarged and painful bladder. Diagnosis is made

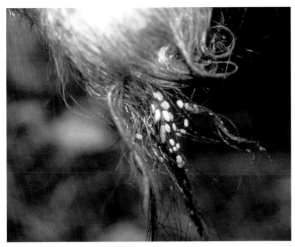

511

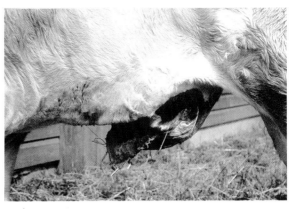

514

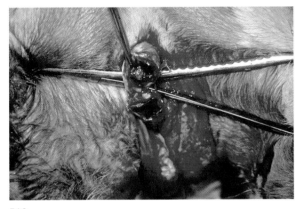

512

The Hereford steer in (513) has a large subcutaneous swelling containing urine as a result of urethral rupture in the sigmoid region. The swelling extends forwards from the sigmoid to the preputial orifice, which is discolored and shows dry preputial hairs covered with crystals. Sometimes the swelling is unusually discretely localized to the peripreputial area. In contrast, in a severe and advanced case the Friesian steer (514) had such severe swelling that ischemic necrosis has caused an extensive skin slough overlying the penis.

In another Hereford steer (515) it is the bladder rather than the urethra that has ruptured as a result of urethral obstruction, and urine has gathered in the ventral abdominal cavity, causing a progressive swelling and distension of the flanks (uroperitoneum).

Postmortem examination of a 6-year-old Shorthorn bull that died as a result of severe uremia following bladder rupture and uroperitoneum, reveals a congested

on the basis of changes in the preputial region. Although preputial crystals (often struvite, i.e., magnesium-ammonium-phosphate hexahydrate) appear in many calves (511), relatively few will develop signs of obstruction, which tends to occur in or just proximal to the sigmoid flexure, or in the distal portion of the penis. An intraoperative view (512) of the perineal region shows the dilated urethra proximal to the sigmoid flexure and the obstructing calculus. Continuing complete urethral obstruction results in either bladder or, more commonly, urethral rupture.

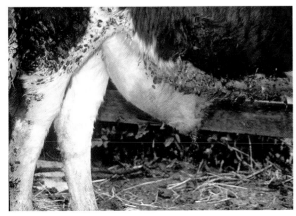

513

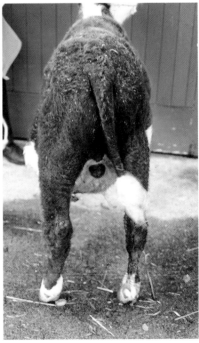

515

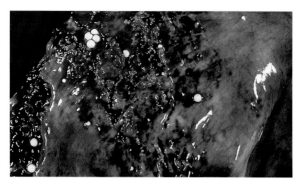

516

and hemorrhagic bladder mucosa (516). Numerous calculi (2–7 mm diameter) and fibrin are seen on the mucosal surface. The peritoneum tends to be diffusely inflamed, but the changes are less severe than those following septic reticuloperitonitis (219, 220). Urolithiasis frequently accompanies cases of severe pyelonephritis (507–509).

Differential diagnosis: in a mature bull this includes penile hematoma (527) or abscess formation, or, in a younger animal, urethral rupture due to faulty application of a bloodless castrator (Burdizzo) some days previously (see p. 157). Differentials for cases with ventral abdominal swelling not localized to the penis and prepuce include ascites (221), intestinal obstruction (218), and generalized peritonitis with massive exudation (220). Other differential diagnoses include cystitis (519), severe balanoposthitis, and severe preputial frostbite.

Management: cases of severe uremia will not pass meat inspection, so if the bladder and urethra are intact, antispasmodics may be tried for a limited period. If blockage persists, a perineal urethrotomy dorsal to the scrotum (512) is a salvage procedure. Urine scald and urethrostomal stricture may be subsequent problems. Rarely, a palpable single calculus can be removed by surgery. Fattening steers with distal urethral rupture and skin slough can also be salvaged to fatten.

Prevention: correction of Ca:P ratio in ration (about 2:1), avoidance of excessive Mg. Many calf rations now include ammonium chloride as a urinary acidifier. Provision of supplementary salt in concentrate feed (2–5%) which drastically increases fluid intake and dilutes urine.

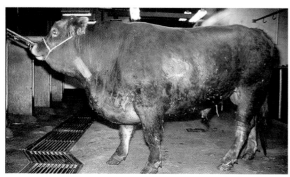

517

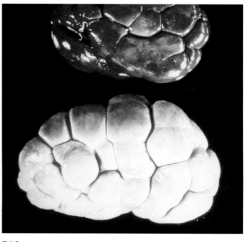

518

Therefore ensure easy access to fresh drinking water. Control possible primary cystitis (see below).

Amyloidosis

Definition: extracellular deposition of abnormal almost insoluble protein, amyloid, in various tissues is a sporadic disease. Reactive amyloidosis is derived from excessive serum protein SAA produced following chronic antigenic stimulation. More common is idiopathic (secondary) amyloidosis associated with chronic suppurative conditions.

Clinical features: the marked presternal edema in the 3-year-old Limousin bull in 517 was caused by severe bilateral renal amyloidosis, which is characterized by polyuria and massive proteinuria leading to pronounced hypoproteinemia.

In a chronic suppurative condition the bull's kidney in 518 is markedly enlarged, pale, waxy and granular in comparison with the normal kidney above it. This degree of enlargement should be detectable on rectal palpation.

Differential diagnosis: diagnosis is difficult, especially in the presence of co-existing disease, and includes pyelonephritis.

Management: amyloidosis is incurable, and cannot be prevented.

Cystitis

Definition: this inflammation of the bladder may be associated with pyelonephritis, urolithiasis or be idiopathic or mechanical in origin.

Clinical features: the 6-month-old heifer in 519 passed urine frequently and in small amounts. The perineal region had a foul odor of stale urine and shows excoriation as a result of urine dribbling. The tail is slightly elevated in-

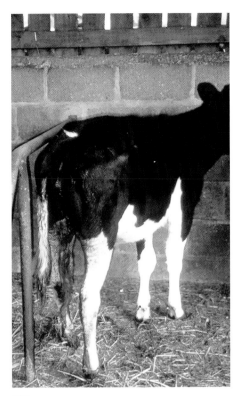

519

dicative of urinary tenesmus. The thickened bladder wall is often detectable on rectal examination of older animals.

Differential diagnosis: urinalysis will differentiate pyelonephritis and urolithiasis.

Management: aggressive parenteral amoxycillin or trimethoprim-sulfa drugs is usually effective in uncomplicated cases.

Male genital tract
Introduction

The anatomical separation of parts of the male genital tract, and their common development with parts of the urinary tract, makes integration of this section difficult. The section starts with congenital conditions, and continues with abnormalities affecting the penis, prepuce, scrotum, and, finally, the epididymis and seminal vesicles. Some congenital anomalies (e.g., persistent frenulum, cryptorchidism and testicular hypoplasia) may not become apparent until breeding age (1–2 years old).

Congenital male genital abnormalities
Pseudohermaphrodite (freemartin)

Definition: an individual with gonads of one sex but with contradictions in the morphological criteria of sex.

Clinical features: the condition is rare. The animal may be mistaken for female at birth owing to the origin of the urine flow. The freemartin condition is illustrated in 543–545.

Persistent penile preputial frenulum

Definition: persistence of or incomplete separation of the penis and prepuce along the ventral raphé during the first year.

Clinical features: in 520 the penile body remains attached to the prepuce by a fine, longitudinal band of connective tissue (A). Persistent penile frenulum causing penile deviation is a congenital anomaly, but signs, such as ventral penile deviation or a failure of complete protrusion, are usually first seen at attempted intromission. In some breeds it is inherited, and surgically corrected bulls should not be used to sire replacement breeding stock.

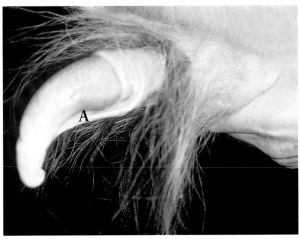

520

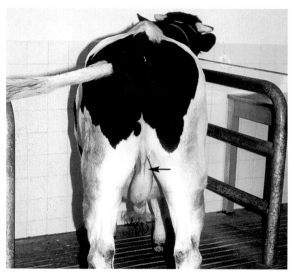

521

Testicular hypoplasia with cryptorchidism

The left testicle is descended and of normal size in the Friesian calf in **521**. The right testicle, which is small and incompletely descended, is in the scrotal neck.

Cryptorchidism

Definition: a condition characterized by incomplete development of one or both testes, including small size and incomplete descent.

Clinical features: bovine cryptorchidism, which is rare, is possibly associated with the polled character. In the 4-week-old Hereford cross calf in **522**, the normal right testicle is in the scrotal sac, but the left testicle is in an inguinal position (A). The misplaced gonad has deviated from the normal course of descent and may be termed an 'ectopic testicle'.

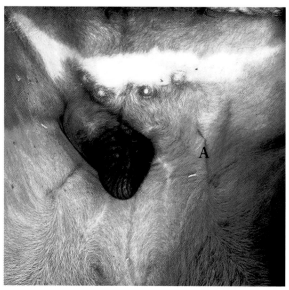

522

Penile conditions
Fibropapilloma ('wart')

Definition: a benign tumor of epithelial and connective tissue caused by a species-specific papovavirus.

Clinical features: the 2-year-old Friesian bull in **523** has several highly vascular, ulcerated masses attached to the glans penis. Caudal to the large mass is a smaller, more sessile fibropapilloma. These are typical sites for such multiple, proliferating masses, which are infectious, and relatively common in groups of young bulls confined in a small area.

Management: large masses may cause persistent penile protrusion and require removal (e.g., by ligation). Smaller tumors regress over time. **524** shows the same bull as in **523** 4 months later and soon afterwards he was used for service. In some cases healing is accompanied by scarring and distortion of the penile tunic, resulting in penile deviation and failure of intromission.

Spiral deviation of penis ('corkscrew penis')

Definition: spiral deviation is due to slipping of the dorsal apical ligament of the penis and may occur intermittently.

Clinical features: a spiral or corkscrew penile conformation is a normal occurrence at ejaculation in the vagina, but premature corkscrewing may be severe enough to prevent intromission. The first case, a 2-year-old Charolais,

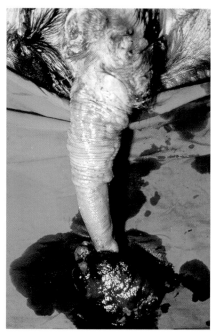

523

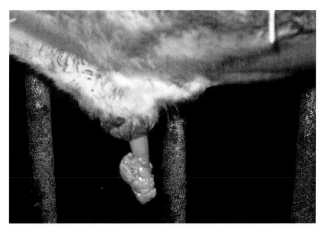

524

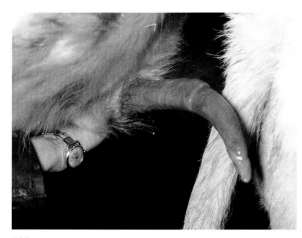

525

shows a 90° ventral curvature (**525**). The second case (**526**) clearly illustrates the spiraling effect, and the difficulty of intromission. In some bulls, an ulcer on the glans penis indicates abrasion from repeated perineal contact. Rarely is the condition traumatic.

Differential diagnosis: persistent penile frenulum in young bulls, scarring following fibropapillomata.

Management: surgical correction is possible, but ethical consideration is important if an inherited condition is suspected.

Penile and parapenile hematoma ('fracture of penis', 'broken penis')

Definition and pathogenesis: a localized collection of blood involves the corpus cavernosum penis (CCP) and is almost always through the dorsal wall of the tunica, just distal to the sigmoid flexure. The tunica albuginea is ruptured, producing a prescrotal hematoma and edema. Rupture occurs at ejaculation, or, less commonly, at intromission when the fully engorged penis is suddenly bent beyond its physiological limits, for example, when the cow or heifer suddenly moves.

Clinical features: a discrete swelling is seen in the Hereford bull in **527**, which also had a secondary prolapse of the penis. He cannot serve. The extent of the ruptured CCP is evident in the postmortem specimen of an affected penis (**528**) in which the sigmoid flexure is just proximal to the mass.

Differential diagnosis: parapenile abscess.

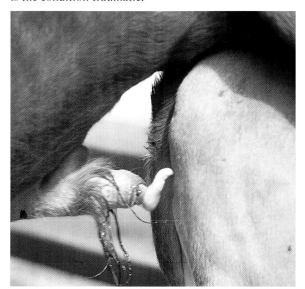

526

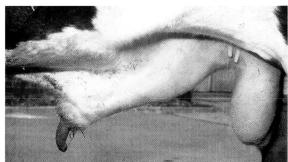

527

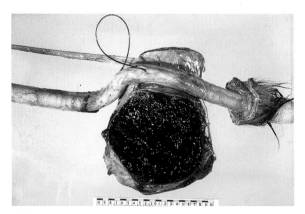

528

Management: small lesions may resolve after 4–6 months' rest in isolation away from cycling females. When service is attempted, some bulls experience further bleeding. Some cases develop into parapenile abscesses, at which stage surgical correction (careful drainage and evacuation) is no longer useful.

Preputial conditions

Prolapsed prepuce (preputial eversion)

Definition: skin lining the preputial cavity prolapses through the preputial orifice.

Clinical features: preputial prolapse occurs as a breed characteristic in *Bos indicus*, e.g., Brahman and Santa Gertrudis, and in polled breeds which are liable to have comparatively weaker preputial muscles. Injury and infection are common causes. A partial preputial prolapse of comparatively recent onset is shown in a 6-year-old Brahman from South Africa (**529**). The mucosa has a granular appearance, with areas of superficial hemorrhage. More severe cases are very prone to secondary trauma and edema.

Management: careful conservative medical management by cleansing, disinfection and replacement of the prolapse

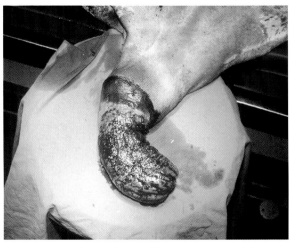

529

and retention by a purse-string suture. Surgical resection is required in severe cases. More serious cases cannot initially be replaced and must be pressure-bandaged, with daily bandage changes.

Preputial and penile abscess

Clinical features: in the 5-year-old Hereford bull in **530**, the penis has been manually prolapsed. The hand holds the prepuce and penis just caudal to the point of attachment of the preputial mucosa (internal lamina) to the body of the penis, shown as a transverse fold. Pus oozes from a mucosal tear incurred when the penis was extended. Deep-red erectile tissue is evident in the defect. Below the wound, the mucosa is smooth and slightly pinkish-gray due to a further abscess pocket.

Management: the prognosis is poor since effective and complete drainage of many abscesses in this area is difficult.

Posthitis and balanoposthitis

Definition: posthitis is an inflammation of the prepuce; balanoposthitis is an inflammation of both prepuce and penis.

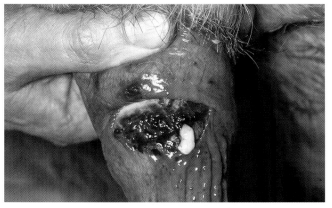

530

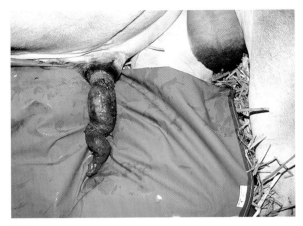

531

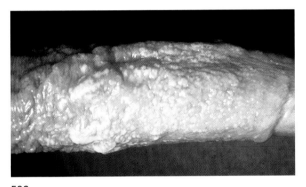

532

Some cases of balanoposthitis are due to genital IBR infection (**532**). This case of herpesvirus (BHV1) balanoposthitis shows multiple pale vesicles, some of which are confluent, in the preputial mucosa. The reflection of the prepuce onto the penis is to the right. Other cases of balanoposthitis have a traumatic origin.

Management: medical. The presence of severe and extensive adhesions is usually not amenable to treatment.

Scrotal conditions

Inguinal hernia

Clinical features: there is a soft, reducible swelling in the inguinal region overlying the two rudimentary teats in this Sussex bull from Zimbabwe (**533**). Neither the scrotal neck nor the body is enlarged, showing that only the inguinal canal is involved. An inguinal hernia may contain omentum, or both omentum and small intestinal loops. Cattle have a genetic predisposition to inguinal hernia, inheritance being recessive.

Differential diagnosis: in over-conditioned animals it can be difficult to differentiate fat deposits from a hernia. Abscessation is also possible.

Management: affected bulls should not be used to sire replacement stock.

Scrotal hernia

Definition: an inguinal hernia which has passed into the scrotum.

Clinical features: in **534** a 6-year-old Hereford bull shows an obvious swelling in the left side of the scrotal neck. It was soft, painless and partially reducible. This scrotal hernia resulted in the production of very poor quality semen due to local hyperthermia. The hernia had been acquired as a result of traumatic injury, and was not congenital. Scrotal hernia is rare in cattle, and seldom results in intestinal strangulation.

Clinical features: the Piedmontese bull in **531** developed a sudden prolapse of the prepuce and penis. Normal pink prepuce is visible at the skin junction. The central region of the prepuce is damaged (posthitis), the distal part of which forms a tight band around the penis, constricting the blood flow. The pink penis is congested and enlarged. The bull recovered well following conservative management.

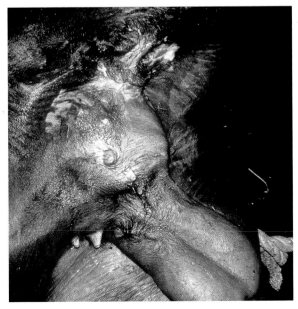

533

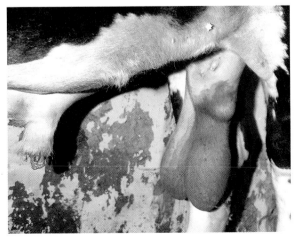

534

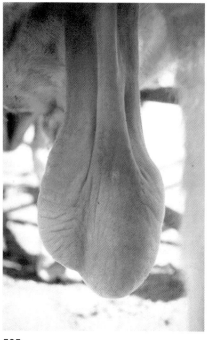

535

Differential diagnosis: unilateral orchitis.

Management: cull, as surgery is problematical.

Orchitis

Definition: inflammation of a testis.

Clinical features: in 535 the scrotum of a 4-year-old Simmental bull shows enlargement of the right testis, which is more dependent than the left. Note that the scrotal neck is not swollen. The testis was painful and

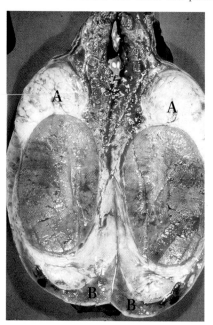

536

sensitive to touch. The etiology of this unilateral orchitis was probably traumatic, although various bacterial pathogens, including *Brucella abortus*, *Mycobacterium bovis* and *Arcanobacterium pyogenes*, have been isolated. In the acute *Brucella* orchitis illustrated in **536**, the inflammatory reaction in the tunics and epididymis caused a severe periorchitis (pale areas (A)), with early testicular necrosis as a result of testicular enlargement, and compression by the tunica albuginea. Ventrally, edematous fluid lies subcutaneously (B).

Differential diagnosis: scrotal hernia, scrotal hematoma.

Management: antibiotic therapy may be attempted in early stages. Recovered animals should be culled.

Scrotal hematoma

Clinical features: scrotal hematoma is common in beef bulls following trauma (**537**). The scrotum is large and relatively painless. The testicle remains normal, despite the large volume of blood on the right side.

Differential diagnosis: orchitis, scrotal hernia.

Management: most cases resolve spontaneously.

Scirrhous cord

Definition: fibrotic infected enlarged stump of spermatic cord following castration.

Clinical features: the scrotum is very swollen in the 4-month-old Friesian calf in **538**. A dried blood clot lies over the ventral scrotal incision (castration). Exploration revealed an enlarged stump of the spermatic cord, which resulted from infection acquired at surgery. Such wounds predispose calves to tetanus.

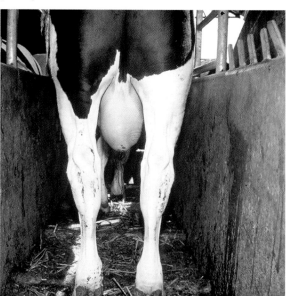

537

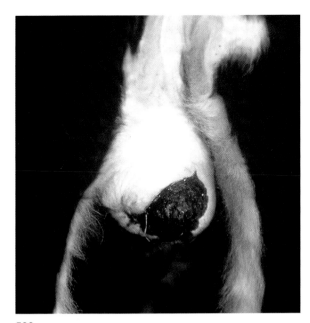

538

Management: in most calves provision of good drainage, cleansing of the stump and systemic antibiotics for 5–7 days is effective. In persisting problem cases amputation of stump of cord including all areas of microabscessation may be needed.

Prevention: clean surgical technique and aftercare (e.g., clean straw).

Scrotal necrosis and gangrene

Clinical features: the Friesian calf in **539** has an irregular necrotic line at the scrotal neck, separating gangrenous from normal tissue. The reaction is a result of faulty application of a bloodless castrator (Burdizzo). A continuous, crushed line encircles the scrotal neck, cutting off the blood supply to the lower skin. The same effect is obtained when a rubber castration ring is placed around the scrotal neck, and all tissue distal to the ring undergoes atrophy. When this is done relatively late, i.e., after

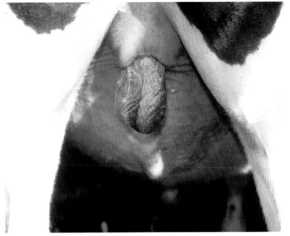

540

1 week old, the reaction is much more severe. In the Friesian calf in **540** the ring was applied at 2 months. Welfare legislation makes this procedure illegal in many countries. Note the considerable swelling proximal to the ring, compared with the shrivelled, dark, necrotic, distal portion.

If a bloodless castrator is applied too high, the urethra may be accidentally crushed, leading to urethral rupture, and a ventral, subcutaneous accumulation of urine similar to that following urethral calculus obstruction (**514**). Many countries have legal (statutory) upper limits on the age at which Burdizzo and rubber ring castration may be carried out.

Differential diagnosis: urolithiasis.

Management: calves with tissue swelling (**540**) should be given prophylactic antibiotics. Other cases may be left to slough naturally.

Scrotal frostbite

Clinical features: moderate frostbite affected the bottom of the scrotum of a 2-year-old Simmental (**541**) following exposure to a temperature of −30°C in Saskatchewan, Canada, 2–8 weeks previously. The semen

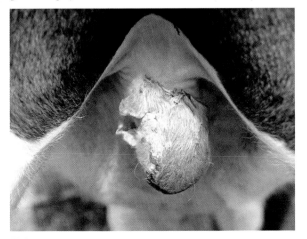

539

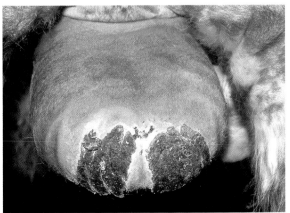

541

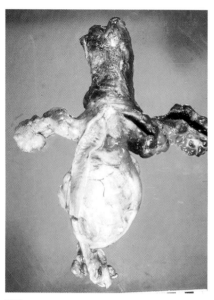

542

quality was poor (<10% live cells). Most cases return to normal semen quality within 2–3 months.

Seminal vesiculitis

Clinical features: although the right seminal vesicle of the bull in **542** is normal and the ampulla has its lumen exposed, the left ampulla is absent and the left seminal vesicle shows cystic, hemorrhagic and mild inflammatory changes. Seminal vesiculitis causes a purulent, preputial discharge after service, or pus may be seen in semen collected for artificial insemination (AI). Common organisms include *Arcanobacterium pyogenes*, *Brucella* and *Escherichia coli*. Young bulls are predominantly involved.

Diagnosis: seminal vesiculitis is diagnosed by rectal palpation and semen examination. Lack of symmetry, firmness and pain are the significant findings.

Management: incurable.

Female genital tract
Introduction

Maintenance of optimum fertility is of major economic importance in both beef and dairy herds. A high life-time output of milk and calves can only be attained if cows breed regularly, and considerable effort is expended on veterinary fertility examinations, health control, disease prevention and optimizing nutrition to achieve this. Much of this work cannot be adequately illustrated. For example, mineral and trace element deficiencies may affect fertility by reducing conception rates or interrupting ovarian cycles, but they cannot be demonstrated pictorially. Poor manage-

ment techniques, particularly heat detection, which is very important, are best demonstrated by an analysis of herd breeding records, and is not discussed in this atlas.

Diseases and disorders of the female genital tract are numerous. This chapter starts with a description of anatomical, congenital and developmental abnormalities, including cystic ovaries and neoplasia of the tract. The latter is comparatively rare. Dystocia is difficult to illustrate. Many conditions are diagnosed and corrected by intra-vaginal and intrauterine manipulation. Postpartum complications include vaginal wall rupture and hemorrhage, prolapse of parts of the genital tract (uterine prolapse is the most common) and metritis, endometritis and pyometra, all of which are sequelae of dystocia, which in turn is commonly the result of poor bull selection. There is often a conflict of interest between the use of a large breed bull to produce valuable offspring and a small breed to facilitate easy parturition. Not all pregnancies reach term and the final section of the chapter illustrates some causes of abortion and premature calving.

Congenital abnormalities

Intersexuality and freemartinism result from placental fusion in early pregnancy. Segmental aplasia of the müllerian duct system is inherited and leads to a range of abnormalities including white heifer disease (imperforate hymen). Ovarian agenesis, ovarian hypoplasia and fallopian tube aplasia have all been reported, but they are rare and, therefore, not illustrated.

Freemartinism

Definition: a sterile female born twin with a male.

Clinical features: in cattle, over 90% of twin calves have fused placentae, with a common blood supply. **543** shows how small the point of fusion may be. The heifer calf starts its development as a female, but, owing to the interchange of embryonic cells and hormones between the 30th and 40th days of pregnancy (i.e., before the stage of sexual dimorphism), many develop male characteristics. The freemartin is probably masculinized by the secretion

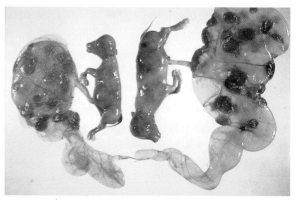

543

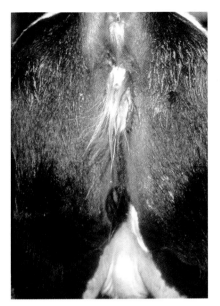

544

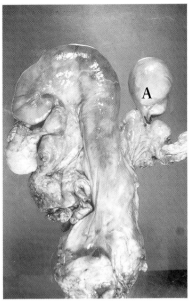

546

from its own gonads. The Friesian animal in **544** has an enlarged clitoris, and excess hair is growing as a tuft from the ventral vulval commissure. On rectal examination, no internal genitalia could be palpated beyond the cervix. Testicles were present in the scrotum, the right side of which is enlarged. Varying degrees of hypoplasia and masculinization may be seen. **545** demonstrates hypoplasia of the anterior vagina (A), an absence of the cervix, vestigial ovaries (B) and testes (C) that are joined to the immature uterine horns by ducts.

Diagnosis: vaginal length can be checked in young heifers using a test tube. Most cases are identified by rectal palpation of non-breeding heifers, and by external genital changes. Blood-sampling for chromosome analysis is possible as a freemartin has white cells containing both XY and XX chromosomes.

Segmental uterine aplasia ('white heifer disease', imperforate hymen)

Definition: segmental uterine aplasia is a developmental defect of the müllerian duct system, in which ovarian development allows normal estrus behavior, but the hymen

is often persistent. Pregnancy may occur in mild cases, with the persistent hymen sometimes leading to dystocia.

Clinical features: in the advanced case shown in **546**, the right uterine horn is aplastic, the residual portion (A) being dilated with cyclical fluid. This could be classified as uterus unicornis. The condition is due to a sex-linked recessive gene, but, despite its popular name of white heifer disease, it is not always related to coat color.

Double cervix (double os uteri externum)

Only the external cervical os is duplicated in this second example of a müllerian duct defect (**547**). An endoscopic view (**548**) illustrates placental membranes, visible through the left (upper dark) os. This relatively common

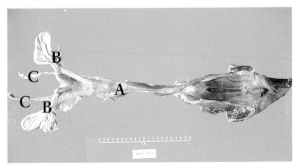

545

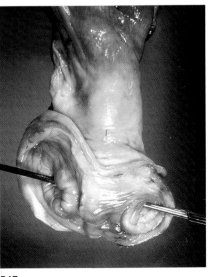

547

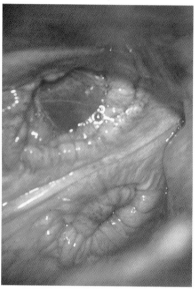

548

congenital condition leads to surprisingly few incidents of dystocia.

Ovarian disorders

Cystic ovaries

Ovarian cysts arise from a failure of ovulation. The anovulatory follicle increases in size to produce a fluid-filled structure greater than 2.5 cm in diameter, and normal ovarian cycles are usually interrupted. Cysts are not incompatible with pregnancy, however, and abattoir studies show a surprising number of pregnant cows with cysts. Stress, deficiencies, feeding for high milk yields and heredity are among the suggested causes. Although classically subdivided into luteal and follicular cysts, there is probably a degree of interchange between the two states. Many cysts resolve spontaneously, whilst others require treatment.

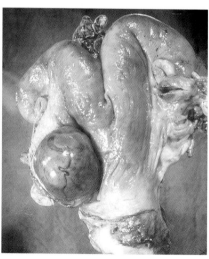

549

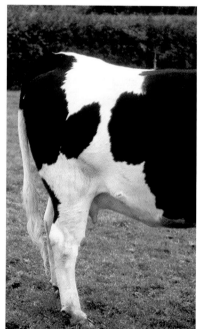

550

Luteal cyst

In **549** a single, large, spherical, thick-walled cyst is present in the left ovary. Luteal cysts secrete progesterone and may lead to prolonged anestrus. The right ovary contains an incised cystic corpus luteum.

Follicular cyst

In **550** the right ovary contains a large, thin-walled follicular cyst. Such cysts are invariably estrogenic and lead to irregular or prolonged estrus periods. Multilocular follicular cysts frequently occur. A corpus luteum, 5–7 days old, is present in the left ovary, suggesting that normal cyclicity can continue in the non-affected ovary. Cows with unresolved follicular cysts may develop both a raised tail head as a result of relaxation of the pelvic ligaments (**551**), and characteristic male behavioral changes, such as deep bellowing and pawing the ground.

551

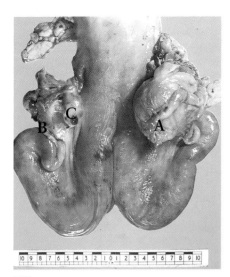

552

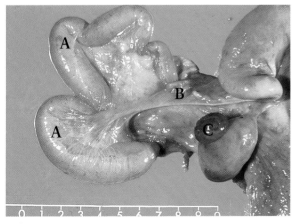

553

Management: control predisposing factors. Treatment with prostaglandin, GnRH or progesterone-releasing devices.

Bursal adhesions and hydrosalpinx

The bursa in **552** is tightly adherent to a large cyst in the right ovary, the oviduct (A) of which is distended with fluid (hydrosalpinx). The small visible portion (B) of the left oviduct is normal and the left ovary contains a 3–5-day-old corpus luteum (C). Bursal adhesions and hydrosalpinx can both result from rough handling of the ovary during, for example, manual rupture of ovarian cysts and enucleation of corpora lutea.

Hydrosalpinx is more pronounced in the oviduct of **553**, which is grossly distended with fluid (A) following a loss of patency. A small segment of normal duct (B) is visible on the bursa, as well as a 6–8-day-old corpus luteum on the ovary (C).

Management: adhesions alone do not necessarily result in infertility, as the fallopian tube may remain patent.

554

Patency can be tested by intrauterine infusion of dye.

Female genital tract tumors

Incidence: granulosa cell tumors are by far the most common ovarian neoplasms, but fibromas, sarcomas and carcinomas have been reported. Uterine fibromyomas, leiomyomas and lymphosarcomas are rare, whilst fibropapillomas (polyps) of the vagina and cervix are not uncommon.

Ovarian granulosa cell tumor

Definition: ovarian stromal neoplasm developing in the solid granulosa cells surrounding the ovum in the developing graafian follicle.

Clinical features: a large cystic neoplasm is seen in the right ovary in **554**. Initially estrogen-secreting, such tumors cause nymphomania. Advanced cases undergo luteinization, leading to anestrus or even masculinization. The incised uterine horn shows endometrial hyperplasia and mucometra.

Management: surgical ovariectomy is a simple procedure, although most cases would be culled.

Uterine lymphosarcoma (lymphoma)

Clinical features: usually seen as one of a number of sites for neoplasia in enzootic (adult) bovine leukosis (EBL), (**717, 718**), including heart, spinal canal (**347**) and liver, such uterine involvement (**555**) is easily appreciated on rectal palpation for pregnancy diagnosis. The mass is firm, smooth and local lymphadenopathy (lumbar nodes) is usually appreciable. Postmortem reveals multiple nodules of soft tan tissue in the uterine wall (**555**). All the masses involve the uterine wall which has been incised at two points to show the thickness.

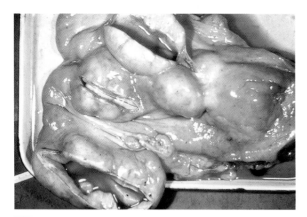

555

Differential diagnosis: early stage pregnancy, other uterine tumor (556).

Management: early cull.

Uterine fibromyoma

Definition: benign tumor containing fibroid elements, or leiomyoma.

Clinical features: seen as a smooth mass involving much of the uterine wall (556), and easily palpable on rectal examination. This type of tumor does not necessarily interrupt pregnancy.

Hydrops allantois (hydrops amnii)

Definition: excess fluid accumulating in allantoic or amniotic sac or both.

Clinical features: in hydrops allantois (hydrallantois) the lower abdomen is grossly and tightly distended bilaterally as a result of excess fluid accumulating in the uterus, usually in the allantoic sac (557). The condition develops in the seventh to ninth months of pregnancy, and is seen initially as a slowly progressive abdominal distention, with

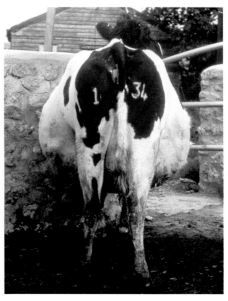

557

weight loss, inappetence, increasing dyspnea, difficulty in rising and eventual recumbency. Fetal death may occur, and hydrops may result in the rupture of the prepubic tendon (131). Fluid volumes of up to 300 liters have been recorded (normal 8–10 liters).

Differential diagnosis: rumen bloat, ascites, large abdominal tumor.

Management: induce parturition with prostaglandin $F_{2\alpha}$ or an analog, or corticosteroids. Shock, uterine inertia, dystocia and retained placenta are common complications, which frequently are fatal. Slaughter without treatment is likely to result in carcass condemnation for edema and emaciation, while welfare considerations prohibit transport in many countries.

Dystocia

Definition: difficult parturition.

Etiology: dystocia in cattle may be due to twins, fetal postural defects, fetal monstrosities (e.g., anasarca, 562, and schistosomus reflexus, 10), maternal problems (e.g., uterine torsion), and disproportion between fetal and maternal size. The latter is the most common cause, especially in heifers, and typically results from small undersized heifers, or from inappropriate bull selection leading to an oversized fetus, or from the restriction of available space in the pelvic birth canal by overfeeding of the dam. The conditions illustrated in this section are chosen as examples. The list is by no means comprehensive.

Management: many management options are available, e.g., traction, manual fetal manipulation (for malpresentation), embryotomy, cesarian section, etc.

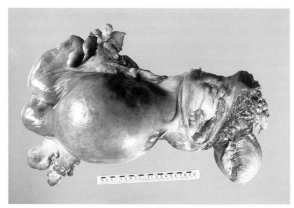

556

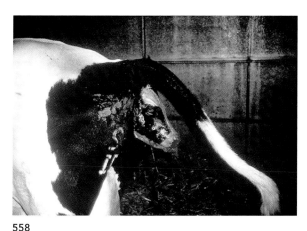

558

Prevention: correct sire selection and maternal nutrition.

Head only presentation

The case in **558** is not a longstanding dystocia, as the head is moist, of normal size, and has no tongue protrusion. The shoulders will be at the pelvic inlet, the forelimbs in the uterus.

Head and one leg presentation

In **559** a more longstanding case of dystocia (leg back) is illustrated. The head is dry and swollen and the protruding tongue is edematous. The enlarged and edematous vulval lips may persist for 24–48 hours after parturition.

Posterior presentation, with fetal dorsoventral rotation

Initial observation of the calf's feet and fetlocks in **560** might suggest a case of anterior presentation, with lateral deviation of the head (head back). Closer inspection shows the hocks at the vulva, but the point of the hock

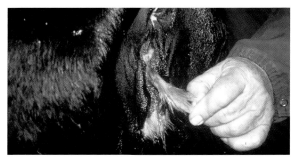

560

(os calcis) is ventral. Rotation facilitated delivery of a live calf.

Breech presentation (hip flexion)

In **561** only the tail is visible and there is no vulval enlargement. Since insufficient fetal mass can enter the birth canal to stimulate abdominal contractions, many breech presentations pass unrecognized for several hours, or even days, and the calf is then often stillborn.

Anasarca

Definition: extensive subcutaneous edema.

Clinical features: note the subcutaneous edema over the head, chest and abdomen in the anasarca calf in **562**. Although many cases can be delivered *per vaginum* by slow traction and lubrication, in this, a neglected case, it led to maternal death from uterine rupture. Fetal anasarca in Ayrshires is hereditary. Other fetal monstrosities leading to dystocia include arthrogryposis (**12**), schistosomus reflexus (**10**), perosomus elumbus (absence of lumbar spine and pelvis) and ascites.

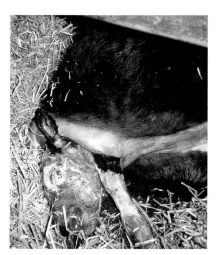

559

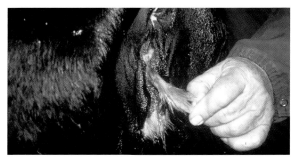

561

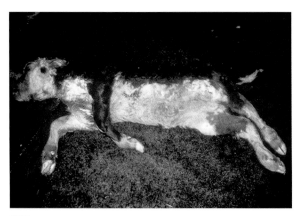

562

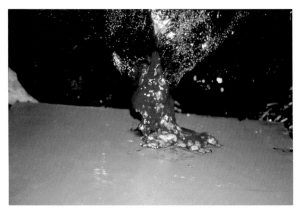

564

Uterine torsion

Clinical features: the anterior vagina can be seen to be rotated clockwise (**563**). About 75% of cases involve an anticlockwise torsion of 90–360°, detected clinically as a spiral effect on the vaginal wall. Torsion develops at the very end of pregnancy, during late first-stage or early second-stage labor, and is usually associated with a large calf. A live calf was delivered from this cow, following correction of the torsion, but many are stillborn.

Management: in most cases correction is by uterine manipulation *per vaginum*, or by rolling the cow in the same direction as torsion. But many cows also have incomplete cervical relaxation, resulting in dystocia, so that cesarian section may then prove the best option.

Postpartum complications

Introduction: normal, unassisted births result in few complications. However, after dystocia, particularly in cases of maternal disproportion involving considerable traction, complications are frequent. The most common is endometritis, which depresses subsequent fertility. Some of the more dramatic, but fortunately less frequent, complications illustrated here include vaginal wall rupture, uterine

and other prolapses, rectovaginal fistula and septic vaginitis. A retained placenta can follow a normal parturition. Manual or endoscopic examination of discharges from the cervix and anterior vagina play an important role in prebreeding examination carried out as part of a herd fertility control program. A range of discharges encountered is illustrated with some gross uterine pathology.

Vaginal wall rupture and hemorrhage

Clinical features: vaginal wall rupture with hemorrhage is a common complication, seen especially in overfat heifers with large calves, insufficient lubrication during traction, and excessively rapid traction that does not permit normal vaginal and vulval dilation. Preventive episiotomy is useful. Typically, the lateral vaginal wall tears approximately 10–20 cm from the vulval lips, dorsal to the external urethral orifice. A large mass of pelvic fat may prolapse through the tear and protrude through the vulval lips (**564**). Rupture of the vaginal artery, a branch of the internal pudendal artery that is easily palpated in the lateral vaginal wall at the point of tearing, can result in severe and often fatal hemorrhage within an hour of parturition (**565**). Fortunately, the blood vessel was identified and ligated in this heifer, although she subsequently developed a severe perivaginitis and localized pelvic peritonitis.

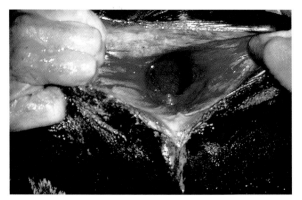

563

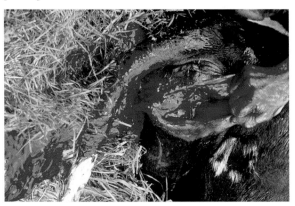

565

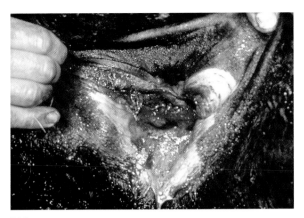

566

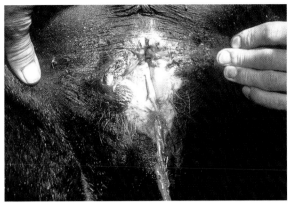

568

Management: prevention is based on avoidance of dystocia (sire selection, dam nutrition) and careful delivery (ample lubricant, slow traction). The early recognition of the potential (episiotomy) or recent problem (vaginal tear, arterial rupture) may lead to corrective surgical steps. Delay, whether resulting from failure of observation or incorrect diagnosis, may result in death.

Rectovaginal fistula

Definition: traumatic connection between rectum and vagina.

Clinical features: rectovaginal fistula is a complication of dystocia, usually resulting from an oversized or mal-presented fetus. In **566** (taken 5 days postpartum) the ventral anal mucosa is torn and there are extensive lacerations to the dorsal vaginal wall. The white material on the vaginal floor originates from intrauterine therapy. In the same cow three months later (**567**) the vaginal and

anal lacerations had healed spontaneously, leaving a small, deformed area. Although fertility is usually reduced, due to development of pneumovagina or aspiration of feces into vagina, this cow became pregnant in each of the next 2 years.

Management: only small fistulae will heal spontaneously. Most require surgical repair. Large fistulae are untreatable. Some untreated cows do, however, remain fertile.

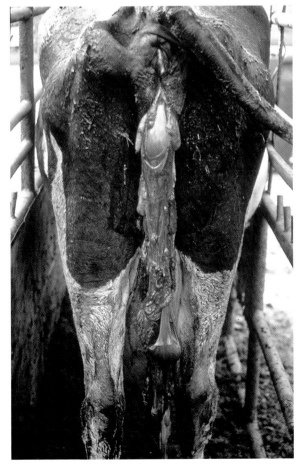

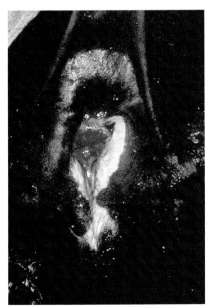

567

569

Septic vulvitis and vulvovaginitis

Clinical features: in 568 small, infected skin fissures are seen around the dorsal margin of the enlarged vulva, 4 days after the difficult delivery of an oversized calf. A length of placenta is seen in the ventral vulva. In severe cases of septic vulvitis the vulva is inflamed and edematous, especially at the ventral commissure, and there is often a purulent hemorrhagic discharge from the vulva. A raised tail and tenesmus indicate discomfort. Although trauma at parturition is the commonest cause of vulval edema and cellulitis, the condition may also be the result of irritant feces caused by acute diarrhea.

Management: parenteral antibiotics, and also NSAIDs if pain and tenesmus are evident.

Retained placenta

Clinical features: a retained placenta (569) is typically associated with factors that interfere with the third stage of labor, such as twins, prolonged parturition, excessive manual interference, abortion and premature calving, cows that are overfat or too thin, and vitamin, mineral and trace element deficiencies as vitamin E and selenium. In 569, taken 4 days postpartum, the placenta is turning pink due to autolysis, and the udder is stained with a foul uterine discharge.

Management: treatment is controversial! Attempt *gentle* traction after a few days, while parenteral antibiotics for any pyrexia will assist resolution.

Prevention: attend to causative factors.

Vulval discharges, endometritis, metritis and pyometra

Clinical features: vulval discharges may be associated with septic vulvovaginitis, a retained placenta, metritis

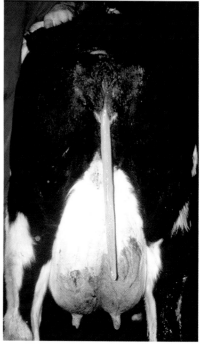

571

and endometritis. The type of discharge depends on the interval from calving to clinical examination, and on the degree of endometritis. Many discharges are normal and do not require treatment. Postestral blood in clear mucus is derived from uterine caruncle hemorrhage (570). A plug of cervical mucus (571), which may be seen immediately prepartum or postpartum, is normal. Discolored mucus containing red-brown material (572), or globules of yellow detritus (573), are examples of lochia that would not normally be treated.

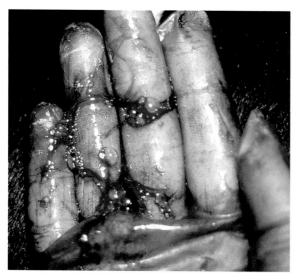

570

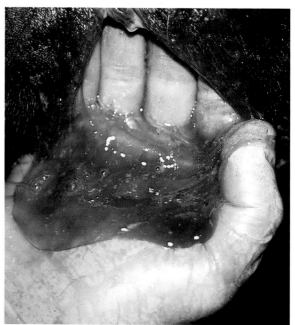

572

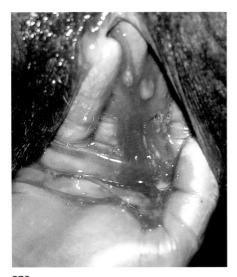

573

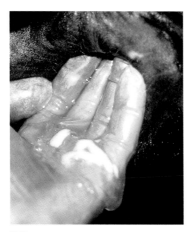

575

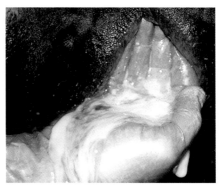

576

Endometritis is first seen by the herdsman as a white purulent vulval discharge from a cow lying in a cubicle, the material often being deposited on the back of the standing (574).

Clear mucus containing white flecks (575) is believed to indicate a low-grade endometritis. A thick, white discharge is typically indicative of a significant endometritis, especially if accompanied by a purulent smell. *Arcanobacterium pyogenes* and *Fusobacterium necrophorum* are commonly involved. Some cases have blood mixed with white globules (576). Metritis is indicated by a stinking, brown discharge (577), particularly when the consistency is fluid and not mucoid. Affected animals often show systemic signs. For example, the cow in 578 was scouring and recumbent, with a sunken eye exposing congested conjunctiva. She died within a few hours as a result of toxemia and severe dehydration.

On postmortem, the incised horn exposed necrotic cotyledons in brown, purulent fluid (579). An area of caseopurulent perimetritis is seen above the incision, with discoloration and inflammation extending over the cervix and onto the pelvic vagina.

Management: vaginal examination and treatment of endometritis, where necessary, is an important part of routine herd fertility control, especially in dairy herds. Reference should be made to appropriate texts for details. Prevention depends on avoidance of dystocia, correct dam nutrition, especially in the periparturient period, control of metabolic disease and proper hygiene at calving.

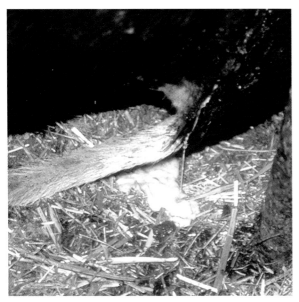

574

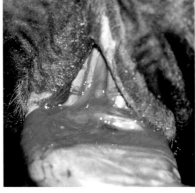

577

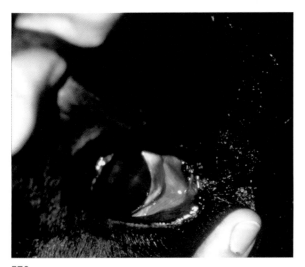

578

Vaginal prolapse

Etiology: although it may occasionally be seen after parturition, vaginal prolapse typically occurs in older cows in late pregnancy. It is associated with excess perivaginal fat, any type of vaginal or rectoanal irritation leading to tenesmus, older cows, estrogenic factors in feed leading

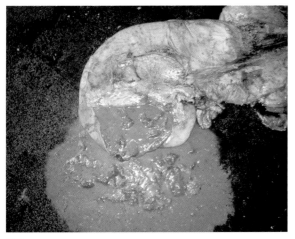

579

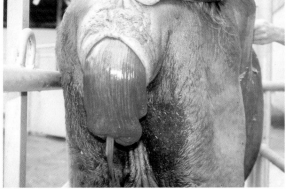

580

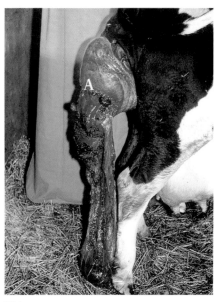

581

to pelvic ligament relaxation, and with certain beef breeds, particularly Herefords.

Clinical features: the fresh, red appearance of the prolapse in **580** indicates that it is recent, with only mild congestion from exposure. A plug of cervical mucus is visible at the lower extremity. Prolonged cases become engorged and irritant, stimulating straining. Prolapse of the vaginal wall with dystocia, as in **581**, is uncommon. The vagina is the large everted structure protruding from the vulva and ending at the cervix (A). The fetus is still within the placenta, its forefoot being palpable through the partially dilated cervix.

Management: in individual cows prepartum prolapse can be controlled by manual replacement and a purse-string suture in the vulva. It is vital to check for the onset of parturition, when the suture should be released. In the case of **581** manual replacement and minimal assistance resulted in a normal birth. In herds with multiple cases the above predisposing factors should be examined carefully.

Cervical prolapse

Cervical prolapse is similar in etiology to vaginal prolapse. Small portions of the external os of the cervix may protrude through the vulva in cows in late pregnancy or early lactation (**582**), often disappearing when they stand. A more advanced case is shown in the postpartum Shorthorn cow in **583**. The external os is edematous and grossly distended. A short length of vaginal wall is exposed between the cervix and vulva. Complete cervicovaginal prolapse may occur.

Management: small prolapses may resolve spontaneously. Larger masses should be cleansed, replaced and held in place with transverse vulval sutures.

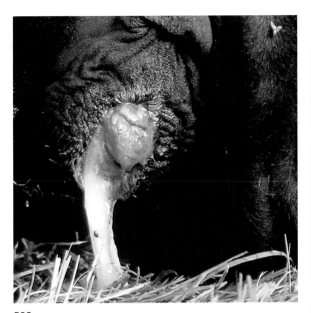

582

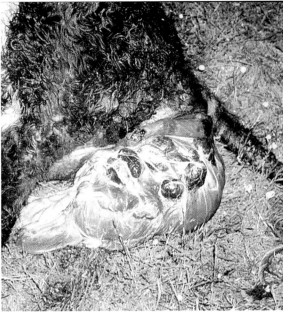

584

Uterine prolapse

Most cases of uterine prolapse occur within a few hours of calving. They are typically seen in older cows following dystocia or delivery of a large fetus, and may be associated with hypocalcemia or a retained placenta. The young Hereford cow in **584** has a prolapse of less than 2 hours' duration. The placenta is still attached and has a moist, fresh appearance. Most animals remain recumbent. Those which do move may traumatize the prolapse, increasing the risk of death from hemorrhage and shock. The Shorthorn cow in **585** has a complete prolapse of the uterus, vagina and cervix. This is a rare condition and, like other cases involving the vagina and cervix, although the prolapse was replaced, she died within 12 hours as a result of shock and internal hemorrhage.

Management: treat as emergency! The uterus can be protected from trauma and contamination by wrapping in a clean sheet, but many cows are best left lying undisturbed. Replace under epidural anesthesia with recumbent cow in ventral recumbency with hind legs extended back, or by lifting hindquarters off the ground. Administer oxytocin, antibiotics, calcium borogluconate, and NSAIDs in possibly shocked cases. Most cows recover well, remain fertile, and recurrence at subsequent parturition is unlikely.

Vaginal and cervical polyps

Although not a postpartum complication, vaginal polyps are sometimes confused with an early prolapse. The vaginal

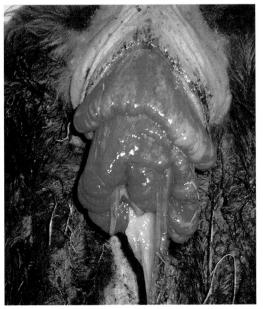

583

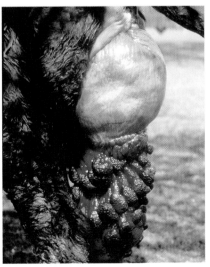

585

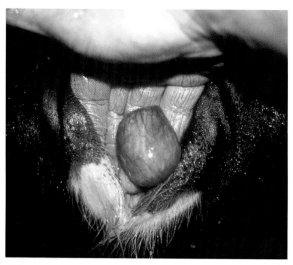

586

polyp in **586** was pedunculated and protruded from the vulva in late pregnancy, disappearing postpartum when abdominal pressure was reduced.

Management: no treatment necessary.

Abortion and premature parturition

Definition: abortion has been defined as the premature expulsion of the products of conception, typically producing a dead calf. Premature calving occurs late in gestation, to give a live but weak calf, or a dead calf which would have been capable of an independent existence. Both phenomena may have similar infectious and noninfectious causes.

Clinical features: possible infectious factors include brucellosis, IBR, BVD, leptospirosis, vibriosis (*Campylobacter*), bluetongue, neosporosis, listeriosis, *Chlamydia*, *Coxiella*, aspergillosis and, important in the Western USA, epizootic bovine abortion. Noninfectious factors

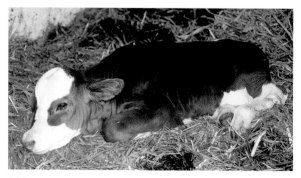

588

include stress, lethal genes (e.g., arthrogryposis), poisons (e.g., locoweed (**737**) and mycotoxins), nutritional deficiencies (e.g., vitamin E, selenium or iodine (**75**)), and physical injuries. The appearance of an aborted fetus (**587** was aborted at 7 months of gestation) often gives little indication of the cause.

Many of the causes of abortion listed above are not illustrated, as they have no specific diagnostic features in the placenta or fetus.

Differential diagnosis: specific diagnostic tests are necessary, but despite careful investigation, the cause of abortion is found in less than 25% of all cases.

Management: dam occasionally needs treatment for endometritis (p. 167). Identify cause. Vaccines are available against BVD, IBR and leptospirosis. Control possible oral ingestion of aspergillus, listeria and toxins. Consider culling carrier cows with neospora.

Premature calf

In addition to a reduced body size, the premature (7 months) Simmental crossbred calf in **588** shows hyperemia (reddening) of the mouth and nostrils, soft hooves and a short, 'staring' coat. Most causes of abortion mentioned previously can also produce premature births. Leptospirosis was the most probable cause in this case as the dam had a titer of 1:1600 to *Leptospira hardjo*.

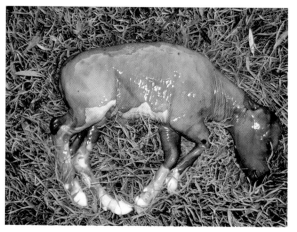

587

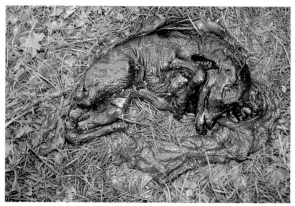

589

Mummified fetus

The fetus in **589** died at approximately 4 months of gestation, but was not expelled until 8 months. Note the sunken eye sockets and the characteristic dry, chocolate-brown color of the decomposing fetus and placenta. BVD and *Neospora* are two common causes of mummification. Stress in early pregnancy may predispose. Certain bulls, especially Jerseys, may genetically produce an increased incidence of mummified fetuses.

Abortion

Brucellosis (contagious abortion, Bang's disease)

Definition: brucellosis is a bacterial infection caused in cattle by *Brucella abortus*.

Clinical features: susceptible cattle ingest material from an infected fetus, placenta or uterine discharge and typically abort between 7 and 8 months of gestation. A marked placentitis may occur in the form of small, white, necrotic foci on the cotyledons and thickening of the intercotyledonary placenta (**590**). Organisms are shed in milk as well as uterine discharges. Most cows only abort once, although they may remain persistent carriers and excrete *Brucella* at subsequent normal parturitions. Retained placenta, endometritis and infertility are common complications.

In the bull, the testicles (**536**) and seminal vesicles may be affected, although infection is only rarely present in the semen. Brucellosis is transmissible to humans, and is a notifiable disease in many countries.

Differential diagnosis: other causes of abortion, e.g., trichomoniasis, leptospirosis, IBR, neosporosis. Diagnosis by blood agglutination tests, milk ring test, CF tests.

Management: many countries have national eradication programs involving testing, elimination of reactors and vaccination in calves.

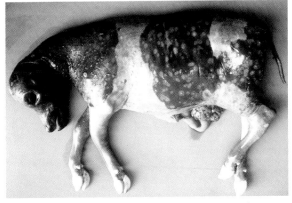

591

Mycotic abortion

Definition: systemic mycoses (aspergillosis, rarely candidiasis and zygomycosis) tend to be sporadic nonspecific syndromes which can lead to abortion.

Clinical features: moldy silage which was accidentally fed to 20 cows in late pregnancy led to systemic aspergillosis. Hematogenous spread, leading to fetal infection, produced three abortions in 10 days. *Aspergillus* was isolated from the fetuses. In some cases, small, circular, ringworm-like lesions (**591**) are seen on the fetal skin.

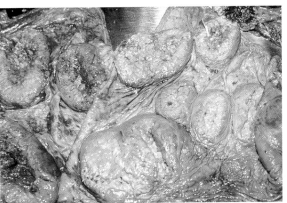

592

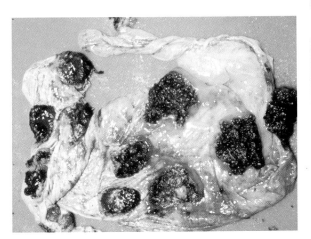

590

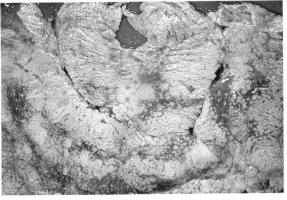

593

There may also be a pronounced thickening of the placenta and necrosis of the cotyledons (592). Abortions tend to occur from 4 months to term, and are commoner in the winter months. *Mucor* species may also be involved, producing a yellow discoloration and degeneration of the serosal surface of the placenta (593).

Diagnosis: based on skin lesions, demonstrations of hyphae in fetal dermatitis, especially on eyelids, placental lesions, bronchopneumonia and possibly abomasal contents.

Management: avoidance of moldy feed.

chapter 11

Udder and teat disorders

Introduction

The dairy cow is bred and fed to produce large volumes of milk. With the metabolic stress of high performance and the physical effects of being milked and handled two or three times daily, it is not surprising that the udder and teats are subject to a wide variety of disorders. The primary disease, mastitis, is of worldwide economic importance and much money is spent on its prevention, treatment and control. The first part of the chapter deals with mastitis in lactating and dry cows, and describes changes that may be seen in milk. The second part illustrates teat lesions, including a wide variety of viral infections, notably bovine herpes mammillitis, cowpox and pseudocowpox, vesicular stomatitis and fibropapillomas (warts). Other systemic diseases that also affect the teats, for example foot-and-mouth disease, are mentioned elsewhere.

Because of their anatomical position, especially in cows with pendulous udders, teats are vulnerable to injuries, eczema and other physical influences. These problems are considered in the third part, although changes associated with photosensitization are covered elsewhere (80). The final part of the chapter includes miscellaneous conditions of the udder.

Mastitis

Summer mastitis

Definition: severe form of mastitis, typically in a dry heifer or cow, liable to lead to extensive parenchymal damage and loss of the quarter, commonly involving *Arcanobacterium pyogenes* and many other organisms, and transmitted by the sheep head fly, *Hydrotoea irritans*.

Clinical features: this endemic form of suppurative mastitis, with a characteristic foul odor, typically occurs

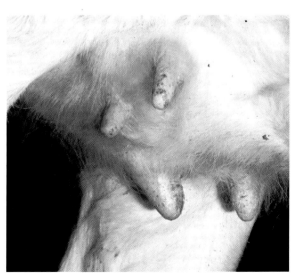

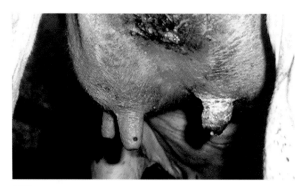

595

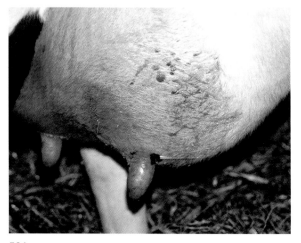

596

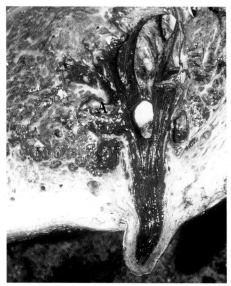

597

sporadically in mid–late summer. It may also arise from a teat sphincter injury in a lactating cow. Mild cases become only slightly ill, whilst the more severely affected cows are dull, pyrexic and anorexic. They may abort, or produce weakly calves at term. Acute, untreated cases may die. Very few quarters recover, although cases are very occasionally mild enough to pass unrecognized until calving, when the affected quarter is nonfunctional ('blind') (see

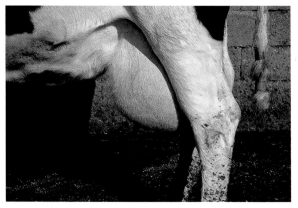

598

also **603**) and the teat is palpably thickened. Occasionally summer mastitis is seen in a bull or a young calf.

The Charolais heifer in **594** is an early case, showing distension of the left hind quarter, which was typically hard and sore, with a prominent, turgid teat. In more advanced cases, the infection may burst through the udder, as shown in the right hind quarter in **595**. A thickening of the central teat canal was palpable, the quarter was very hard, and yellow pus with a pungent odor was discharging from the teat and udder.

Management: parenteral treatment with antibiotics possibly and NSAIDs will reduce the systemic effects. Local antibiotic treatment of the quarter is rarely successful, but frequent stripping or surgical drainage may prevent udder abscessation.

Control includes dry cow therapy with longacting intramammary antibiotics, fly repellents, and keeping cattle away from known fly areas. In high-risk areas fly repellents should ideally be applied to the udder weekly. Teat sealants are also used as a protective film.

Acute mastitis

Introduction: peracute and acute mastitis are most commonly seen in the first few weeks after calving, and may result from recrudescence of dormant dry period infections, although cases can occur throughout lactation. In most

599

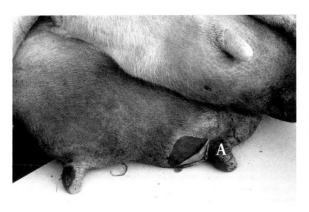

600

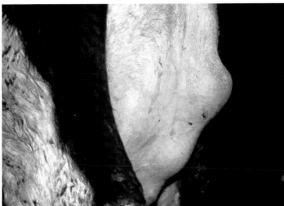

602

cases, peracute mastitis with toxemia results from coliform infections. Similarly, in acute mastitis, environmental organisms such as coliforms (e.g., *Escherichia coli*) or *Streptococcus uberis* are frequently involved. Immune suppression occasionally leads to acute disease from 'contagious' mastitis organisms such as staphylococci, which are carried on the skin or in the udder of affected cows and transmitted to other cows during milking.

Clinical features: the most prominent sign of acute mastitis is an enlarged, hard, hot and painful quarter. This may be apparent before any changes are visible in the milk. In some cases, a brown serous discharge may be seen on the surface of the affected quarter and teat, as in the lactating Friesian cow in 596. In a section of an affected udder (597), deep red inflammation of the teat cistern and teat canal mucosa is seen. There is prominent subcutaneous edema and the skin at the tip of the teat is congested. Changes of this nature can lead to gangrene. The yellow foci (A) in the udder parenchyma are pockets of pus. In 598 the teat skin, which was still warm and soft, and the affected quarter, are encircled by a ring of black gangrene, with red erythema at the periphery. The cow was severely ill with an eventually fatal toxemia.

Such cases should not be confused with udder bruising (599). In this cow the forequarter is obviously enlarged, the front teat deviates medially, and a blue discoloration is seen on the lower half of both quarters. The cow was,

however, bright and alert, there were no visible changes in the milk, and the skin remained warm.

Advanced gangrene (600) leads to cold, damp teat skin. Although mastitis was limited to the left fore quarter (A), the entire udder was blue, edematous, and cold to the touch. Adjacent to the affected teat is a skin slough and red exudate. The secretion from the udder was a deep port-wine color and was mixed with gas. The cow had been normal when milked 12 hours previously, indicating the peracute onset of disease. In cases of nonfatal, gangrenous mastitis the overlying skin (601), or even the entire affected quarter, sloughs in a process which may take 1–2 months.

Management: intramammary antibiotics are the primary treatment for individual quarters, combined with parenteral antibiotics, fluid therapy and NSAIDs for more acute cases. Continual stripping of affected quarters, and parenteral oxytocin allegedly improves recovery rate. Prevention depends on reducing pathogen concentration at the teat orifice and correct machine function. Environmental hygiene, correct pre-milking teat preparation, avoidance of mechanical trauma to the teat sphincter (623, 624), and minimization of teat end impacts are all important points. Standard texts give details.

Chronic mastitis and blind quarter

Definition: *Streptococcus agalactiae*, *S. dysgalactiae*, *S. uberis*, staphylococci, *Arcanobacterium pyogenes* and other bacteria can produce a chronic mastitis, manifested as 'clots' in the milk (606), with or without palpable udder changes.

Clinical features: the Friesian cow in 602 shows large, hard nodules protruding from the udder, with two in the right quarter and one in the left. These are chronic, intramammary, staphylococcal abscesses. Staphylococci were cultured from the milk, which had a high cell count and gave a strongly positive reaction to the California mastitis test. Such advanced cases, which are usually unresponsive to treatment, are dangerous carriers and should

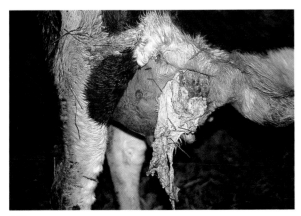

601

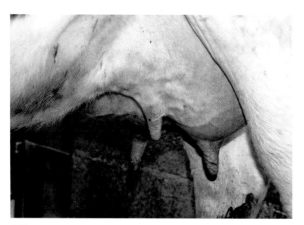

603

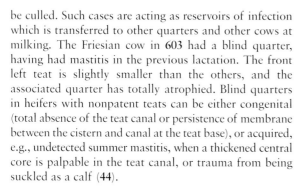

605

be culled. Such cases are acting as reservoirs of infection which is transferred to other quarters and other cows at milking. The Friesian cow in **603** had a blind quarter, having had mastitis in the previous lactation. The front left teat is slightly smaller than the others, and the associated quarter has totally atrophied. Blind quarters in heifers with nonpatent teats can be either congenital (total absence of the teat canal or persistence of membrane between the cistern and canal at the teat base), or acquired, e.g., undetected summer mastitis, when a thickened central core is palpable in the teat canal, or trauma from being suckled as a calf (**44**).

Management: treatment options are as for environmental infections. Control of contagious mastitis rests on reducing cow-to-cow spread of infection during the milking process. Milking hygiene (gloves, liners, paper towels, etc.), early detection and treatment of cases, thorough post-milking teat disinfection, correct milking machine function, dry cow antibiotic therapy and culling are important control measures. Raised cell counts in the bulk tank milk may lead to financial penalties.

Mastitic changes in milk

Milk is thicker and more viscous during the dry period and immediately postpartum (i.e., colostrum). Its character

also changes in mastitis. Although specific types of mastitic infection frequently lead to similar changes in milk, the appearance of the milk is *not* pathognomonic, and bacteriological examination is required to confirm the causative organism and to determine the antibiotic sensitivity.

Blood in milk

Clinical features: true blood clots are the characteristic feature of blood in milk. They may be present in slightly pink-tinged milk (**604**) or, in more severe cases, in a secretion that is almost totally red (**605**). Seen only in newly calved cows, or after trauma, the condition usually resolves spontaneously. Herd outbreaks of unknown etiology may occur.

Management: no treatment has been found to be consistently useful. Incomplete milking leading to increased intramammary pressure is believed to assist in hemostasis, but as this increases the risk of a new quarter infection, antibiotic cover should be given.

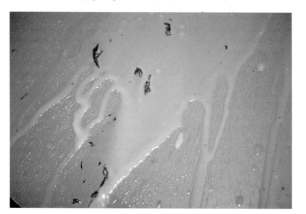

604

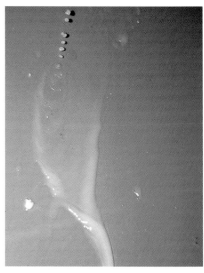

606

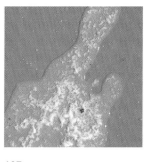

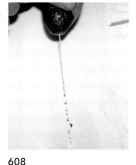

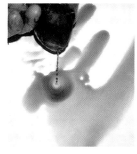

607 608 609

Mastitic milk

Clinical features: watery, translucent milk with occasional clots (**606**) is typical of a mild mastitis such as that caused by *S. agalactiae* or *dysgalactiae*. Normal milk may be totally absent in severe staphylococcal (**607**) or *Arcanobacterium pyogenes* infections, when the secretion consists of thick clots suspended in a clear, serous fluid. Summer mastitis (often *Actinomyces*) invariably produces a thick secretion with a characteristic pungent odor.

A brownish, serum-colored secretion is typical of *Escherichia coli* infection (**608**), while acute gangrenous mastitis (e.g., acute staphylococcal) may produce a red or brown homogenous secretion (**609**), often mixed with gas.

Infectious teat conditions

Introduction: teats are affected by two pox viruses, pseudocowpox (paravaccinia), a mild infection that occurs throughout the world, and cowpox (vaccinia), which is now extremely rare. Both are transmissible to man. The parapoxvirus of pseudocowpox is related to bovine papular stomatitis (**155, 156**). Bovine herpes mammillitis (BHM) is a much more severe infection and may be confused clinically with the teat changes associated with necrotic dermatitis (udder seborrhea). Other viral infections producing teat lesions include vesicular stomatitis (**617, 618**), fibropapillomas (**620–622**), bluetongue (**661**), foot-and-mouth disease (**646**) and rinderpest (**652**). Teats are also subject to physical injury, chapping and eczema often exacerbated by cold, wet conditions and poor milking machine function. Examples include hyperkeratosis and 'black spot' of the teat sphincter (**629**), summer (licking) sores (**630**), trauma, and photosensitization (**80**).

Bovine herpes mammillitis (BHM)

Definition: infectious ulcerative dermatitis of teats and udder skin caused by bovine herpes virus 2.

Clinical features: BHM initially produces fluid-filled vesicles, seen in the center and towards the tip of the teat in **610**. The overlying epithelium is tense and white. The initial vesicles rupture easily to expose raw, ulcerated areas (seen between the two vesicles in **610**), which coalesce and later become covered by thick scabs (**611**). The condition is so painful that it is often impossible to milk affected cows (compare pseudocowpox, **612–615**). BHM tends to occur in outbreaks, most commonly in first calving heifers soon after calving, and secondary mastitis is a major problem. Calves sucking affected cows can develop ulcers on the muzzle, buccal mucosa and tongue, may become febrile and lose weight. Many cases occur in the first few weeks postpartum and are thought to result from immune suppression in the periparturient carrier cow. Persistent herd infection is possible. Lifelong immunity follows recovery.

Differential diagnosis: necrotic dermatitis (**640**), bluetongue (**661**), FMD (**649**) and pseudocowpox (**612**).

Management: iodophor teat disinfectants help to prevent spread. Isolation has not been helpful.

Pseudocowpox (parapox)

Definition: teat infection caused by a paravaccinia virus.

Clinical features: pseudocowpox is a worldwide infection, spreading slowly within a herd. Both the teats

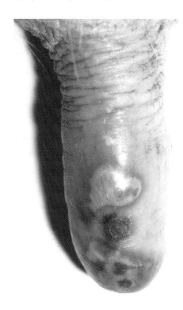

610

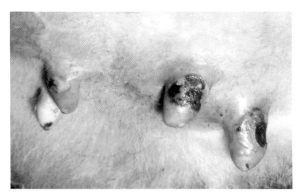

611

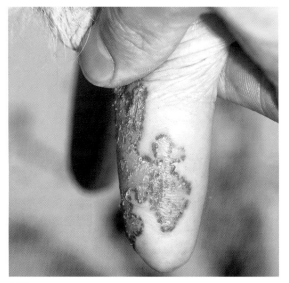

613

(primarily) and the udder may be affected and 'milker's nodules' may occur on the fingers of man. An individual cow may remain clinically affected for several months and, as immunity is short-lived, repeated attacks can occur every 2–3 years.

The disease starts as a small, painless papule affecting the superficial layers of the skin (**612**). After 7–10 days the lesion enlarges from the periphery to produce characteristic circular or horse-shoe-shaped areas, delineated by small, red scabs (**613**). The affected area feels rough, but is not painful, and milking is not usually impeded. Scabs slowly resolve in the healing phase (**614**). In rare cases, the lesion develops a very rough, slightly moist, papilliform appearance, with several elevated and confluent masses (**615**).

Differential diagnosis: bluetongue (**661**), cowpox (**616**), vesicular stomatitis (**617, 618**) and bovine herpes mammillitis (**610, 611**).

Management: milking hygiene, use of good-quality teat dips with emollients, and reduction of teat skin trauma help to prevent the spread of infection.

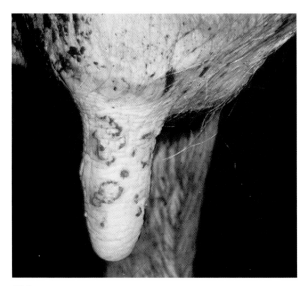

614

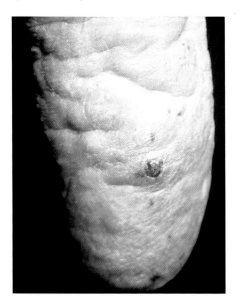

612

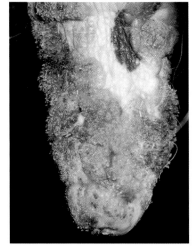

615

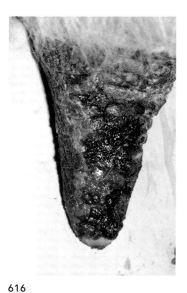

616

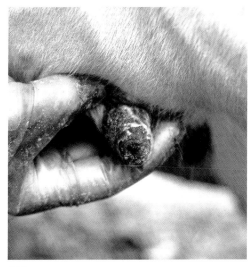

618

Cowpox (bovine orthopox)

Definition: benign contagious teat infection caused by an Orthopox virus closely related to smallpox in man.

Clinical features: cowpox produces vesicles on the skin of the teats and the udder. **616** illustrates three teat skin vesicles which have ruptured, exposing the underlying granulation tissue. As with the two previous conditions spread is by teat cups and milkers' hands. Cowpox is now extremely rare and the infection is limited to Western Europe.

Differential diagnosis: pseudocowpox, BHM, vesicular stomatitis, necrotic dermatitis.

Management: general measures as for BHM.

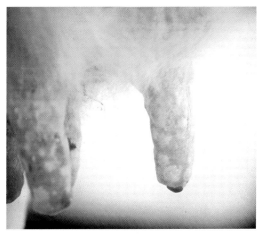

619

Vesicular stomatitis

Definition: infectious viral (*rhabdovirus*) disease causing stomatitis (**153**), sometimes with lesions on the udder, teats, coronary band and interdigital space.

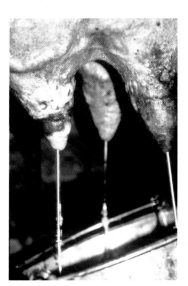

617

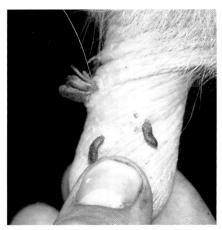

620

Clinical features: vesicular stomatitis is found only in North and South America and is transmitted by mosquitoes and biting flies. The reservoir hosts are American forest ground mammals. Excessive salivation is frequently the first sign. It primarily produces mouth lesions (**153**), but lesions can also occur on the teats. Multiple, irregular-shaped, white vesicles, some of which have ruptured, cover much of the teat skin in **617** and **618**. Uncomplicated cases heal within 2 weeks. Recovered animals are immune for 12–18 months.

Differential diagnosis: foot-and-mouth disease (**646–650**), bovine papular stomatitis (**155, 156**). Diagnosis is usually by ELISA and CF tests.

Management: disease should be notified to national animal health authorities. Symptomatic treatment and restriction on animal movement are usual.

Foot-and-mouth disease

Clinical features: though not a primary clinical sign, cows with FMD in the acute phase may develop multiple vesicles on the teats, in some cases becoming almost impossible to milk. **619** shows multiple teat vesicles in a Kuwait cow (see also p. 187).

Fibropapillomas (warts)

Clinical features: caused by different strains of papovaviruses, warts are common among groups of pregnant and first lactation heifers, typically over the lower part of the teat. Some have a 'feathery', keratinized and papilliform appearance (**620**) and can be easily pulled off. Others are more nodular (**621**) and tightly adherent to the skin. Mixed infections may occur (**622**). Fibropapillomas close to the teat orifice and sphincter (**622**) interfere with milking and predispose animals to teat stenosis and mastitis. Flies are considered to be important vectors for transmission. Warts also occur on the skin (**109**), eye (**467**) and penis (**523**).

Management: 'feathery warts' and those with a distinct stalk can be pulled off surprisingly easily and produce

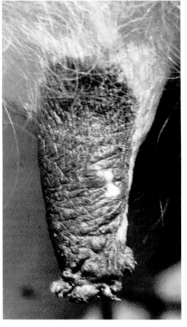

622

minimal hemorrhage. No vaccines are very effective though autogenous products seem better than commercial vaccines. Many warts slowly resolve in the first lactation.

Noninfectious teat conditions

Introduction: the teats are susceptible to trauma from the milking machine, the environment and physical factors. Any damage is of considerable economic importance as it predisposes to mastitis.

Teat end callosity (hyperkeratosis or canal eversion)

Clinical features: in the normal bovine teat, the canal sphincter and orifice should show minimal protrusion from the teat end. Teat end callosity and subsequent hyperkeratosis, i.e., protrusion of keratin fronds or filaments, is always the result of a faulty milking machine and is more common in pointed than in cylindrical teats. In **623**

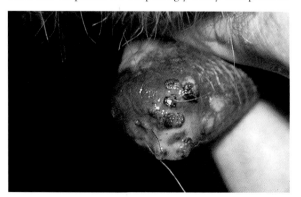

621

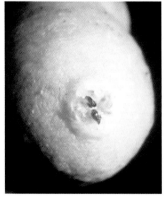

623

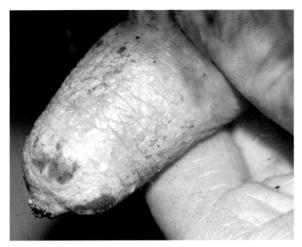

624

the teat canal is seen as a raised, pale, bulbous swelling of the circular sphincter area, with small, protruding fragments of dry, keratinized material. This indicates a grade 2 hyperkeratosis (grades 0–5 indicate normal to severe change: other scoring systems are also used). **624** shows a grade 3 callosity, with keratin fronding around the entire everted teat canal circumference. Milking machine trauma also produced the dry, circular, hemorrhagic areas seen at the teat apex. Advanced cases, which predispose to mastitis, show severe keratinization (**625**, grade 5), which may precede black spot.

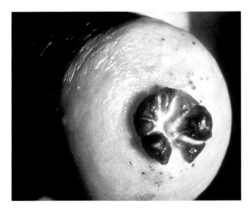

625

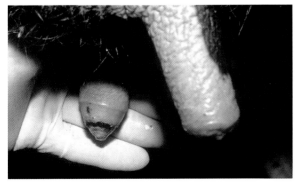

626

Teat end slough

Clinical features: much less common than teat end callosity, this condition (**626**) is also caused by milking machine trauma. Initial changes of hyperemia and thickening (right teat) of the teat skin may progress following ischemic necrosis, to a superficial slough over the teat canal, extending some 10–15 mm dorsally (**626**, left). Only superficial skin layers slough, and although the circumferential slough is remarkably symmetrical, healing is quite rapid once the milking machine trauma has been removed, leaving an obvious skin change similar to a burn.

Chaps, fissures and 'black spot'

Clinical features: 'teat chaps' are skin fissures. They may result from repeated exposure to wet, cold winds, inappropriate post-milking teat disinfectants, teeth damage caused by a suckling calf, or irritant chemicals. Chaps, as in **627**, may affect the whole of the teat, and when skin defenses are compromised in this way, mastitis organisms such as *Staphylococcus aureus* and *Streptococcus dysgalactiae* may proliferate. Skin fissures or 'chaps' at the teat orifice (**628**) may be caused by over-worn liners (inflations) producing a 'slapping' effect on the teat end during pulsation, as the liner always opens and closes in the same horizontal plane.

Black spot describes a proliferative necrotic dermatitis of the teat end around the sphincter, seen extending to the left in **629**. Black necrotic tissue is clearly visible. The lesion often starts as an environmental trauma (e.g., overmilking, excessive vacuum fluctuation, liner slap, wet

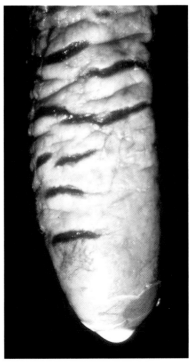

627

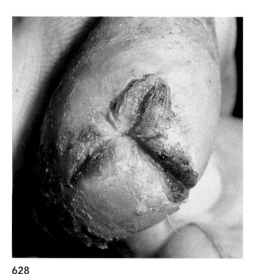

628

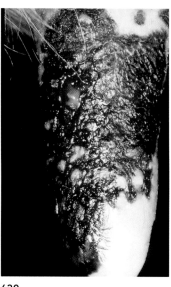

630

teats exposed to a chilling wind), leading to damage of the teat orifice, which is then secondarily infected with *Fusobacterium necrophorum* (see also **633**). The skin fissure adjacent to the black spot lesion in **629** is a teat chap.

Management: where multiple teats in several cows are involved, teat end callosity/hyperkeratosis will invariably be caused by defective milking machine function, e.g., excessive vacuum, prolonged milking times, poor udder preparation leading to delayed let-down, etc. Healing takes place after correction of the fault(s). Healing of black spot and chaps benefits from teat emollients, topical antibiotics or antiseptics and debriding agents.

Summer sores and teat eczema

Clinical features: summer sores are eczematous lesions that result from excessive licking, and may be secondary to irritation caused by flies. First seen as irregular-shaped areas of moist, wet eczema at the teat base, they may spread to involve almost the entire teat (**630**), when they can be very painful. **630** shows islets of residual epithelium in the granulation tissue, especially towards the tip of the teat, and there is a serous exudate. Simple sunburn producing a thickening of teat skin may also occur (**79**).

Differential diagnosis: from bovine herpes mammillitis (**611**) and necrotic dermatitis (**638**) is difficult at the stage seen in **630**.

Management: fly preventive measures, emollients.

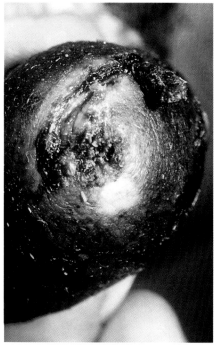

629

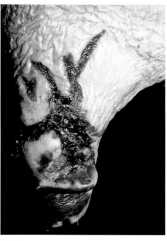

631

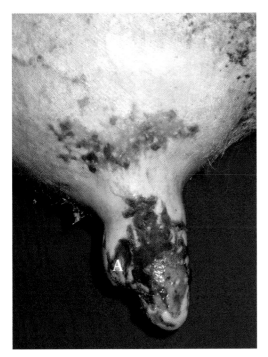

632

Teat trauma

Clinical features: because of their position, teats are very prone to injury, especially in cows with turgid or pendulous udders. Barbed wire often produces multiple lacerations and may leave a horizontal flap of skin (**631**). This flap tends to be pulled downwards when the teat cups are removed at milking, thus retarding healing. Amputation of the skin flap promotes healing. Superficial epidermal abrasions (**632**) cause few problems, although this teat had been injured in a previous lactation, leaving a fistula (A) of the cistern at its base. Trauma can cause complete loss of a large area of teat skin, but this often heals surprisingly well. Injuries such as a contaminated flap involving the teat sphincter, or localized ulceration (**633**), in this case with secondary infection causing black spot, carry a high risk of both mastitis and stenosis of the orifice.

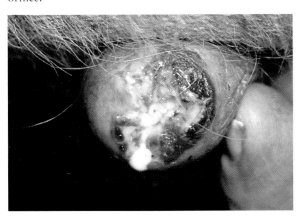

633

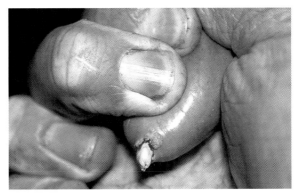

634

Teat cistern granuloma ('pea')

Definition: discrete fibrogranulomatous mass which may float free in teat cistern or be attached to the endothelium.

Clinical features: free-floating, irregular, rubbery masses of fibrocollagenous material ('peas') may develop in the teat cistern and pass down to the sphincter, thus obstructing the milk flow. As in **634**, some can be manually expressed from a surgically dilated teat orifice. Others remain attached to the teat mucosa, cannot be so easily removed and may continue to block the teat canal. A variety of shapes, sizes and colors is found (**635**). All have a rubbery texture, about 5–10 mm long and, as many are red, they probably originate from blood clots.

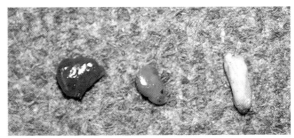

635

Supernumerary teats

Clinical features: supernumerary teats are a congenital condition. They may be found between the front and rear teats, and/or attached to the udder behind the rear teats (**636**), or to the base or side of one of the main teats, where they can interfere with milking. Typically, they are shorter than normal teats, and have thinner walls. They may connect to the sinus of an existing teat, or, more commonly, have a separate supernumerary gland.

Management: as such teats are unsightly, may interfere with milking and can develop mastitis, they are normally removed with curved scissors early in life. Care is necessary to identify the correct teat.

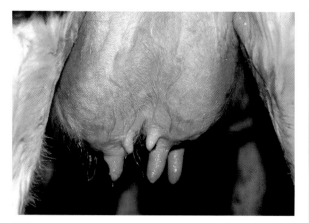

636

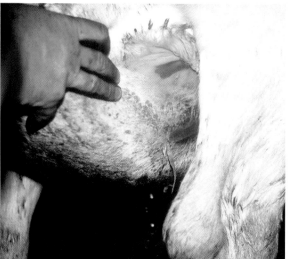

638

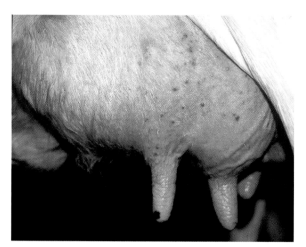

637

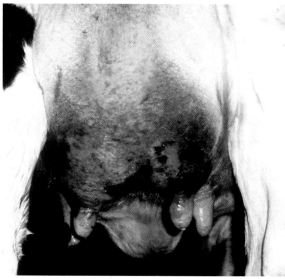

639

Conditions of the udder skin and subcutis

Udder impetigo (udder acne)

Definition: a staphylococcal dermatitis of the teats and udder skin.

Clinical features: small, red papules are seen on the udder of the Friesian in **637**. They sometimes coalesce to produce an exudative dermatitis that can spread onto the teats and may develop a foul odor. A coagulase-positive *Staphylococcus* was isolated in this case.

Differential diagnosis (of advanced teat cases): bovine herpes mammillitis (**610**) and necrotic dermatitis (**638**).

Management: topical antibiotic therapy is surprisingly effective.

Necrotic dermatitis (udder seborrhea)

Clinical features: this dermatitis occurs in the first 1–2 weeks after calving, especially in heifers, and is associated with excessive prepartum udder edema, leading to skin ischemia and necrosis. Mild cases (**638**) develop a moist and often foul-smelling superficial dermatitis laterally in the contact area between the udder and thigh. In more advanced cases (**639**) the ischemic udder skin turns reddish-purple and produces a dirty, serous exudate, similar to some cases of acute or peracute mastitis (**596**). A dry, scaly dermatitis (**640**) may lead to extensive thickening of the teats, and some animals become impossible to milk. Note the residual cutaneous edema cranial to the udder in this heifer.

In mature cows a common site of the dermatitis is the area of skin between the two forequarters and the ventral body wall. The lesion, also called intertrigo, which may persist for several weeks or months, is a deep, moist and exudative dermatitis with a pungent odor (**641**). Necrotic debris is seen in the center. Organisms closely resembling the spirochaetes of digital dermatitis have been identified in the lesions.

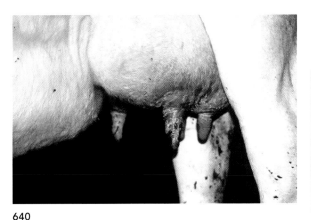

640

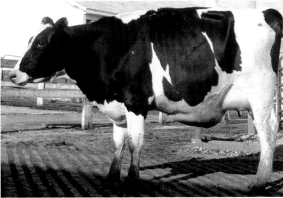

642

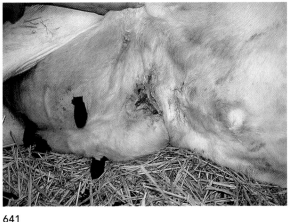

641

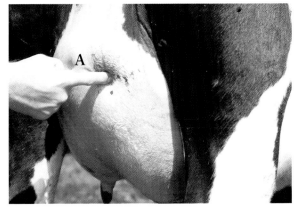

643

Differential diagnosis: severe udder impetigo (staphylococcal dermatitis) (**637**), bluetongue (**661**), bovine herpes mammillitis (**610**).

Management: cleanse lesions, removing debris, apply topical antibiotics or antiseptics.

Prevention: careful transition feed management and increase exercise to avoid mammary edema.

Ventral abdominal edema

Clinical features: a physiological periparturient condition, extensive subcutaneous edema is seen cranial to the udder of the Holstein heifer in **642**, 2 days after calving. In advanced cases it may extend to the sternum.

Typically, edema is demonstrated as 'pitting' when pressure is applied. Digital pressure on the rear of an edematous udder (**643**) creates a depression (seen to the left of the finger (A)) which persists for 30–60 seconds after the finger has been withdrawn.

Differential diagnosis: abscess, hematoma.

Management: overfeeding, excessive salt and other mineral intakes, an overfat prepartum condition, heredity and lack of exercise are among the factors contributing

to excess edema and require appropriate measures. A sudden onset of edema in one or more quarters in mid-lactation cows, with unknown etiology, has recently been reported.

Rupture of udder ligaments ('dropped udder')

Introduction: the suspensory apparatus of the udder consists of superficial and deep lateral ligaments, anterior ligament and a fibroelastic median ligament. Any can stretch or rupture.

Clinical features: rupture of the median and lateral suspensory apparatus. The 6-year-old Guernsey cow in **644** had calved 4 weeks previously, and had suddenly developed a grossly pendulous udder as a result of sudden rupture of both the lateral and median suspensory apparatus (ligaments) of the udder. Note that the ventral udder surface is considerably below the level of the hock. The outward direction of the teats is a mechanical result of the loss of the median ligamentous support of the udder. There was no evidence of mastitis. Postmortem examination revealed a massive hematoma surrounding the ligamentous rupture between the ventral body wall and the gland parenchyma.

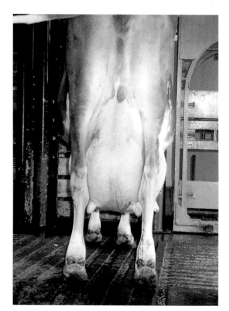

644

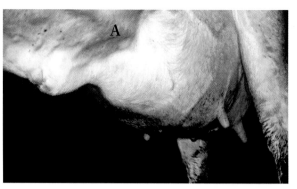

645

is impossible. The milk vein runs along the top of the picture, and may occasionally rupture internally leading to quite severe anemia.

Differential diagnosis: acute mastitis, ventral abdominal rupture (prepubic tendon (**131**), or rectus abdominis muscle), hematoma and severe udder edema (**643**).

Management: incurable condition. Moderate cases can often be kept for the remainder of the lactation, but are best housed in straw yards rather than cubicles (free stalls). Cluster attachment is often difficult due to teat displacement and the engorged udder. Breeding and prepartum overfeeding that leads to excessive udder engorgement are predisposing factors.

Rupture of the anterior ligament is seen in the freshly calved Friesian cow (**645**) which suddenly developed this massive midline swelling cranial to the udder, filling the normal space between the forequarters and ventral body wall. Note that the front teats are so splayed that milking

chapter 12

Infectious diseases

Introduction

Infectious diseases are a major limiting factor in cattle production in many parts of the world. In tropical Africa, with its 160 million cattle, the major diseases, i.e., rinderpest, foot-and-mouth disease (FMD), contagious bovine pleuropneumonia, theileriosis and trypanosomiasis, are all infectious. Such limitations on livestock production lead to shortages of meat, milk, draught animals and manure, and to the necessity to import from developed countries such as North America and Australia, and the European Community. These imports in turn discourage domestic livestock production, while the presence of infectious diseases bars the export of cattle and cattle products to developed countries.

Viral diseases

Several major bovine diseases, endemic in many parts of the world, have a viral etiology. They are characterized by their highly contagious nature and the variety of their cloven-footed hosts. Early recognition of suspicious signs and confirmation of the disease in the laboratory, together with prompt and effective control measures, are essential for their eradication.

Foot-and-mouth disease (FMD)

Definition: highly infectious disease with a short incubation period caused by aphthovirus of the family *Picornaviridae* with seven serotypes. List A disease of OIE.

Clinical features: cattle infected with foot-and-mouth disease are dull, off feed, and drool saliva. Some are lame. On opening the mouth (**646**), large areas of epithelial loss, that are the result of recently ruptured FMD vesicles, are seen on the tongue and hard palate, as in this animal from Zimbabwe. An unruptured vesicle on the dorsum of the tongue is seen in **647**.

In a steer infected experimentally, in as little as 2 days initial vesicles have ruptured to reveal ulcers which are seen along the lower gums and inside the lower lip, together with ruptured tongue vesicles (**648**). Two days later the lesions on the tongue, lower lip and gums have become secondarily infected (**649**). A vesicle on the coronary band and dorsal part of the interdigital space has ruptured. On the seventh day, (**650**) the interdigital space shows widespread ulceration along its entire length. A vesicle on the soft skin above the heel has ruptured in another cow (**651**). Lameness may be the first sign of FMD. These interdigital lesions easily become secondarily infected. Multiple teat vesicles are shown in **619** (p. 179).

Differential diagnosis: includes vesicular stomatitis (**153**), BVD/MD (**145**), bovine papular stomatitis (**155**, **156**) and rinderpest (**656**), digital dermatitis (**315–318**), interdigital dermatitis (**321**).

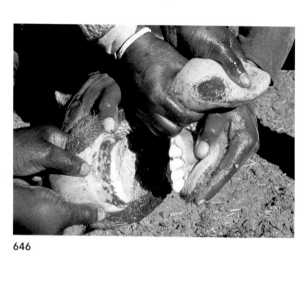

646

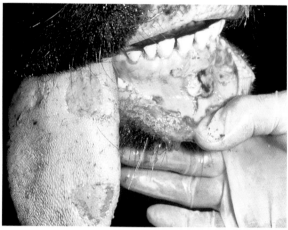

649

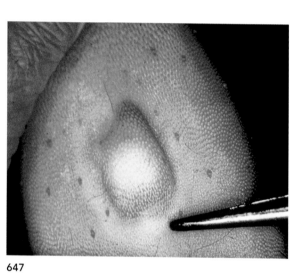

647

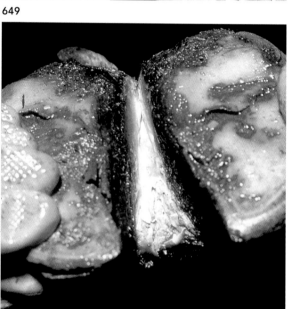

650

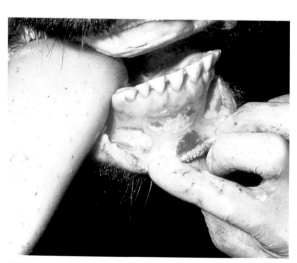

648

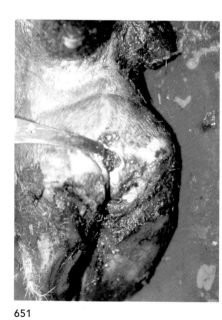

651

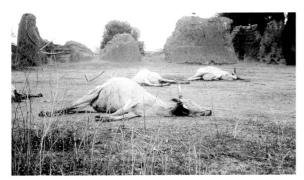

652

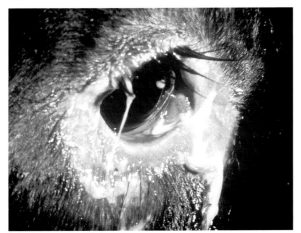

653

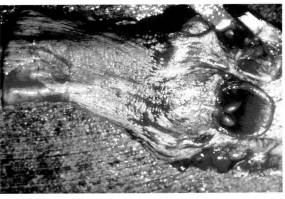

654

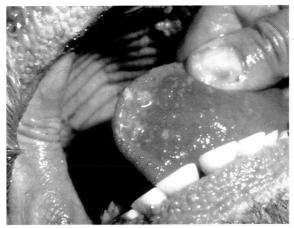

655

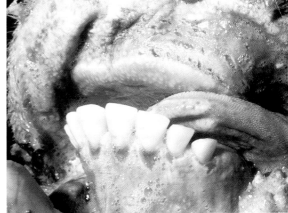

656

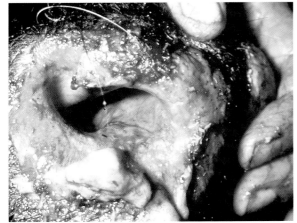

657

Management: slaughter policy in FMD-free countries, and elsewhere isolation, quarantine and ring vaccination, where disease is endemic.

Rinderpest ('cattle plague')

Definition: infectious disease caused by a Morbillivirus having variable virulence and a wide ungulate host range.

Clinical features: virgin-soil epizootics (652) fulminate rapidly and frequently escalate into panzootics whereas enzootic rinderpest spreads slowly, even inapparently, for months in immature and young adult stock free of maternally derived antibodies.

Clinical diagnosis in fresh epizootics is relatively easy: after a prodromal onset of fever, illness is evident in 48 hours. The affected animals are restless and have dry muzzles and staring coats. Milk yields fall, respirations are shallow and rapid, visible mucous membranes are congested, while tears (653) and nasal fluids (654) flow profusely. The appetite is impaired and constipation occurs.

The emergence of mucosal erosions 2–5 days later is the first sign suggestive of rinderpest: raised pinheads of necrotic epithelium reminiscent of oatmeal coat all visible mucous membranes (655). They are abraded readily to reveal shallow erosions with a hemorrhagic layer of intact

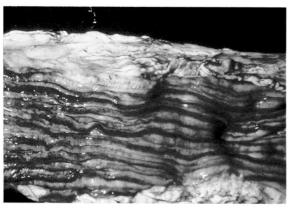

658

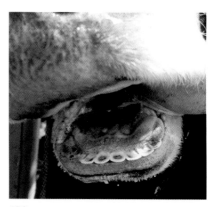

659

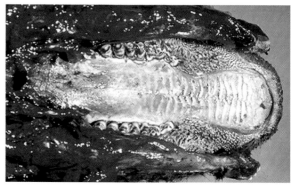

660

basal cells (**656**). The erosions enlarge and coalesce throughout the alimentary tract from the mouth (**657**) to the rectum. Salivation is profuse. The affected cattle are now obviously sick, drink excessively and pass soft feces. In 2–3 days the fever regresses and diarrhea starts. The brown fluid feces contain necrotic debris streaked with blood. Dehydration is rapid and the frequent straining reveals the capillary stasis in the rectum known as zebra stripes (**658**). Breathing is labored and painful. Most die within 6–12 days of the onset of overt illness. Pregnant cows abort during convalescence that lasts for months. In contrast, enzootic rinderpest is difficult to diagnose clinically. Adult cows are immune and passively immunize their sucking progeny, protecting them for up to 9 months. Thereafter they are at risk. The clinical signs are muted and often one or more of the cardinal features of the classic epizootic syndrome such as fever, erosions, mucopurulent nasal and ocular discharges, and diarrhea are absent. Most affected animals survive and suspicions of rinderpest are not roused. The illustrations are from Saudi Arabia, Yemen and Nigeria.

Differential diagnosis: lesions are indistinguishable from those in BVD (**145**). Other similar diseases are FMD (**646–651**), IBR (**235**) and malignant catarrhal fever (**662–664**).

Management: the incidence of rinderpest has declined spectacularly following massive international vaccination campaigns financed by Europe and USA and organized in Africa and Asia by the Food and Agricultural Organization of the United Nations (FAO) and OIE. Today, there are only a few pockets of known infection that are held behind vaccinated cordon sanitaires where broad-spectrum antibiotic therapy may be justified to reduce the severity of secondary infections. Elsewhere, vaccination is forbidden. Previously infected countries are actively following OIE regulations (List A disease) leading to total eradication of rinderpest. The global freedom target date is 2010. Early recognition and notification of new outbreaks are vital.

Bluetongue

Definition: disease is caused by an orbivirus with many serotypes and is transmitted by windborne midges (*Culicoides*).

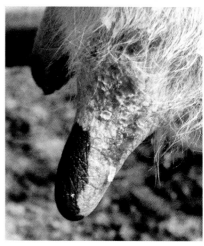

661

Clinical features: bluetongue causes initial hyperemia of the muzzle and lips, followed by inflammatory and erosive lesions. Necrotic areas may be seen in the gums and the dental pad (**659**), and hard palate (**660**) and there may be irregular, superficial erosions on the teats (**661**). Clinical lesions in cattle are allegedly mediated by an IgE hypersensitivity reaction. While endemic on the African continent, bluetongue is sporadic in many other parts of the world, including Eastern Europe and the Mediterranean Basin. In North America it is a mild clinical condition and differential diagnosis is difficult. Infection is more common than disease.

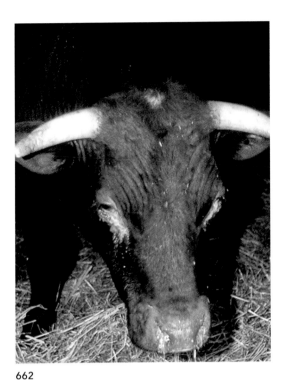

662

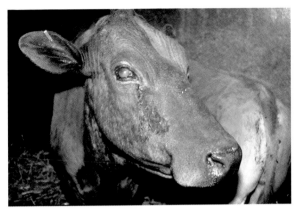

663

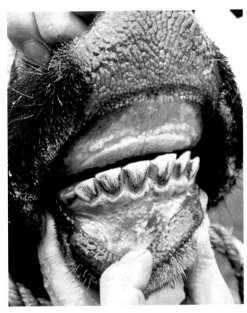

664

Differential diagnosis: photosensitization (**79, 80**), BVD (**145**), IBR (**236**), vesicular stomatitis (**153**) and FMD (**646**). Mycotic stomatitis is also caused by the bluetongue virus. Diagnosis is by PCR and AGID assay and by virus isolation.

Management: individual cases should receive supportive therapy. Vaccine is available for herds in epidemic areas. Attempt to reduce exposure to *Culicoides*.

Malignant catarrhal fever (MCF, bovine malignant catarrh, malignant head catarrh)

Definition: a worldwide sporadic, herpesvirus infection, almost invariably fatal. One (wildebeest-associated) form is caused by alcelaphine herpesvirus-1, the other (sheep-associated) by ovine herpesvirus-2.

Clinical features: malignant catarrhal fever causes marked pyrexia, anorexia and profound depression, with catarrhal and mucopurulent inflammation of the upper respiratory and alimentary epithelia, keratoconjunctivitis following a characteristic initial peripheral keratitis, and lymphadenopathy. MCF herd outbreaks are seasonal and occur predominantly in Africa. Elsewhere (North America and Europe), only sporadic cases are seen. The 'head and eye' syndrome of the Devon cow in **662** includes a purulent oculonasal discharge, mild keratitis, and hyperemia of the nostrils. Note the almost pathognomonic hypopyon in the cross-bred Charolais suckler cow in **663**. There is a marked ocular discharge and pus is settling towards the base of the anterior chamber. Iridocyclitis may lead to photophobia. The nasal discharge is, unusually, not particularly severe. Areas of dry necrosis and ulceration are seen on the gums and dental pad of **664**. Similar changes are commonly seen on the nostrils. Clinical cases in cattle are not infectious, but if they survive they are infected for life and may infect their calves *in utero*.

Differential diagnosis: rinderpest (**652**), bluetongue (**659–661**), East Coast fever (**689**), IBR (**235**), BVD/MD (**143**), Jembrana disease (Indonesia) (**698–701**) and bovine iritis (**460**).

Diagnosis: by clinical picture, gross pathology, and confirmed in outbreaks by ELISA serology and PCR of viral DNA in host lymphocytes.

Management: despite occasional reports of success with cortisone and antibiotics, most cases are best culled as soon as the diagnosis is confirmed. Inactivated wildebeest-associated MCF vaccine is available in some countries. List A disease of OIE.

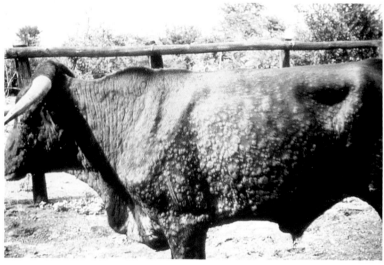

665

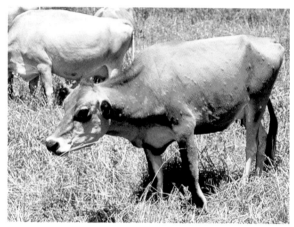

666

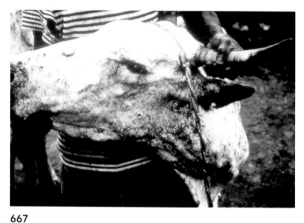

667

Lumpy-skin disease

Definition: a capripoxvirus disease of cattle first reported in Northern Rhodesia (Zambia) in 1929, now widespread in Africa, including Egypt, with recent spread into Israel. Biting flies are the main vectors.

Clinical features: initially a fluctuating fever, lacrimation and inappetance for 2 weeks, during which circumscribed nodules appear in the skin (**665**) and mucous membranes of the mouth and respiratory tract, genitalia (orchitis) and conjunctiva. The nodules (**666**) are discrete, firm, raised and painful, and contain hard gray-yellow material. Regional nodes are enlarged (prescapular in **666**). Some nodules resolve rapidly, others become a firm necrotic sitfast (**665** body and **667** head and neck) that heals slowly, and drops out leaving a scar. Secondary infection can lead to suppurating ulcers and abscesses. A few nodules may persist for years. Subclinical cases develop isolated nodules which are often missed.

Mortality rates in endemic areas are 1–3%, but in virgin-soil epidemics may approach 100%. In South Africa lumpy-skin disease is the most serious cause of economic loss in cattle, due to prolonged debility, milk loss, infertility in both cows and bulls, abortion and hide damage.

Differential diagnosis: ulcerative lymphangitis (pseudotuberculosis) (**113**), pseudo-lumpy-skin disease (Allerton herpes virus infection) (**668, 669**), and dermatophilosis (streptothricosis) (**107**).

Management: good nursing, sulfonamides or antibiotics for secondary infections, use of attenuated virus vaccine (Neethling strain). Slaughter policy of affected and contact cattle, coupled with vaccination of at-risk cattle before likely disease spread into a previously free area or country. List A disease of OIE.

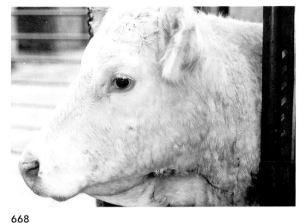

668

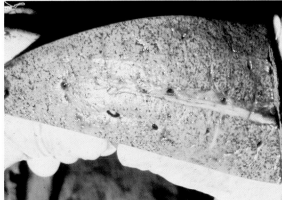

670

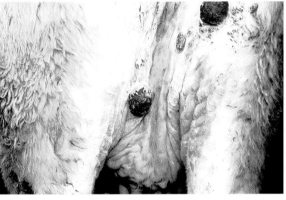

669

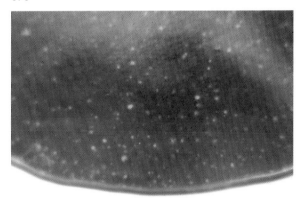

671

Pseudo-lumpy-skin disease (Allerton virus infection)

Definition: one of two bovine herpes virus-2 syndromes (see also bovine herpes mammillitis (p. 177)), pseudo (false)-lumpy-skin disease is characterized by transient moderate fever and exudative cutaneous plaques.

Disease occurs primarily in southern Africa, and very occasionally in USA, Australia and UK.

Clinical features: initial fever and mild lymphadenopathy are followed within a few days by emergence of numerous circular or oval superficial cutaneous plaques about 1–2 cm diameter. These are hard, firm and have a red margin and enlarge to 3–5 cm, becoming umbilicated. The centers are depressed and exude to form brown crusts (**668**). The skin beneath the crusts dies within 2 weeks to reveal smooth new skin and fresh hair grows within 2 months. Lesions are frequently on the face, neck, back and perineum (**669**), as in this pedigree Charolais heifer in the UK. Clinical recovery is uncomplicated.

Diagnosis depends on clinical appearance and demonstration of herpes virus-2 from peripheral lesions (skin scraping or punch biopsy). Biopsy will also reveal eosinophilic intranuclear inclusion bodies.

Differential diagnosis: lumpy-skin disease (**666**), urticaria (**76, 77**), dermatophilosis (**106–108**).

Management: nursing care.

Rift Valley fever (RVF)

Definition: acute febrile disease of cattle and sheep readily communicable to humans, and caused by a mosquito-borne phlebovirus (*Bunyaviridae*). Previously confined to Africa, including Egypt (1977–78), a major epidemic (2000) in Saudi Arabia and Yemen resulted in severe cattle losses and numerous human deaths.

Clinical features: calves usually die after a short peracute illness with high fever, severe dyspnea and terminally lateral recumbency with extended legs and neck. Cows, following a transient fever, icterus, leucopenia and inco-ordination, abort and may die. Non-pregnant adults experience a low-grade fever. Epidemics of RVF are linked to wet years in which hatching of larger numbers of infected mosquito eggs occurs (*Aedes linneatopennis*).

Postmortem changes in calves and fetuses include a spectacular bright orange-yellow and diffusely necrotic liver (**670**), while adult cattle show discrete focal necrotic hepatic lesions (**671**). Diagnosis depends on viral isolation from aborted fetuses or blood. Veterinarians are at particular risk when handling infected tissues.

Differential diagnosis: ephemeral fever (**672, 673**), rinderpest (**652**), brucellosis (storm).

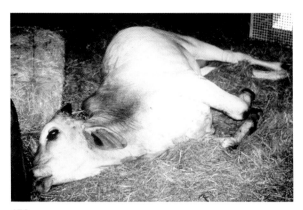

672

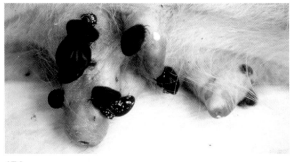

674

Management: control depends primarily on strict prohibition of the import of susceptible cattle and other species from endemic parts of the African continent and adjacent regions. Zoonotic spread from country to country by human carriers is possible. Attenuated killed virus and mutagen-attenuated vaccines are practical and economic control measures. List A disease of OIE.

Ephemeral fever ('three-day sickness')

Definition: infectious, rarely fatal disease caused by a rhabdovirus transmitted by *Culicoides* (midges) and mosquitoes. Wind-borne dissemination occurs.

Clinical features: mild cases remain reasonably bright but are pyrexic, stiff or slightly lame and lactating cows have a pronounced drop in yield. Severe cases of ephemeral fever are initially seen in sternal recumbency and later in lateral recumbency (**672**) with signs of flaccid paralysis. Other features include rumen atony, loss of the swallow reflex and tongue tonus (**673**), and partial paralysis of the lower jaw (**672**), resembling botulism. Atypical interstitial pneumonia, and lymphadenopathy may occur. Death is rare. The disease occurs in Africa, Asia and Australia.

Differential diagnosis: botulism (**709**), pneumonia, severe toxemia, physical injury, Rift Valley fever (**670**) and rabies (**494–496**).

Diagnosis: clinical signs and serology (CF, AGID and ELISA).

Management: supportive care, e.g., NSAIDs and calcium solutions may benefit recumbent cows. Prevention by annual vaccination and fly control.

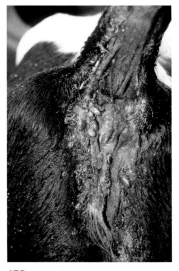

675

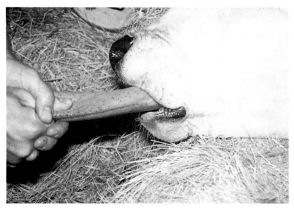

673

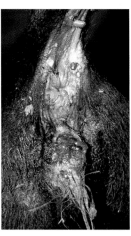

676

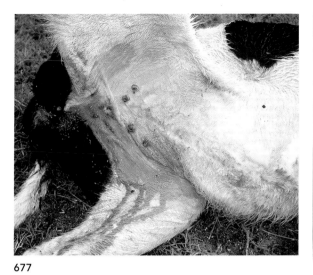

677

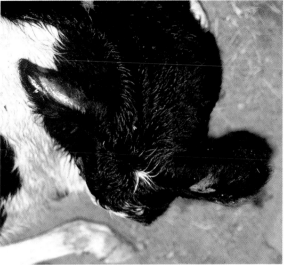

678

Tick-borne diseases (protozoal and rickettsial infections)

Introduction: in the tropics, ticks are very important owing to their impact on the cattle industry. Tick infestations depress productivity as a direct result of their feeding activity. This is primarily through reduced live-weight gain. Other consequences include anemia, skin wounds that are susceptible to secondary bacterial infection or screw-worm infestation (**121**), and toxic reactions to tick saliva (e.g., sweating sickness, **677**) Indirectly however, they have a far more significant role as vectors of diseases such as theilerioses that are widespread in subtropical Europe, Africa and Asia.

Other tropical tick-borne diseases that limit cattle production include babesiosis, anaplasmosis, heartwater (cowdriosis) and dermatophilosis. Ticks parasitic on cattle can be divided into two families, the Ixodidae or 'hard' ticks and the Argasidae or 'soft' ticks, depending on the presence or absence of a hard, dorsal scutum. These families also have many other differences.

Tick infestations

Clinical features: taken in Antigua, West Indies, **674** shows *Amblyomma variegatum* (tropical African bont) ticks feeding on teats. These species are mainly found in the tropics and subtropics, causing disease both directly and by parasite transmission. Mixed tick infections do occur. Their large mouthparts can cause serious wounds that are liable to secondary infection. The scrotum is also a common region for tick feeding. In **675** *Amblyomma* species are seen in varying stages of engorgement, feeding around the perineum and anus of a 4-month-old Friesian heifer from Zimbabwe. White larvae along the edge of the tail indicate early myiasis lesions. These changes are more pronounced in **676**, where tick damage has resulted in an enlarged vulva, with raw, bleeding areas. Early myiasis is again visible. Myiasis lesions are also shown in **121** and **122**.

Cowdria ruminantium, the ehrlichial rickettsial agent of heartwater is carried by *A. variegatum*.

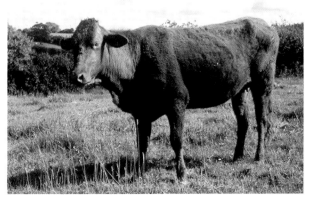

679

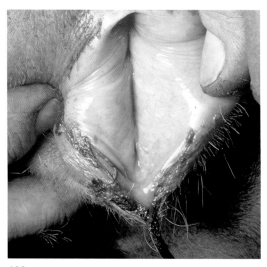

680

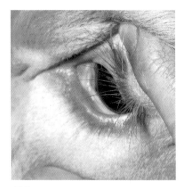

681

Tick toxicosis

There are two tick toxicoses, tick paralysis and sweating sickness.

Definition: tick paralysis is a widespread affliction of calves induced by at least three tick species, *Ixodes* spp., *Dermacentor* spp., and *Haemaphysalis* spp. The toxin causes an ascending paralysis that spreads from the hind limbs to the fore limbs. Death follows respiratory failure.

Definition: sweating sickness is an acute non-infectious disease of calves caused by bites of female *Hyalomma* spp. ticks, whose saliva apparently contains an epitheliotropic toxin. The female *Hyalomma truncatum* appears to be infectious at a weight of 25–50 mg. The tick must feed for 5–7 days before sufficient toxin has entered the host calf.

Clinical features: sweating sickness is seen in Central and Southern Africa and India. As in the Friesian calf from Zimbabwe (**677**), the moist dermatitis (sweat) typically affects the inguinum, the perineum and the axilla, producing a sour smell. Note the early myiasis ventral to the vulva. Young calves are usually affected and immunity lasts for 4–5 years. Hair loss, which may be total, occurs secondary to the initial moist dermatitis. Hair may be pulled off when the animal is handled, for example over the ears (**678**). Secondary skin infection often develops. Lacrimation and salivation may occur because all mucous membranes are affected.

Diagnosis: demonstration of the vector tick. Differentials include cerebral babesiosis (**679–682**), cerebral theileriosis (**689**), meningitis (**484, 485**), encephalitis, rabies (**495, 496**).

Management: NSAIDs and broad-spectrum antibiotics to relieve dermatitis, and acaricides to control secondary myiasis. Tick control to prevent further cases. In endemic areas cattle may have to be dipped weekly during the season of risk. No vaccine is available.

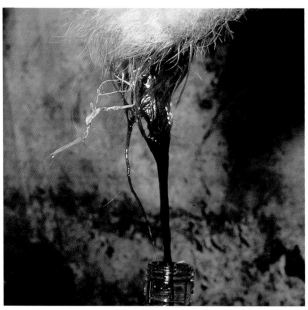

682

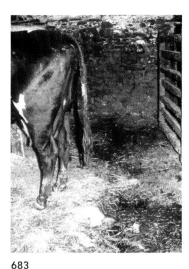

683

Babesiosis ('redwater fever', 'Texas fever')

Clinical features: the term 'redwater' originates from the hemoglobinuria that is seen following a hemolytic anemia produced by protozoa of *Babesia* species, *B. bovis* and *B. divergens* being the most important. They may occur singly or together, and in combination with *Anaplasma* to produce fatal 'tick fever'. The South Devon cow in **679** has lost condition. She has a dejected appearance, with drooping ears, half-closed eyes and the front legs abducted to maintain balance. Her flank is hollow, indicating lack of rumen fill. There is extreme pallor of the vulval mucosa (**680**) and the conjunctiva is both anemic and jaundiced (**681**). Dark, port wine-colored urine, as seen in the South Devon steer in **682**, often produces a characteristic golden yellow froth as it hits the ground (**683**). Affected cattle are febrile and develop anal sphincter spasm, producing 'coiling' of feces which are voided under pressure (**684**). Some animals may die suddenly after 24 hours of acute illness, others may abort. *Ixodes ricinus* is the common vector for *Babesia bigemina*, the major form of

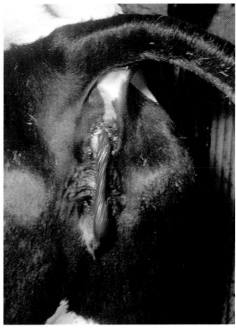

684

babesiosis in the UK. Disease caused by babesiosis is distributed worldwide wherever there are ticks.

Differential diagnosis (of redwater): includes anaplasmosis (**685**), theileriosis (**689**), bracken poisoning (**721**), kale poisoning (**728**), leptospirosis in calves, bacillary hemoglobinuria and nitrate poisoning (**745**). Diagnosis is by examination of blood smear.

Management: individual treatment involves protozoal destruction by babesicides such as imidocarb or amidocarb, and possibly blood transfusions in severe cases.

Prevention: eradication of ticks, (e.g., by pasture improvement), regular dipping and possibly vaccination or chemoimmunization.

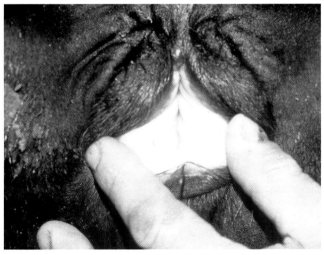

685

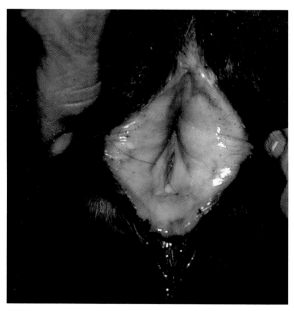

686

Tick-borne fever

Definition: a benign rickettsial disease caused by *Ehrlichia phagocytophila*, which parasitizes white blood cells. Tick-borne fever is limited to temperate regions of Europe, Africa and Asia. Natural tick vectors are *Ixodes ricinus* (Europe) and *Rhipicephalus haemophysaloides* (Asia), hence outbreaks are seasonal.

Clinical features: compared with babesiosis (p. 197) tick-borne fever is much less severe. Milking cows lose production and may abort, especially if recently introduced to the area. Cows are febrile, off feed and appear stiff. Pregnant heifers in their second grazing season ('pasture fever') may experience a high fever, can cough, have drooping ears and may abort. A depressed defense mechanism can result in secondary infection such as postparturient sepsis.

Differential diagnosis: babesiosis (**679–683**), brucellosis (**590**); diagnosis is usually based on typical geographical location and tick activity. Giemsa-stained blood film 2–8 days after onset of fever can be diagnostic.

Management: avoid placing naïve heifers and cows in late pregnancy onto tick-infested pastures. Tetracyclines are effective in treatment and control.

Anaplasmosis ('gall sickness')

Definition: anaplasmosis is caused by a tick-borne ehrlichial parasite *Anaplasma marginale* which leads to disruption of host erythrocytes.

Clinical features: gall sickness is endemic in tropical and subtropical regions of Africa, Asia, Australia and the

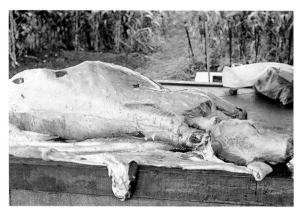

687

Americas. Transmission is by ticks (*Boophilus* and *Dermacentor* species), biting flies, or iatrogenically, for example, during mass vaccination. Calves infected remain infected throughout life. Most appear healthy, but if stressed will develop clinical signs. Adult cattle are more severely affected. After initial pyrexia and anorexia, anemia develops, as shown on the vaginal mucosa in **685**, and later jaundice (**686**). Hemoglobinuria is absent. In the occasional peracute case in a dairy cow severe pyrexia and dyspnea may be associated with hyperexcitability. Mortality may reach 50%.

On postmortem examination (**687**), the carcass is pale, anemic and slightly jaundiced. Unclotted blood can be seen on the hide adjacent to the spine. The liver is enlarged and mottled (**688**), the distended gallbladder contains thick bile, and there is splenic enlargement. Recovered animals may remain carriers for life. These illustrations are from Zimbabwe and from Queensland, Australia.

Differential diagnosis: babesiosis (**679–684**), bacillary hemoglobinuria (**227–228**), theileriosis (**689**), trypanosomiasis (**703**). Diagnosis is on examination of a blood smear.

Management: treatment is with tetracyclines or with imidocarb dipropionate, possibly blood transfusion in very anemic cases. Prevention by insect control is not practical in many regions but an acaricide dip at weekly intervals

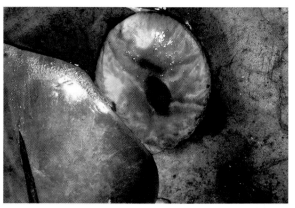

688

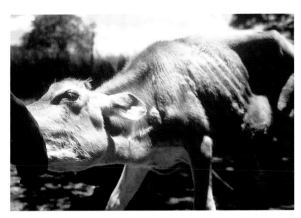

689

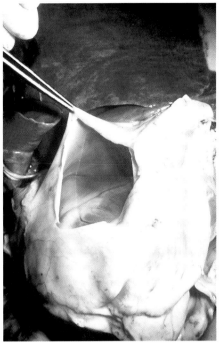

692

in endemic areas controls tick. Avoidance of iatrogenic transmission (syringes and needles). Vaccination regimes are currently controversial.

Theilerioses

Definition: *Theileria* species are tick-borne protozoal parasites that multiply in lymphocytes and then enter erythrocytes.

Clinical features: theileriosis is common in tick-infested areas throughout the world. *T. parva* (East Coast fever,

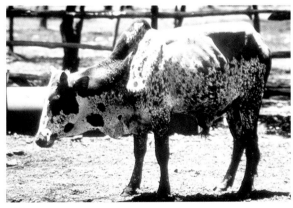

690

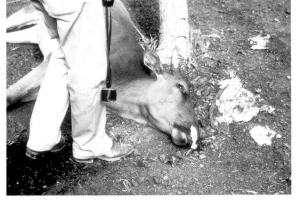

691

ECF), transmitted by *Rhipicephalus appendiculatus*, is a serious problem in Central and East Africa. *T. annulata*, transmitted by *Hyalomma* species, occurs in North Africa, southern Europe, the Middle East, India and Asia. Its pathogenicity varies but can result in mortality rates up to 90%. In **689**, the Jersey heifer from Zimbabwe is in poor condition and shows gross enlargement of the parotid and prescapular lymph nodes, a rough coat (particularly dorsally), and matted hair over the face due to epiphora. Affected animals are pyrexic and anemic. On postmortem examination, splenic enlargement, severe pulmonary emphysema and edema, and generalized lymphoid hyperplasia are the most striking changes.

Differential diagnosis: trypanosomiasis (703), cowdriosis (690–693), malignant catarrhal fever (662–665).

Management: use of resistant cattle breeds, acaricides, vaccination (infection and treatment methods).

Cowdriosis ('heartwater')

Definition: caused by the ehrlichial rickettsia *Cowdria ruminantium*, heartwater is transmitted from reservoir wildlife hosts (e.g., wildebeest) to susceptible cattle by *Amblyomma* (bont) ticks, producing severe damage to the vascular endothelium, and results in pyrexia, hydropericardium and nervous signs.

Clinical features: the disease is common in many parts of Africa and the Caribbean; the cattle illustrated are from Mali. Peracute disease produces rapid death. Acute cases are initially dull, pyrexic and anorexic, diarrheic,

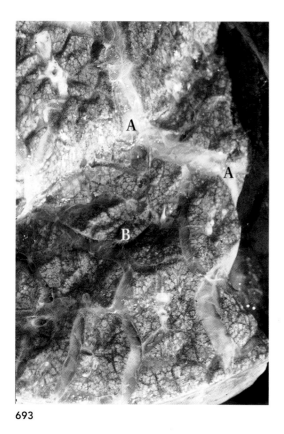

693

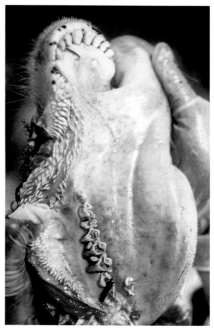

695

with a 'tucked up' abdomen, as seen in the Zebu steer in **690**. Nervous signs, convulsions, maniacal behavior and death in extensor spasm may follow rapidly, with a frothy discharge from the nostrils (**691**). Increased vascular permeability produces a generalized circulatory failure, seen as lung congestion, hydrothorax and hydropericardium (**692**, where the forceps raise the margin of the incised pericardium). In **693** the cut surface of an affected lung shows massive interlobular edema (A) and congestion (B). Disease is sometimes mild or inapparent.

Differential diagnosis: anthrax (**713**), rabies (**495, 496**), cerebral babesiosis (**679**), cerebral theileriosis (**689**), meningitis (**484, 485**). Clinical signs in susceptible cattle

(often imported) are usually diagnostic. Confirmation by demonstrating ehrlichial colonies in brain capillary endothelium.

Management: oxytetracyclines to clinical cases. Prevention by vaccination, tick control and chemoprophylaxis.

Q fever

Definition: a worldwide zoonosis caused by *Coxiella burnetii*, a Gram-negative obligate intracellular parasite,

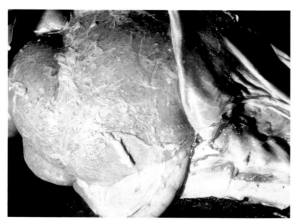

694

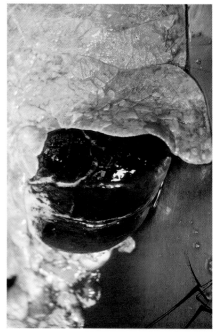

696

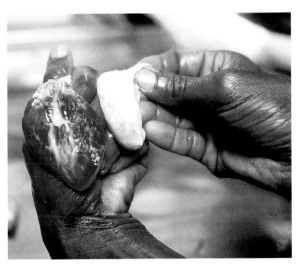

697

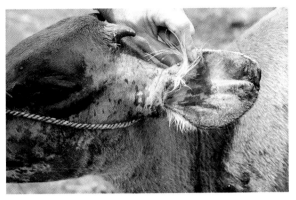

698

which appears either as a small compact rod or large pleomorphic organism inside vacuoles of the cytoplasm, causing abortion in cattle.

Clinical signs: infection is usually subclinical. Spread is by aerosol spray, direct contact, ingestion of infected placenta, or milk. Major risk is to pregnant humans.

The uterus can develop a mild to severe placentitis. The organism can localize in the udder, drainage lymph nodes, placenta and uterus, and can be shed at subsequent parturitions.

Differential diagnosis: other causes of abortion: diagnosis depends on demonstration of the organism (e.g., in placenta).

Management: need for treatment with tetracyclines rarely arises. Isolation of aborting cattle and destruction by burning of infected material, aborted fetuses, (discharges, bedding).

Sporadic bovine encephalomyelitis (SBE, 'Buss disease', transmissible serositis)

Definition: SBE is caused by *Chlamydia psittaci*. A recently described paramyxoviral SBE is a separate entity.

Clinical features: also known as transmissible serositis, it is an uncommon systemic infection with a worldwide distribution and causes a generalized inflammation of blood vessels, serous membranes and synoviae. The calf in **694** shows a chronic fibrinous exudative peritonitis. Pleurisy and pericarditis were also present. The epidemiology and pathogenesis resemble MCF (**662–665**) but the mortality rate is low. Encephalitis develops secondarily to the mesenchymal damage.

Differential diagnosis: bovine malignant catarrh, listeriosis (**477, 478**), rabies (**494–496**), lead poisoning (**747**) and pneumonic pasteurellosis (**241–242**).

Diagnosis: Giemsa-stained tissue impression smears, brain histopathology, or isolation of organism by tissue culture.

Management: possibly broad-spectrum antibiotics in early stages.

Bovine petechial fever (Ondiri disease)

Definition: the causal rickettsia is *Ehrlichia ondiri*. The natural mode of transmission is unknown but is likely to be a tick. The rickettsia is not contagious.

Clinical features: the organism is present in circulating granulocytes and monocytes during the clinical syndrome and later localizes in the spleen and other organs. Disease is confined to altitudes above 1500 m in Kenya and possibly neighboring Tanzania. Indigenous cattle do not develop clinical signs when infected. Newly arrived exotic cattle develop dramatic signs with sudden fever, often missed as cattle eat and behave normally. Dairy cows lose all milk production. Within 24 hours numerous petechiae emerge in visible mucosae, for example beneath the tongue (**695**) as well as internal organs such as epicardium (**696**) and the enlarged lymph nodes (**697**). Epistaxis, melena and hyphema occur in severe cases. Hair follicles ooze blood and a straw-colored fluid which dries into a scurf. Scleral and conjunctival hemorrhages may occur and occasionally free blood is present in the lower segment of the aqueous humor. The eyeball is tense, protruding through swollen everted conjunctival sacs, as the so-called 'poached egg eye'. Snorting cattle trying to clear airways of blood and catarrhal exudate usually die, especially if pulmonary edema is present. The visible mucosae are white at death.

Diagnosis: demonstration of organisms in blood during febrile phase, typical history and signs.

Management: systemic oxytetracycline in early stages of clinical disease. Recovered cases may remain latent carriers. Areas of previous outbreaks should ideally be avoided.

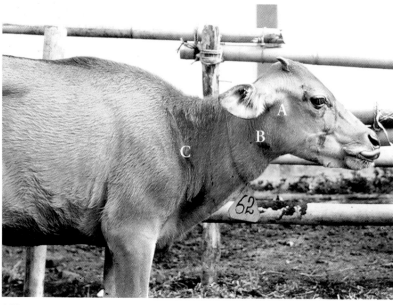

699

Jembrana disease

Definition: an immunosuppressive hemorrhagic diathesis of domesticated banteng (*Bos sondiacus*, syn. *Bos javanicus*) in the Jembrana region on the island of Bali. Etiology is uncertain, possibly a Boophilus tick-borne ehrlichiosis, or a lentiviral infection (spread by close animal contact).

Clinical features: first seen in 1964, when 61% of 31,000 banteng died, the disease has now spread to other Indonesian islands. Bali disease is another form, characterized by peripheral necrosis (e.g., ears **698**) as a result of a generalized vasculitis. Early signs in virgin-soil epidemics include fever, anorexia, lethargy and reluctance to move, as well as behavioral changes, severe generalized lymphadenopathy (**699**) and pallor. The cow shows enlarged parotid (A), retropharyngeal (B) and prescapular nodes (C). Feces may contain blood from intestinal hemorrhage (**700**). Pregnant animals may abort. Postmortem changes include severe hemorrhages in all organs including the hard and soft palate (**701**), and the serosal surface of the intestine. Proliferative changes are present in the lymphoreticular system, GI tract, liver, kidneys and lungs. Endemic cases are milder and have about 20% mortality rate.

Differential diagnosis: rinderpest (**652**), hemorrhagic septicemia.

Management and control: recovered animals remain persistent carriers and are immune. Considerable risk of disease transmission mechanically during mass vaccination against hemorrhagic septicemia. ELISA and AGID tests are available for survey work, but not useful for diagnosis. Supportive treatment including tetracyclines may be helpful. No specific control is available.

Ehrlichiosis (Nofel syndrome)

Definition: *Ehrlichia bovis* is a persistent parasite of circulating monocytes of low pathogenicity in healthy

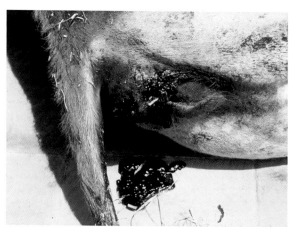

700

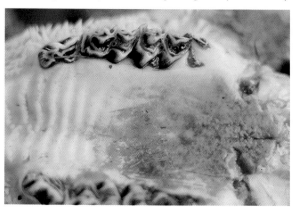

701

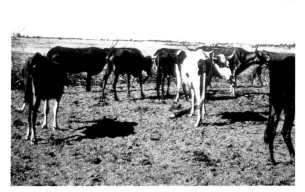

702

cattle reared on tick-infested land where the parasite is endemic. Vectors are *Hyalomma aegypticus* (North Africa), *Amblyomma variegatum* (West Africa), *Rhipicephalus* (Southern Africa) and *A. cajennense* (Brazil).

Clinical features: naïve imports develop primary infection with fluctuating fever, anorexia and diarrhea, lose condition and may show nervous signs. Mortality is low. Another form (Nofel) is an exacerbated *E. bovis* infection in over-stressed transhumant cattle which develop marked lymphadenopathy, enormous edema in drooping ears, purulent oculonasal discharges, anorexia and constipation. Most cattle die rapidly unless treated.

Differential diagnosis: cowdriosis (690–693).

Management: avoid introduction of susceptible naïve cattle; practise regular dipping. Tetracyclines in severe cases.

Trypanosomiasis (Nagana or African trypanosomosis)

Introduction: of all animal diseases, the most important constraint on animal production in the sub-humid and humid tropics is trypanomiasis, which in Africa alone affects animals in an area one-third larger than the continent of the United States. Annual losses may be as high as US$5 billion.

Definition: an acute, subacute or chronic disease caused by blood parasites called trypanosomes. These are of various species: *Trypanosoma congolense* and *T. brucei* occur only in the areas of Africa where the vector, some 20 species of tsetse flies (*Glossina*), is found. *T. vivax* occurs not only in tsetse areas but also in the non-tsetse areas of Africa, Asia and South and Central America. The parasites are cyclically transmitted biologically by tsetse but may be transferred mechanically during interrupted blood meals by other biting flies such as *Stomoxys*, *Tabanidae*, *Lyperosia* and *Hippoboscidae*. The overwhelming majority of clinical infections of African trypanosomiasis are due to tsetse-transmitted *T. congolense*, and *T. vivax*. *T. theileri*, a cosmopolitan species occurring in cattle, is non-pathogenic.

Clinical features: infection of cattle takes place through skin puncture and migration to the bloodstream via lymph nodes. The incubation period is 1–4 weeks. Clinical signs are non-specific and include a staring coat, intermittent fever, dullness, anemia, lowered milk production and loss of weight and condition (702, 703). Abortion and reproductive failure occur. There is a variable mortality rate although the chronic course may continue for months or years. There is also a peracute, hemorrhagic form associated particularly with strains of *T. vivax* in East Africa. Postmortem features are also non-specific but include lymphadenopathy, depletion of fat and anemia (pale and watery carcass). Hemorrhages may be seen in acute *T. vivax* cases as serosal lesions.

Diagnosis: livestock owners rely on clinical signs and response to treatment. Demonstration of parasites in stained blood and lymph gland smears or the centrifugation and examination of the buffy coat in fresh blood samples is definitive. The number of circulating parasites varies greatly so repeat sampling on an individual or herd basis may be necessary to demonstrate infection. Various serological tests involving immunological or molecular technology, which may indicate the degree of past exposure, are available.

Differential diagnosis: chronic wasting conditions such as fascioliasis, helminthiasis e.g., schistosomiasis, babesiosis (679–684) anaplasmosis (685–688), East Coast fever (689), chronic CBPP, tuberculosis, malnutrition (energy, protein or mineral deficiencies) and a combination of old age and repeated pregnancies. Acute hemorrhagic cases must be distinguished from hemorrhagic septicemia, bovine petechial fever or Ondiri disease (695–697) and anthrax (704).

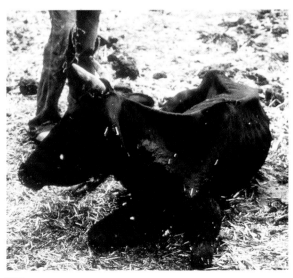

703

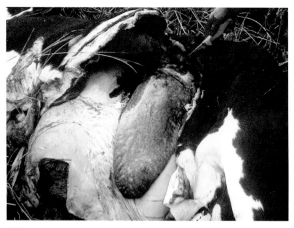

704

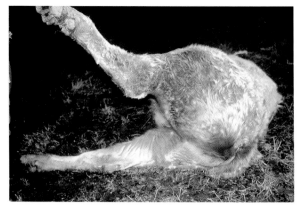

705

Management: treatment of clinical cases with diminazine aceturate (Berenil), isometamidium (Samorin or Trypamidium), quinapyramine sulfate (Trypacide and Triquin), homidium bromide (Ethidium) and chloride (Novidium). Drug resistance is an increasing problem.

Prevention: varying degrees of prophylaxis can be achieved by judicious use of isometamidium and homidium. Seasonal herding practices can reduce exposure to tsetse, habitat modification and strategic application of insecticides either to vegetation, as pour-on formulations to cattle or on traps and insecticide-impregnated targets can reduce tsetse populations. Maintenance of trypanotolerant breeds, particularly the N'dama and Muturu in West Africa is another strategy.

Bacterial diseases
Anthrax (splenic fever)

Definition: peracute disease caused by *Bacillus anthracis*.

Clinical features: most cases are seen as a sudden death in a previously healthy individual. A few cases in terminal septicemia are ataxic and have nasal, oral or anal hemorrhage. Dark blood may be passed from anus and vulva terminally. The characteristic postmortem feature of anthrax is an enlarged, dark, soft-textured spleen, as seen in **704** in the specimen from a crossbred Hereford cow in Zimbabwe. Cattle may be infected through contaminated pastures (e.g., those flooded sporadically with river water carrying tannery effluent), or by eating contaminated artificial or natural feedstuffs. Cattle suspected as possible anthrax cases should not undergo postmortem examination, and diagnosis should be based initially on a blood smear. Anthrax is a notifiable disease in many countries. BSE regulations, which prohibit the feeding of meat and bone meal, have reduced the incidence of anthrax in the UK.

Differential diagnosis: other causes of sudden death, e.g., lightning strike (**503**), bloat (**197, 198**), clostridial diseases,

anaplasmosis (**685–688**), and bacillary hemoglobinuria (**227, 228**).

Management: aggressive systemic penicillin or oxytetracycline therapy in early stages. Vaccination in endemic areas.

Clostridial diseases

Introduction: clostridia are natural inhabitants of the soil and of the gastrointestinal tract of man and animals. Pathogenic effects in cattle arise either from ingestion or from wound contamination. One group of clostridia produces disease by active invasion and toxin production leading to death (gas gangrene), the second produces toxins within the gut (enterotoxemia), or in food or carrion outside the body (botulism). One clostridial disease, malignant edema, caused by *C. septicum*, is illustrated in the alimentary chapter (**180, 181**) to aid in differential diagnosis from other conditions leading to swelling of the head. A range of combined clostridial vaccines is widely available and very effective in preventing disease.

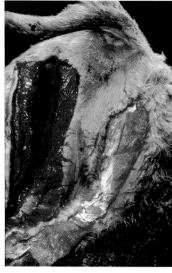

706

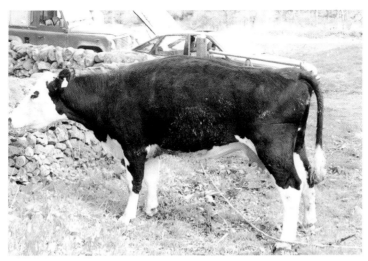

707

Blackleg (*Clostridium chauvoei*)

Definition: an acute febrile necrotizing myositis caused by *C. chauvoei*, characterized by emphysematous swelling.

Clinical features: blackleg develops spontaneously without a history of open wounds, although bruising may be a predisposing factor by producing anaerobic conditions in muscles that are harboring the organism. Occasionally fattening cattle are found dead without showing clinical signs. Most cases end fatally after signs of acute depression and lameness. The crossbred Charolais calf at pasture was severely lame with massive gluteal swelling of the left leg (705). Postmortem examination (706) shows the necrotic muscle compared with the normal right leg. The hindquarters usually have the most severe changes, seen as infiltration of the musculature with gas bubbles that have a characteristic rancid smell, although any part of the body, including heart muscle may be affected. Often, severely affected muscle (dark) lies adjacent to normal tissue (706).

Differential diagnosis: malignant edema (181), anthrax (704), lightning strike (503–505). Gross pathological changes are usually characteristic, and laboratory confirmation is by fluorescent antibody staining.

Management: if not moribund, cattle may be treated with penicillin, NSAIDs and possibly surgical debridement to expose surrounding tissues to atmospheric air. Vaccination on enzootic farms.

Tetanus (*Clostridium tetani*, 'lockjaw')

Definition: tetanus toxemia is produced by a specific neurotoxin of *C. tetani*, usually as a disease passing up the nerve tracts to spinal cord and brain.

Clinical features: introduced into deep, anaerobic skin wounds (e.g., castration, 539), *C. tetani* causes progressive nervous signs as a result of neurotoxin production. Cattle show a generalized stiffness. The Hereford cross suckler cow (707) has an arched back and raised tail, extended head and neck, erect ears, 'Chinese eyes' and flared nostrils. The third eyelid may be prolapsed. Ruminal bloat is common. This cow was hyperaggressive, then fell over and was unable to rise again. The disease progresses into severe extensor rigidity (708) with progressive respiratory failure. Rigidity is so severe that the upper feet remain off the ground. The tail is overextended. Note the severe opisthotonos. This calf had been castrated 2 weeks previously.

Differential diagnosis (in early cases): meningitis (484), cerebrocortical necrosis or polioencephalomalacia (468), hypomagnesemic tetany in calves (471), strychnine poisoning, and acute muscle dystrophy (410).

Management: antisera, antibiotics, muscle relaxants and supportive therapy in a quiet environment. Prevention by maintenance of proper skin and instrument disinfection at castration, and by vaccination.

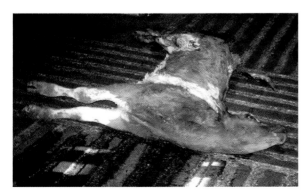

708

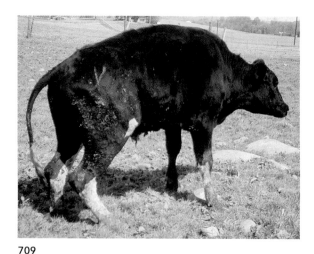

709

Botulism (*Clostridium botulinum*)

Definition: a rapidly fatal motor paralysis, caused by a *C. botulinum* neurotoxin (usually type D).

Clinical features: the toxin is produced as a result of proliferation of the bacteria in decomposing animal matter, for example, chicken manure spread onto pasture subsequently grazed by cattle. The toxemia results in initial posterior ataxia and progresses to paraparesis (**709**). The stance may be straddled (base-wide) and the hind fetlocks may be knuckled. Motor paralysis of the tongue (**710**) causes difficulty in prehension, chewing and swallowing. This cow could not hold its head up. Saliva may contain partially masticated feed material which cannot be swallowed (**711**). Death is from respiratory paralysis. In some countries the major cause of botulism is the ingestion of decomposed animal carcasses. This depraved appetite (pica) is stimulated by a phosphorus deficiency (**420, 421**). Up to 3% of cattle in endemic areas may die from botulism annually. Poultry manure and ensiled poultry litter utilized as cattle feed, as well as

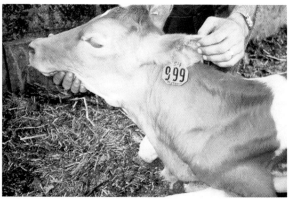

711

poultry litter used as cattle bedding, have been implicated as a clostridial source.

Differential diagnosis: organophosphorus toxicity (**744**), thromboembolic meningoencephalitis (**489**), BSE (**498**), SBE (**694**), paralytic rabies and trauma.

Management: correction of dietary deficiency, removal of source material, possibly immunization in problem areas with types D and/or C toxoid.

Miscellaneous

Bovine leukosis (bovine viral leukosis, bovine lymphosarcoma)

Introduction: leukosis occurs in four forms. The calfhood, thymic and skin types are all termed sporadic leukosis. Bovine leukosis virus cannot be cultured from, nor antibodies be detected in, these three forms. The fourth type, the adult form, is known as enzootic bovine leukosis (EBL) and is caused by the bovine leukosis virus (BLV).

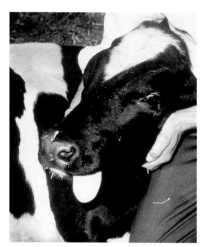

710

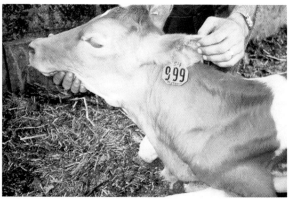

712

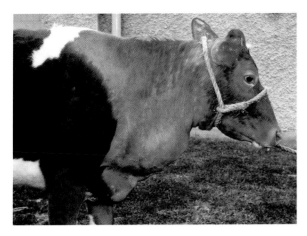

713

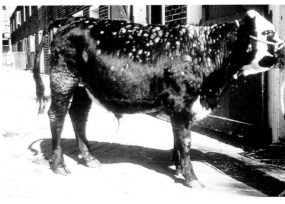

715

Calfhood multicentric lymphosarcoma

The Guernsey calf in **712** showed generalized lymphadenopathy with gross symmetrical enlargement of the prescapular, submandibular, parotid and retropharyngeal nodes. Palpation revealed that the lymph nodes were smooth, painless and freely moveable, not involving the skin. Widespread tumor metastases are present in such cases, usually <6 months old. Like other forms of bovine leukosis, calfhood leukosis has a low and sporadic incidence.

Thymic lymphosarcoma

A large, firm, smooth mass is present in the presternal region of the yearling Guernsey heifer in **713**. Edema is also present. Most cases are seen in the 6–24 months age group. Generalized lymphadenopathy was absent. Some cases have bloat as a result of esophageal obstruction. As in the multicentric form, a cross-section (**714**) of the discrete tumor from a 15-month-old crossbred Angus reveals pale yellow material without granulomatous contents.

Skin lymphosarcoma

Skin leukosis is rare and is seen in immature animals aged 6–24 months. The crossbred Hereford in **715** has gray-white nodules over the neck, back and flanks, which extend deep into the subcutis. There is also a generalized lymphadenopathy with prominent precrural nodes. In **716** another animal has skin leukosis limited to large, ulcerated lesions around the head. This is the only non-fatal lymphoid tumor in cattle and these cutaneous masses regress after some months.

Differential diagnosis: actinobacillosis (**175**), actinomycosis (**177**), and fibropapillomata (warts) (**109**).

Enzootic (adult) bovine leukosis (EBL), bovine lymphosarcoma

Definition: fatal systemic malignant neoplasia of reticuloendothelial system caused by an exogenous C-type oncovirus (BLV).

Clinical features: enzootic bovine leukosis produces a generalized lymphadenopathy with symmetrical enlargement of most peripheral nodes, often with other signs. The Angus cow in **717** had enlarged submandibular, parotid (shaved for needle biopsy before photography) and prescapular nodes. Lymphosarcoma was also found in the heart and uterus. Some cases (20%) have a predilection, usually unilateral, for the orbit. The neoplasia is generally retro-

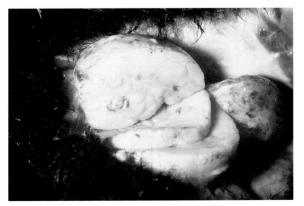

714

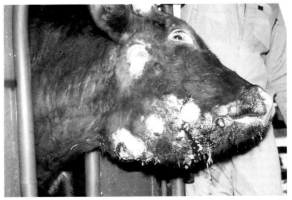

716

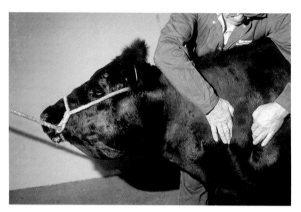

717

bulbar. Exceptionally, the adult cow in **718** has massive bilateral exophthalmos and protrusion of granulation tissue as a result of lymphomatous infiltration into the orbit. Other sites of lymphosarcoma include the globe itself (**466**), the spinal canal and cord, causing progressive posterior paresis as a result of spinal cord compression (**346**), and the abomasum (**210**).

Differential diagnosis of EBL: sporadic bovine leukosis, traumatic pericarditis and congestive heart failure, lymphadenitis due to TB or actinobacillosis.

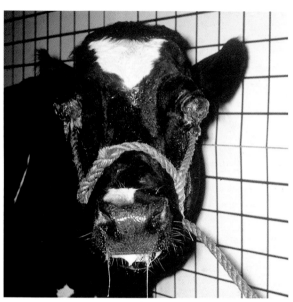

718

Diagnosis: histological examination of enlarged node.

Management of EBL: serological testing of herd at 3-month intervals and culling of positive cases.

chapter 13

Toxicological disorders

Introduction

Illustrations of toxicological disorders in cattle present problems. The clinical signs may be transient, with death occurring within a few minutes, such as in yew (*Taxus baccata*) poisoning. In other cases, the signs may be nonspecific. Where the effects are confined largely to one system, the description has been given in the appropriate section, for example, ergot and fescue foot are dealt with under locomotor disorders (**414–416**). In this chapter, toxicoses have been broadly grouped into plant, organic and inorganic chemical sections.

Plant toxicoses

Bracken (bracken fern)

Definition: acute or chronic worldwide toxicity following ingestion of large quantities of bracken (bracken fern), which contains several bone marrow toxins (aplastic anemia factor) which kill precursor cells in the bone marrow.

Clinical features: bracken (*Pteridium aquilinum*) is usually a cumulative poison, acting in two ways. Firstly, after ingesting large quantities for a few weeks, cattle may show an acute syndrome resulting from aplastic anemia and thrombocytopenia. Sudden death is occasionally seen. In **719** the vulva of the crossbred Angus cow is pale from severe anemia. The pinpoint hemorrhages are a result of thrombocytopenia. Hemorrhages elsewhere can cause epistaxis, hyphema (**720**) (bleeding into the anterior chamber) or hematuria from bladder mucosal hemorrhage (**721**).

Secondly, ingestion of considerable quantities of bracken for several months can lead to a chronic syndrome of enzootic hematuria. A carcinogen causes bladder neoplasia, resulting in enzootic hematuria and malignancies such as hemangiosarcoma (**722**). Numerous discrete masses are seen protruding from the mucosal surface. These masses bleed readily as the bladder distends and contracts. Some mucosal areas (top right, lower left) appear normal. The

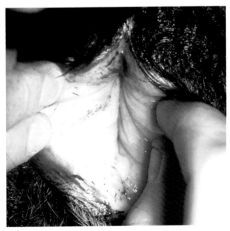

719

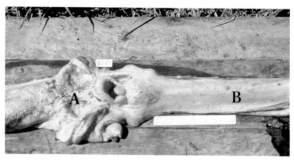

723

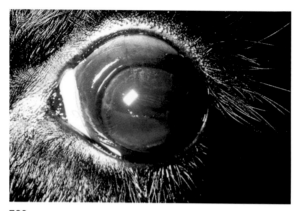

720

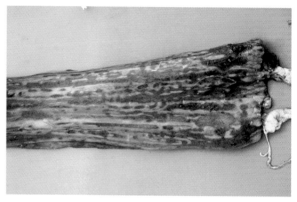

724

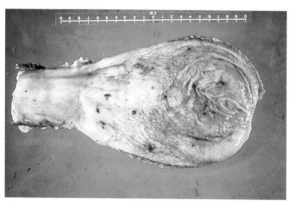

721

Management: treatment of individual cases is usually hopeless, possibly blood transfusion (5–10 L); pasture and grazing management.

Oak (acorn)

Definition: Oak (*Quercus* species) containing a gallotannin, may cause toxic signs following several days ingestion of acorns (autumn) or young leaves (spring).

Clinical features: the toxic principle causes renal and gastrointestinal changes. The signs include abdominal pain, often with a hemorrhagic diarrhea, thirst, polyuria and ventral edema as a result of subacute and chronic toxicity. The esophageal mucosa can be hemorrhagic (724). The enlarged swollen kidneys (725) show scattered

hemangiomata can develop into ulcerating tumors of various types. Alimentary tract neoplasms include squamous cell carcinomas and papillomas affecting the pharynx and esophagus respectively. 723 shows pharyngeal squamous cell carcinomas (A) and esophageal papillomas (B) from Brazil. Bracken toxicosis is widespread in several continents. Bovine papilloma virus (types 2 and 4) may be involved in upper alimentary neoplasms.

Differential diagnosis: acute syndrome: anthrax (704), septicemic pasteurellosis (242), PPH syndrome (161), mycotoxicosis; chronic cases: pyelonephritis (507, 508), cystitis or babesiosis (682).

Diagnosis: a history of exposure to bracken, clinical signs of severe anemia and pancytopenia and low platelet counts.

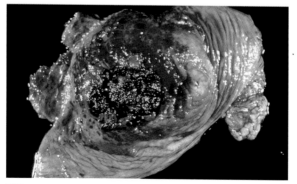

722

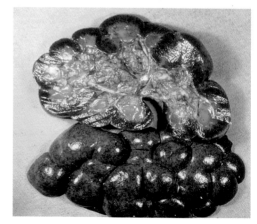

725

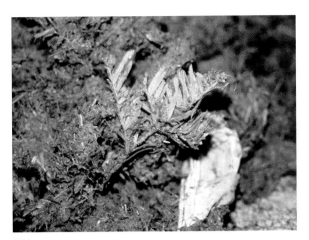

726

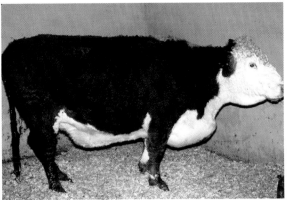

727

hemorrhages and a nephrosis, which accounts for the ventral edema, ascites and hydrothorax seen in cases with renal failure.

Diagnosis: history of known access to young oak leaves or acorns, postmortem features.

Management: symptomatic treatment (NSAIDs and fluid therapy). Prevent sudden access, e.g., following violent storms.

Yew

Definition: Yew (e.g., *Taxus baccata* – English yew, *T. cuspidata* – Japanese yew) contains a cardiotoxic alkaloid, taxine, as well as cyanide.

Clinical features: the opened rumen in **726** shows normal ingesta mixed with needle-like yew leaves. Cattle usually die minutes after ingesting a few mouthfuls of yew twigs or berries, typically encountered as fresh or dried clippings thrown over a graveyard hedge into a bare winter pasture. The lethal dose in adult cattle may be as little as 1 kg of leaves.

Management: oral B_{12}, sucrose and also atropine have been suggested for treatment. Emergency rumenotomy may be considered for valuable animals.

Ragwort (seneciosis)

Definition: Ragwort (*Senecio jacobea*) contains a pyrrolizidine alkaloid, jacobine, that causes acute and chronic liver disease.

Clinical features: early signs include dark-colored diarrhea, photosensitization, jaundice, abdominal pain and central nervous system abnormalities. Prolonged ingestion results in progressive weakness, weight loss and liver failure due to cirrhosis, and severe lung disease. In the mature Hereford cow in **727**, the resulting right heart failure led to the edema affecting the ventral body wall, brisket and head.

Management: as the period from ingestion to the onset of clinical signs may be 4–6 months, diagnosis can be difficult. The fresh plant is bitter and usually avoided. Intoxication occurs following incorporation into conserved forage.

Rape and kale

Definition: some forms of forage of the *Brassica* family, such as kale and rape, contain S-methylcysteine sulfoxide, and can cause a hemolytic (Heinz body) anemia following production of dimethyl disulfide by ruminal bacteria.

Clinical features: cattle develop hemoglobinuria, voiding dark-red urine (**728**), and are anemic and weak. Postmortem examination of fatal cases reveals pallor and jaundice of the liver (**729**) and heart (**730**).

Differential diagnosis: postparturient hemoglobinuria, bacillary hemoglobinuria (**227**), nitrate/nitrite poisoning

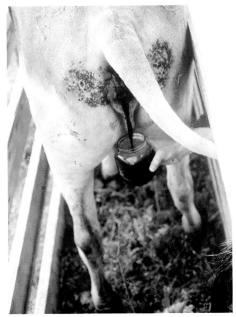

728

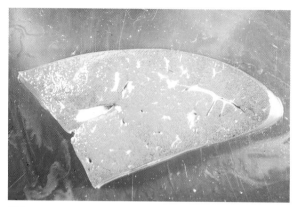

729

(745, 746), hypomagnesemia (472), babesiosis (679–684), anaplasmosis (685–688) and acute bracken poisoning (719–721).

Management: clinical signs are only seen following prolonged high intakes, e.g., 40–50 kg per day. Treat symptomatically for anemia.

Lantana

Definition: *Lantana camara* is a shrub containing toxic triterpenes that causes hepatitis in cattle, producing signs of photosensitization, jaundice, rumen stasis and depression.

Clinical features: in 731 the Holstein steer from Zimbabwe shows severe skin lesions (typical of photosensitisation in that only the white areas are affected), depression, and tenesmus resulting from constipation. See also Chapter 3, photosensitization (p. 24), and facial eczema (p. 214).

Differential diagnosis: photosensitization (78–83) and facial eczema (740–742).

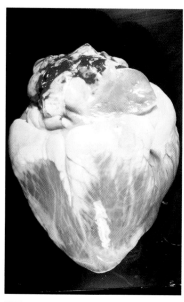

730

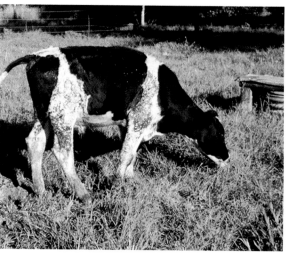

731

Management: avoid access. Unless seen in the early stages of skin edema, treatment (e.g., with NSAIDs) is of limited value and the skin slough will run its course.

Solanum malacoxylon and *Trisetum flavescens* (enzootic calcinosis, enteque seco, Naalehu, espichamento)

Definition: *Solanum malacoxylon* (South America) or *Trisetum flavescens* (Bavaria) acts by increasing calcium absorption from the gut through a metabolite of 1,25-dihydroxycholecalciferol, the active principle of vitamin D, leading to a chronic syndrome of excessive deposition of periosteal new bone and to calcification of blood vessels.

Clinical features: This periosteal new bone and vascular calcification may be appreciated on rectal palpation (aorta) and on the lower limb (distal arteries). In 732 the crossbred cow from Mato Grosso, Brazil, is typically emaciated, stiff and stands on the toes of the forefeet. Walking was typically slow and awkward. The endo-

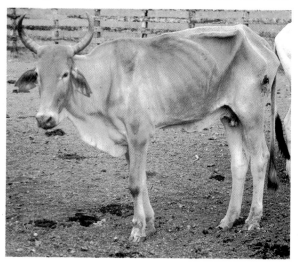

732

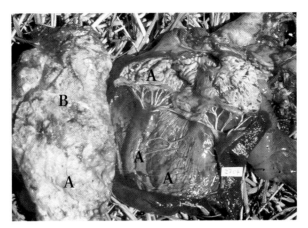

733

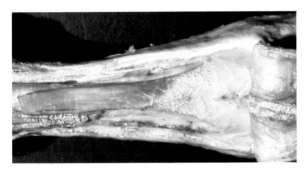

734

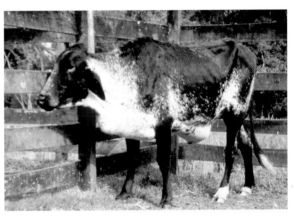

735

cardium and lungs of another cow (733) have areas of calcification (A), and the lungs have patches of ossified tissue (B). Calcification of the deep flexor tendons and blood vessels is present in this German cow (734) with *T. flavescens* toxicity.

Other *Solanum* species can cause cerebellar degeneration or 'crazy cow syndrome' in Africa. The nightshade group (e.g., *Solanum nigrum*, deadly nightshade) can produce gastrointestinal irritation and nervous signs.

Diagnosis: may be difficult in early stages. Later signs and postmortem evidence of calcification of soft tissues (heart, major vessels, pleura, lungs) is diagnostic.

Management: removal from affected pasture, if feasible.

Tetrapteris species (peito inchado)

Definition: *Tetrapteris* species (*T. multiglandulosa* and *T. acutifolia*) cause a widespread cardiomyopathy in south-eastern Brazil.

Clinical features: cattle develop ventral, especially brisket edema (hence peito inchado or swollen breast), jugular venous distension and cardiac arrhythmia, as seen in a 5-year-old crossbred Zebu cow (735). The disease, usually subacute, is sometimes chronic, but rarely peracute. Post-mortem lesions include myocardial pallor with some whitish streaking, and increased firmness suggestive of

fibrosis, as seen in another mature Zebu cow in 736. *Tetrapteris* poisoning has been reproduced by feeding fresh or dry plant material for 9–50 days. The same plant may be responsible for stillbirths.

Selenium toxicity (locoweed, selenosis, 'alkali disease', 'blind staggers')

Definition: enzootic disease resulting from toxic amounts of Se incorporated in specific plants.

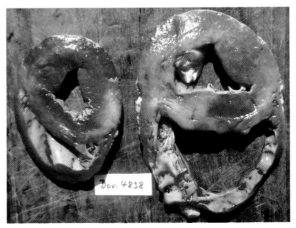

736

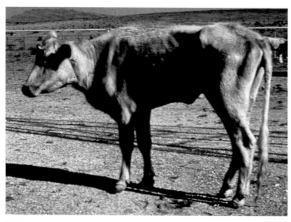

737

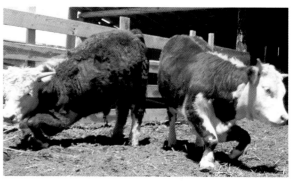

739

Clinical features: selenosis occurs in specific areas of North America, Ireland, Canada, Israel, Australia and South Africa where the soils contain a high level of Se. Clinical signs, which are similar to swainsonine toxicity (**737**), include emaciation, hair loss and claw deformities, resulting from prolonged ingestion of excessive selenium (exceeding 5 ppm in diet) incorporated in *Astragalus* species, which are selenium accumulator plants. A horizontal band starts below the coronary band and moves slowly distally. Pain, producing severe lameness, results from the movement of wall horn over the exposed sensitive laminae (**738**). Affected cattle may be forced to graze in a kneeling position. Another toxic syndrome is 'blind staggers'. Other toxins can also contribute to the clinical picture. Occasionally, as a result of careless Se supplementation, acute Se poisoning occurs and causes diarrhea, dyspnea and death.

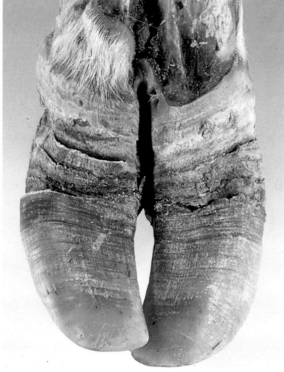

738

Differential diagnosis: diagnosis is based on clinical signs, postmortem and laboratory evidence of high Se levels in diet.

Management: elimination of source, symptomatic support.

Lupine toxicity (crooked calf disease)

Definition: crooked calf disease is a generalized congenital defect caused by the neurogenic quinolidizine alkaloid anagyrine in *Lupinus caudatus* and *L. sericeus*, in some cases the alkaloid being in an aphis on a lupinus plant. Reduction of fetal movement is the cause of the teratogenic signs (e.g., joint contracture, torticollis, scoliosis).

Clinical signs: deformed calves, with variable degrees of malalignment of the long bones, are born to cows that have ingested large quantities of these lupine plants and *L. sericeus* during pregnancy. The calves in **739** were born to cows fed lupines from the 40th to the 70th day of gestation. Lupine species can also cause liver toxicity. See Chapter 1 (**15**) for other forms of arthrogryposis (e.g., BVD/MD virus infection).

Management: cows should not be grazed on lupine pastures during the period when they are liable to be 40–120 days pregnant.

Mycotoxicoses

Mycotoxicosis is a poisoning due to the ingestion of a fungal toxin. Ryegrass staggers is seen as an ataxia, initially in the hind legs, later progressing to the forelimbs and recumbency. The toxin Loitrem B, produced by the fungus *Acremonium lolii*, which is found in dry conditions in ryegrass swards, is the cause. Aflotoxicosis is another example. One or more systems may be affected. The photodermatitis associated with the fungus *Pithomyces chartarum* is the selected example for description.

Facial eczema (pithomycotoxicosis)

Definition: a photomycotic disease of grazing cattle caused by sporidesmins, which are secondary metabolites of a saprophytic fungus, *Pithomyces chartarum*.

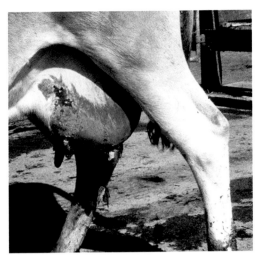

740

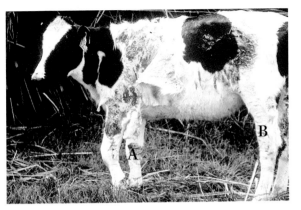

741

Clinical signs: facial eczema is an important disease in New Zealand, and also occurs in Australia, France, South Africa and South America. The fungus produces a hepatotoxic agent, which is commonly associated with ryegrass pastures. The clinical signs include lethargy, anorexia, conjunctivitis, jaundice and a photosensitive dermatitis. At an early stage, the thin skin of the udder of the Jersey cow in **740** had lost its hair, and a moist dermatitis and hyperemia were evident. The skin in the upper left denuded area was starting to slough and the teats were also involved. Affected cows may lick this area of mild chronic irritation.

A late stage of facial eczema (**741**) shows a Friesian heifer with an extensive skin slough, typically confined to the white area. Note the involvement of the forelimbs (A), where carpal flexion has caused sloughing, and the thickened, wrinkled appearance of the skin extending down the hind legs (B). In a Brazilian Zebu herd, a 1-month-old male calf (**742**) had an extensive photodermatitis involving the ventral neck fold and chest wall and flank. The same fungus, *Pithomyces chartarum*, was consumed by the dam from a pasture of *Brachiaria decubens*, sporidesmin being ingested through the milk. The dam is normal.

Differential diagnosis: other forms of photodermatitis. Exposure to ryegrass, sunshine, typical signs and characteristic appearance of the liver are pathognomonic.

Management: avoidance of exposure at critical times, pasture control such as sowing clover, and use of fungicidal sprays to reduce the build-up of *P. chartarum* spores. NSAIDs may be helpful in early stages.

Other examples of mycotoxicoses are illustrated in Chapter 7 (fescue foot, **414**; ergot, **415**, **416**). Photosensitization is covered in Chapter 3 (**78–83**).

Organic toxicoses
Chlorinated naphthalenes

Definition: naphthalenes, formerly extensively used as lubricants and wood-preserving compounds are agents that cause hypovitaminosis A by interfering with the conversion of carotene to vitamin A.

Clinical features: hyperkeratosis of skin, emaciation, and possibly death, result when they are ingested over a long period. In **743** the head of the South African Friesian cow shows thickening, scaliness and wrinkling of skin. The hindquarters also had severe changes over the gaskin, hock, and metatarsus.

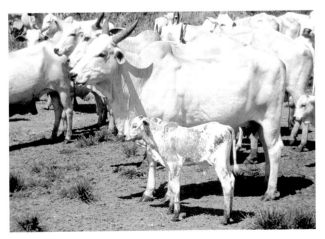

742

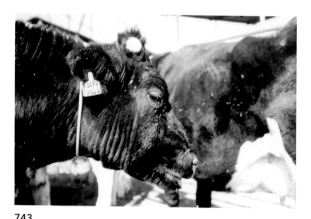

743

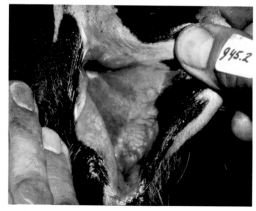

745

Carbamate and organophosphorus compounds

Definition: these organophosphates inactivate cholinesterase, causing a rise in tissue acetylcholine and increased parasympathetic activity.

Clinical features: since the toxic signs of carbamate and organophosphorus tend to be similar, both organic groups can be discussed together. Poisoning is relatively common.

The crossbred Angus cow in **744** had ingested a carbamate insecticide powder (carbofuran or 'Furadan') from a half-empty bag about 6–16 hours previously. Initial generalized muscle twitching, depression and locomotor incoordination were accompanied by hypersalivation. The cow then became semicomatose. Still salivating profusely, she showed miosis, severe dyspnea and pronounced bradycardia, and died 2 hours later. Her calf (**744**) was healthy throughout.

Differential diagnosis: nitrate and gyanide poisoning (**745**), acute grain overload (**192**), acute interstitial pneumonia or 'fog fever' (**259**), acute anaphylaxis, and urea toxicity.

Diagnosis: exposure to agent in feed or environment.

Management: in early acute disease massive doses of atropine (0.25 mg/kg) and possibly also oximes.

Inorganic chemical toxicoses
Nitrate/nitrite

Definition: nitrates form nitrites before or after ingestion and cause respiratory distress because methemoglobin formation leads to an anoxic anemia.

Clinical signs: nitrites are about 10 times as toxic as nitrates. The sources of nitrate/nitrite are numerous and variable in type, and include cereals, certain weeds (e.g., thistles, docks, Johnson grass), specific plants, and both organic and inorganic fertilizers. A characteristic feature of this type of poisoning is the color change in the vaginal mucosa. Levels of 22% (**745**) and 60% (**746**) methemoglobin are illustrated. Clinical signs include tachypnea, muscle tremors and ataxia. They appear at a level of about 20% conversion of hemoglobin to methemoglobin, while death follows at 60–80%.

Differential diagnosis: silo gas poisoning, sodium chlorate poisoning, acute rape or kale toxicity (**728**), and cyanide, carbon dioxide, cobalt or chronic copper poisoning (**751**).

Management: treatment with intravenous methylene blue and fluid therapy is effective in many cases.

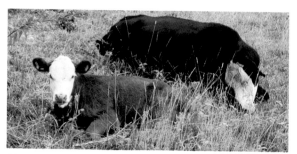

744

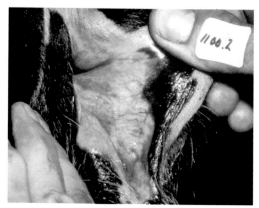

746

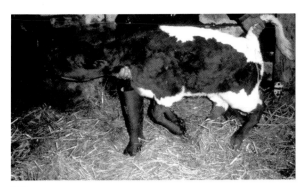

747

Lead (plumbism)

Definition: acute or chronic lead poisoning results from lead deposition in various tissues, including bone, where it is in an inert form. Lead adversely affects sulfhydryl-containing enzymes and tissues rich in mitochondria, leading to cerebellar hemorrhage and edema.

Clinical signs: in lead poisoning the major signs of central nervous system (CNS) involvement are depression, blindness and, often, head-pressing. Some cases exhibit maniacal behavior. The 1-month-old Gloucester calf in 747 shows severe CNS signs. Unable to stand, its head and neck are extended to push against the brick wall. It was also blind and anorexic. Lead is a common toxicological problem in younger cattle. The source, usually environmental, is often paint from old doors, as in this calf, although crankcase oil from farm machinery, lead batteries, contaminated feedstuffs and golfballs are other sources.

Differential diagnosis: polioencephalomalacia (CCN) (468), listeriosis (477) and meningitis (484).

Management: individual therapy consists of calcium EDTA i.v. or s.c. for several days, plus oral magnesium sulfate to render any remaining lead unavailable as lead sulfate, and also thiamine. Note that meat withhold times in recovered cases may be several months to allow excretion of stored lead. Lead is excreted into milk.

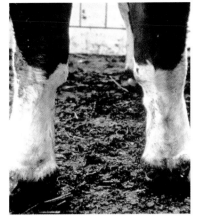

749

Iodine (iodism)

Definition: excess oral intake of inorganic and organic iodine compounds.

Clinical features: common sources are ethylene diamine dihydroiodide in a feed additive (for footrot prevention) and potassium iodide for treatment of actinobacillosis. Iodism in this calf (748) is manifested by a dry seborrheic dermatitis primarily affecting the head and neck. Recovery followed removal of the excess element.

Fluorosis

Clinical features: Fluorosis usually results from the prolonged ingestion of fluorine in high fluorine-phosphatic supplementary feeds, or from herbage ingested from pastures contaminated by industrial emissions. Deep wells are important sources of fluorine poisoning in Australia and South America. Two forms of chronic toxicity occur: osteofluorosis and dental fluorosis. The absorption capacity is much higher in young animals and on high-concentrate diets, both of which predispose to toxicity. Large periosteal plaques form on long bones. 749 shows several enlargements that are firm and smooth to the touch on the medial aspects of the metatarsi. In 750 the extensive periosteal plaques, which do not involve the

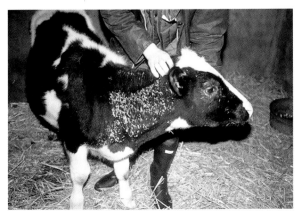

748

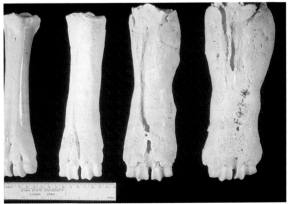

750

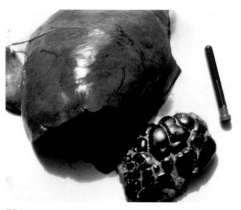

751

articular surfaces, are seen next to normal metatarsi (to the left). Cattle may become lame owing to osteoporosis, osteomalacia and periarticular bone proliferation. Another sign of chronic disease is mottling of the temporary incisors (see **168**). Temporary teeth can be damaged while *in utero*, the permanent dentition exposed to intoxication before their eruption.

Differential diagnosis: degenerative joint disease (**373**), aphosphorosis (**420**), selenosis (**737**) and enzootic calcinosis (**732–734**).

Management: difficult in affected cattle, but oral aluminum salts and parenteral calcium are used. Prevention by altering water supply and grazing regime.

Copper

Definition: excessive ingested copper is suddenly released from its liver store causing lipid peroxidation, intravascular hemolysis and severe clinical signs.

Clinical features: copper toxicosis in cattle tends to be chronic, although the onset of clinical signs may be acute and associated with stress. The source may be an error of copper supplementation, or ingestion of pasture with an abnormal level of copper (from slurry or fertilizer top-dressing) and the sudden onset of clinical signs of depression, weakness, thirst and jaundice may be due to a hemolytic crisis. Affected animals have dark urine due to hemoglobinuria. The major postmortem changes include a large, friable, icteric liver and a characteristic bluish-black ('gunmetal') coloring of the kidneys (**751**). Note color of urine in adjacent tube.

Differential diagnosis: calfhood leptospirosis (**510**), necrotic hepatitis (**227**), babesiosis (**679–684**), anaplasmosis (**685–688**) and other causes of hemolytic anemia.

Management: individual treatment of sick cattle is usually hopeless. Ammonium molybdenate and sodium sulfate reduce the copper content of tissues and increase its fecal excretion. Symptomatic treatment, e.g., gastrointestinal sedatives, may be given. Control by eradication of plants causing phytogenous or hepatogenous copper poisoning may prove impossible, but top-dressing pastures with molybdenum at 70 g/ha or molybdenum dietary supplementation may be feasible.

Molybdenum

Definition: molybdenum toxicity is related to copper, molybdenum and inorganic sulfate, molybdenum and sulfur giving rise to thio-molybdenates, with which copper reacts in the rumen to produce a poorly absorbed and insoluble complex.

Clinical features: molybdenum toxicosis tends to involve a relative copper deficiency. The cow from China (**752**) is thin and shows depigmentation of the normally dark coat. Note the grayish hairs around the eyes. Alopecia is present over the neck, shoulder and withers. Note also the combination halter and nose-ring used in Jiangxi Province. Many cattle with molybdenum toxicity show a persistent diarrhea also typical of the high-molybdenum 'teart' pastures in parts of England. Cattle respond to copper supplementation.

Differential diagnosis: copper deficiency (**423**) and cobalt deficiency (**429**).

Management: use of 1% copper sulfate in salt may control molybdenosis in areas where forage molybdenum is >5 ppm. Higher levels of copper may be given. Use of drenching or pasture top-dressing has also been advised as preventative. Injection of copper glycinate may aid recovery in some clinical cases.

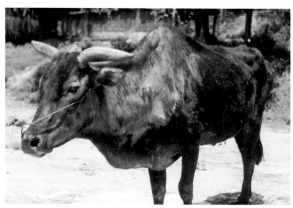

752

Index